DSM-IV-TR CASEBOOK

A Learning Companion to the
Diagnostic and Statistical
Manual of Mental Disorders,
Fourth Edition,
Text Revision

Edited by

Robert L. Spitzer, M.D.
Miriam Gibbon, M.S.W.
Andrew E. Skodol, M.D.
Janet B. W. Williams, D.S.W.
Michael B. First, M.D.

DSM-IV-TR CASEBOOK

A Learning Companion to the Diagnostic and Statistical Manual of Mental Disorders, Fourth Edition, Text Revision

Edited by

Robert L. Spitzer, M.D.
Miriam Gibbon, M.S.W.
Andrew E. Skodol, M.D.
Janet B. W. Williams, D.S.W.
Michael B. First, M.D.

Columbia University
and the
New York State Psychiatric Institute

American Psychiatric Publishing, Inc.

Washington, DC
London, England

Copyright © 2002 American Psychiatric Publishing, Inc.
ALL RIGHTS RESERVED
Manufactured in the United States of America on acid-free paper
First Edition   06   05   04   03   02   5   4   3   2   1
New ICD-9-CM codes effective October 1, 2000, incorporated.

American Psychiatric Publishing, Inc.
1400 K Street, N.W., Washington, DC   20005
www.appi.org

Library of Congress Cataloging-in-Publication Data
DSM-IV-TR casebook : a learning companion to the Diagnostic and statistical manual of mental disorders, Fourth edition, text revision / edited by Robert L. Spitzer . . . [et al.]. — 1st ed.
       p.   cm.
     Includes index.
     ISBN 1-58562-058-0 (alk. paper) — ISBN 1-58562-059-9 (softcover : alk. paper)
     1. Mental illness—Classification—Handbooks, manuals, etc. 2. Mental illness—Diagnosis—Handbooks, manuals, etc. I. Title: DSM-IV-TR casebook. II. Title: DSM-4-TR casebook. III. Spitzer, Robert L. IV. Diagnostic and statistical manual of mental disorders.
     [DNLM: 1. Mental Disorders—diagnosis—Case Report. 2. Diagnosis, Differential—Case Report. 3. Mental Disorders—classification—Case Report. WM 15 D536 2000 Suppl. 2002]
     RC455.2.C4 D536 2000 Suppl.
     616.89'001'2—dc21

                                                                2001053738

British Library Cataloguing in Publication Data
A CIP record is available from the British Library.

Contents

Appendix C

Appendix D

Acknowledgments

Thanks are due to Betty Appelbaum, copy editor for DSM-III, DSM-III-R, and the original *Case Book,* for her meticulous copy editing of this book.

We gratefully acknowledge the contributions of case material supplied by our colleagues listed below.

CONTRIBUTORS OF CASES FROM ENGLISH-SPEAKING COUNTRIES

Gene Abel, M.D.
Henry David Abraham, M.D.
Jacob Abraham, M.D.
Hagop Akiskal, M.D.
Rena Appel, M.D.
Lorian Baker, Ph.D.
Mark S. Bauer, M.D.
Steven Bauer, M.D.
Fred S. Berlin, M.D., Ph.D.
Howard C. Blue, M.D.
Angela Bonavoglia, M.S.W.
John M. W. Bradford, M.B.,
    F.R.C.P.C., D.A.B.P.N.,
    F.R.C.Psych.
Joan Brennan, Ph.D.
Allan Burstein, M.D.
Deborah Cabaniss, M.D.
Eve Caligor, M.D.
Dennis Cantwell, M.D.
Michelle O. Clark, M.D.
David E. Comings M.D.
Anthony J. Costello, M.D.
George C. Curtis, M.D.
Robert L. Custer, M.D.

Pedro L. Dago, M.D.
Carlo C. DiClemente, Ph.D.
Park Elliott Dietz, M.D., M.P.H.,
    Ph.D.
Norman Greenspan Doidge, M.D.
Steve Dummit, M.D.
Julia Eilenberg, M.D.
Armando R. Favazza, M.D.
Alan Felix, M.D.
Max Fink, M.D.
Leslie M. Forman, M.D.
Allen J. Frances, M.D.
Richard Friedman, M.D.
Andrew J. Freinkel, M.D.
Abby J. Fyer, M.D.
Martha Gay, M.D.
Paul H. Gebhard, Ph.D.
Donald Goodwin, M.D.
Arthur H. Green, M.D.
Richard Green, M.D.
Stanley I. Greenspan, M.D.
Ezra E. H. Griffith, M.D.
John G. Gunderson, M.D.
Katherine Halmi, M.D.

Deborah Hasin, Ph.D.
Joseph A. Himle, A.C.S.W.
John R. Hughes, M.D.
Steven Hyler, M.D.
Richard L. Jenkins, M.D.
Edwin E. Johnstone, M.D.
David Kahn, M.D.
Helen S. Kaplan, M.D., Ph.D.
Sandra J. Kaplan, M.D.
Kenneth S. Kendler, M.D.
Otto Kernberg, M.D.
Robert Kertzner, M.D.
Donald Klein, M.D.
Rachel Klein, Ph.D.
S. David Kinzie, M.D.
Richard Kluft, M.D.
Bessel A. van der Kolk, M.D.
Harold S. Koplewicz, M.D.
Robert F. Kraus, M.D.
Robert S. Lampke, M.D.
Cynthia G. Last, Ph.D.
Eve Leeman, M.D.
Jerome H. Liebowitz, M.D.
Harold I. Lief, M.D.
Thomas F. Liffick, M.D.
Z. J. Lipowski, M.D.
Joseph LoPiccolo, Ph.D.
Patrick J. McGrath, M.D.
Salvatore Mannuzza, Ph.D.
Karen S. Marder, M.D.
Randall Marshall, M.D.
Lynn Martin, R.N., M.S.N.
Gary J. May, M.D.
David M. McDowell, M.D.
Patrick McKeon, M.D.
Heino F. L. Meyer-Bahlburg, Dr. rer. nat.
Thomas W. Miller, Ph.D.
John Money, Ph.D.
J. Lawrence Moodie, M.D.

Frank Mucha, M.S.
Alistair Munro, M.D.
Philip Muskin, M.D.
Kathi Nader, M.S.W.
Yehuda Nir, M.D.
Arlene Novick, A.C.S.W.
Maria Oquendo, M.D.
Roger Peele, M.D.
Gerald C. Peterson, M.D.
Katharine A. Phillips, M.D.
Daniel Pine, M.D.
Harrison G. Pope, Jr., M.D.
Michael Popkin, M.D.
Lloyd J. Price, M.D.
Joaquim Puig-Antich, M.D. (deceased)
Robert Pynoos, M.D.
Judith L. Rapaport, M.D.
Quentin R. Regestein, M.D.
Phillip J. Resnick, M.D.
Richard Ries, M.D.
Norman E. Rosenthal, M.D.
Neal D. Ryan, M.D.
Carla Sadik, M.S.W.
Diana Sandberg, M.D.
Benjamin Seltzer, M.D.
Sally K. Severino, M.D.
David Shaffer, M.D.
Arthur Shapiro, M.D.
Elaine Shapiro, Ph.D.
Lawrence Sharpe, M.D.
Michael Sheehy, M.D.
Miriamne Singer, M.D.
Stephan Sorrell, M.D.
David A. Soskis, M.D.
David Spiegel, M.D.
Laurie Stevens, M.D.
Alan Stone, M.D.
Michael Stone, M.D.
Ludwik S. Szymanski, M.D.

Stuart W. Taylor, M.D.
Susan Vaughan, M.D.
Fred R. Volkmar, M.D.
B. Timothy Walsh, M.D.
Arnold M. Washton, Ph.D.
Paul A. Wender, M.D.

Katherine Whipple, Ph.D.
Lorna Wing, M.D.
George Winokur, M.D.
Ronald Winchel, M.D.
Ken Winters, Ph.D.
Kenneth J. Zucker, Ph.D.

CONTRIBUTORS OF INTERNATIONAL CASES

The following clinicians contributed cases to the International Cases chapter. They are listed along with the countries in which their cases were seen.

Renato D. Alarcon, M.D., M.P.H., Peru
Alv A. Dahl, M.D., Norway
Joop T. V. M. de Jong, M.D., Ph.D, West Africa
Ovidio A. deLeon, M.D., Panama
Peter M. Ellis, F.R.A.N.Z.C.P., New Zealand
Yutaka Honda, M.D., Japan
S. T. C. Ilechukwu, M.D., Nigeria
Arthur Kleinman, M.D., People's Republic of China
Carlos A. Leon, M.D., Colombia
Werner Mombour, M.D., Germany
Vernon M. Neppe, M.D., Ph.D, South Africa
Charles Pull, M.D., Luxembourg
Nils Retterstol, Dr. Med., Norway
Hsien Rin, M.D., Taiwan, Republic of China
Shekhar Saxena, M.D., India
Michael von Bose, M.D., Germany
Hans Ulrich Wittchen, Ph.D., Germany
Xu Youxin, M.D., People's Republic of China
DerSon Young, M.D., People's Republic of China
Michael Zaudig, M.D., Germany
Boris Zoubok, M.D., Russia

Introduction and How to Use This Book

INTRODUCTION

This collection of cases grew out of our experience in teaching DSM-III and DSM-III-R and participating in the development of DSM-IV. Reading these accounts of real patients, edited to focus on information relevant to differential diagnosis, has proven to be an effective and enjoyable way for clinicians and students to get experience applying the principles of differential diagnosis to a wide range of patients.

We have chosen focused, edited descriptions of patients, since in standard case summaries discussions of diagnosis often get bogged down in a swamp of details not relevant to the purpose of establishing a diagnosis. (Nondiagnostic information, such as details of childhood and family relationships, however, is often necessary in actual clinical records.) In addition, routine case summaries often inadvertently omit crucial diagnostic information, whereas the cases in this book have been prepared to ensure that all available information necessary for making a diagnosis has been included.

These cases have been drawn from our own experience and from the practices of a large number of clinicians, among them many well-known experts in particular areas of diagnosis and treatment. The identities of the patients have been disguised by altering such details as age and occupation and, occasionally, locale. Often we needed to go back to the contributors of the cases to obtain diagnostically crucial information; we have avoided the temptation to manufacture the missing details. Sometimes, as in the real world, this has led to diagnoses that had to be made provisionally or noted as part of the differential diagnosis.

Following Freud's example, we have provided names for the cases in order to make them easier to refer to. We have included a number of historical cases from the writings of such great nosologists as Emil Kraepelin, Eugen Bleuler, and Sigmund Freud himself. We have made no effort to disguise the identities of these historical patients; we have, however, taken the liberty of providing appropriate names for those who lacked them.

Each case is followed by a discussion of our differential diagnosis, made according to the diagnostic criteria in the text revision of the fourth edition of the American Psychiatric Association's *Diagnostic and Statistical Manual of Mental Disorders* (DSM-IV-TR). (To aid the reader we have noted in parentheses the page number of the diagnostic criteria in the DSM-IV-TR manual.) These discussions include important diagnostic considerations, such as the rationale for making each particular diagnosis, other disorders to be considered in formulating each diagnosis, and, in some cases, recognition of diagnostic uncertainty because of inadequate information, ambiguity in the clinical features, or problems in the classification itself.

These discussions are focused on differential diagnosis, not on the treatment implications of the diagnosis. However, for some of the cases we have been able to obtain follow-up information, which usually includes response to treatment. Often the follow-up information confirms the original diagnosis; occasionally, it raises doubts or leads to a change in diagnosis.

Some degree of ambiguity in diagnosis is still inevitable, despite the increase in reliability made possible by the use of diagnostic criteria. The reader, who may not always agree with our assessment, should understand that we sometimes disagreed with each other about the correct diagnosis. We trust that he or she will seriously consider our formulations, but not regard them as infallible.

These cases can be used for a variety of purposes. They should be of value to experienced clinicians, facilitating their understanding of the concepts and terminology in DSM-IV-TR. All clinicians, regardless of their level of experience and training, may benefit from reading descriptions of cases that are examples of diagnostic categories rarely seen in their treatment settings. Teachers and students of abnormal psychology in the disciplines of psychology, psychiatry, social work, and psychiatric nursing will find these cases useful as illustrations of various types of psychopathology. Similarly, other professionals, such as primary care physicians, internists, and attorneys, may find them instructive.

These cases should prove helpful to professionals studying for specialty examinations, such as the psychiatry boards; they can serve as a means of testing one's knowledge of diagnosis. Research investigators can use them to assess the level of diagnostic expertise and the reliability with which members of their staff can make diagnostic assessments. Finally, these cases provide a historical point of reference as illustrations of diagnostic concepts in the United States at the beginning of this century and, by means of the historical cases, a comparison with diagnostic concepts of the past.

There are five chapters dealing, respectively, with adults, children and adolescents, multiaxial assessment, international cases, and historical cases. The international cases are grouped by geographic region, and the historical cases by their authors.

The original *DSM-III Case Book* was published in 1981, a year after the publication of DSM-III, and revised in 1988, a year after the publication of DSM-III-R. As with the DSM-III-R revision, in the *DSM-IV Casebook* we eliminated some of the earlier cases and added a large number of new cases (these are the first cases in Chapters 1 and 2). The new cases enabled us to expand the coverage of disorders so that we now have at least one example of virtually every diagnostic category in DSM-IV.

HOW TO USE THIS BOOK

The reader who chooses to begin with Chapter 1 and read straight through the book will find cases in no particular diagnostic order. Those who are interested in examples of particular diagnoses (e.g., mood disorders) should consult Appendix D, Index of Cases by DSM-IV-TR diagnoses. Readers who are interested in cases from any of the following categories should consult Appendix B, Cases by Special Interest: forensic, difficult or unusual differential diagnosis, physical disorder, or medical setting.

Appendix A, Index of Case Names, will be useful to the reader who remembers cases by their names. Appendix C, DSM-IV-TR Classification, can be used to see how a particular diagnosis fits into the rest of the classification.

Our own residents in the Department of Psychiatry at Columbia University, College of Physicians and Surgeons, who reviewed the cases in the previous casebook, tell us that they found the cases not only very educational but also fun to read. We hope you will as well.

September 2001

Robert L. Spitzer, M.D.
Miriam Gibbon, M.S.W.
Andrew E. Skodol, M.D.
Janet B. W. Williams, D.S.W.
Michael B. First, M.D.

Chapter 1

Mental Disorders in Adults

BRUJERIA

Celia Vega is a 21-year-old woman, born in Puerto Rico, who is brought, by the police, to the emergency room of a city hospital in handcuffs and leg chains. She is interviewed by an attending psychiatrist, called by the emergency room staff for a consultation. Ms. Vega is a tiny, appealing, childlike woman with dyed red hair who is dressed in hospital clothes. Her face and arms are covered with bruises and scratches from the events of the night before. She is smiling and seductive, rolling her eyes, crossing and recrossing her legs.

The interview takes place in a small, windowless interviewing room into which are crowded the attending psychiatrist, five psychiatric residents, and two social workers. The attending psychiatrist asks her to describe what happened to her, and she says she was washing dishes at her boyfriend's house, where she had been living, and began to have chest pains. Her boyfriend's mother told her to lie down, and the next thing she remembers, she was in the emergency room in chains. The family told her that she "got wild" and tried to bite people. She explains that this has happened many times before, since she was 17. Her boyfriend, who has seen many prior episodes, called the police this time because, as he told her, she had a knife and he was afraid she might kill him.

She has been told that during these episodes she screams, bites, and kicks, and sometimes has tried to get a knife to cut herself. The interviewer asks her, "What do you call these attacks or spells that keep happening to you?" She then says she doesn't want to talk with all the people in the room. She could talk to two or three people, but not eight. The interviewer tries to convince her that these are all people who can help

1

her, and the more the better. She refuses. He then asks if she understands how fortunate she is to be in a famous teaching hospital. She has never heard of it and will not budge. He tells her that these people can help her if she is able to talk to them about what's troubling her. No response. He says, "You have a lot of secrets." More silence.

The interviewer changes tactics. "I'm just going to ask you some questions, and you answer those that you want to."

Interviewer: Do you cry a lot?
Patient: Yes. (Her eyes fill up.)
Interviewer (on a hunch): Bad things have happened to you, right? (She nods.)
Interviewer: Do you ever tell people about the bad things that have happened?
Patient: No. I don't tell nobody nothing.
Interviewer: Do you dream about bad things that have happened?
Patient: Yes, but in the dream it happens to my sister.
Interviewer: What happens? (Silence.) Were you very young when it happened?
Patient: Yes.
Interviewer: 12, 13, 14?
Patient: No.
Interviewer: 15, 16?
Patient: No, the other direction.
Interviewer: 10, 9?
Patient: Yes. When I was 9. Someone did something to me. It changed me. From then on I was different. (She cannot say in what way she was different, and she still will not say what happened.)
Interviewer: Was it someone in your family?
Patient: No. Someone in the neighborhood.
Interviewer: Did it happen over and over?
Patient: No, just a few times.
Interviewer: Did you tell anyone about it?
Patient: No, but my sister told my mother. It happened to my sister too.
Interviewer: What did your mother do?
Patient: Nothing.
Interviewer: Did you feel like it was your fault?
Patient: No. I dream that it happens to my sister, and I wake up crying.

Interviewer: Do you think what happened then has anything to do with these things that happen to you now? What do you call them . . . these attacks, spells?

She says, embarrassed, that they are called *brujeria* (witchcraft). She explains that she was married to a Dominican boy who was a drug dealer. He was sent to prison. His mother blamed her, told her that she would pay for it. After that, 4 years ago, she began having these spells. She now adds that they usually last about 2 hours and that during them she often sees a man's face on the wall.

Interviewer: Who is he? (No answer.) Is he the person who hurt you?

She begins to cry, covers her face with hair, gets very tense. She looks extremely upset, and everyone in the room thinks she's going to have an attack on the spot. The interviewer, recognizing that it would be unwise to pursue this subject further in a group setting, suggests that she now talk to her doctor alone.

Ms. Vega remained in the emergency room overnight and, during several interviews with a social worker, revealed the following additional history. When she was age 9 she and her sister were repeatedly raped by an uncle who used to pick them up from school. Her sister told her mother, who did not believe it and did nothing about it. She acknowledged that the face she saw during the attacks was her uncle's.

She was married at age 14 and had two children, but says that she has never been able to enjoy sex and can have intercourse only if she is high on drugs. During intercourse she often sees the face of her uncle. After her husband went to prison for selling drugs, her mother-in-law got custody of her two children. Why this happened she was unable to explain. She now says that although she loves her children, she gets "nervous" when she has to spend a lot of time with them.

She has not been able to get her life together and finish school or stick with a job. She now lives with her boyfriend's family and spends most of her time watching soap operas. She acknowledges often being quite irritable. She frequently has trouble sleeping and often awakens from bad dreams. Since she had an abortion several months ago, she has been depressed and has had thoughts that she would be better off dead.

Discussion of "Brujeria"

The report that this patient was aggressive, out of control, and brought to the emergency room in restraints suggests either a psychotic episode or drug intoxication. During the interview it appears that neither is likely, and the key question is the nature of the recurrent episodes that the patient has been having for several years. The fact that her behavior during the episodes is so at variance with her normal behavior, and the fact that she does not remember much of what occurs, suggests that she is experiencing recurrent dissociative episodes, or possibly an unusual manifestation of temporal lobe epilepsy. Evidence of the dissociative nature of these episodes emerges as she tells the social worker that the face she sees is that of her uncle who repeatedly raped her when she was a child. (We acknowledge that we have only the patient's report that she was raped, yet we see no reason to doubt her veracity. She has nothing to gain from telling this story, and her distress in speaking about it seems entirely genuine.)

One wonders whether the dissociative episodes may represent a switching to another identity, as in Dissociative Identity Disorder (Multiple Personality Disorder) (see "Mary Quite Contrary," p. 56). However, that diagnosis requires that the alternate personalities have their own relatively enduring pattern of perceiving, relating to, and thinking about the environment and self, and there is no evidence that this occurs during Ms. Vega's dissociative episodes.

We are not surprised to learn later that this patient has many of the symptoms of Posttraumatic Stress Disorder (PTSD). The rapes meet the entry criterion for a traumatic event. The dissociative episodes represent the reexperiencing of the trauma (i.e., fighting off her uncle's sexual advances) as do the dreams and recurrent recollections during sex. PTSD also requires three symptoms of avoidance of stimuli associated with the trauma and numbing of general responsiveness. She clearly avoids sex, and her inability to finish school or work suggests that she may also have markedly diminished interests and a sense of a foreshortened future, which would be evidence of avoidance or numbing. Her difficulty sleeping and irritability satisfy the criterion requirement of increased arousal.

The diagnosis of PTSD is easier to make when a single trauma seems to result in a markedly changed level of functioning. In this case the effect of the trauma is hard to disentangle from the other noxious environmental features of her life. We do not know whether she would have finished school, found a job, and had more satisfying interpersonal relationships if she had not experienced the rape trauma. Still, with all of this uncertainty, our best guess is that the dissociative episodes, which were the ticket to her admission to the mental health system, are symptoms of the more pervasive disorder, Posttraumatic Stress Disorder (DSM-IV-TR, p. 467).

Follow-Up

Ms. Vega was released from the emergency room to live at her sister's house and was visited the next day by the psychiatric resident, along with a social worker from the mobile crisis team. The resident arranged a family meeting with the mother, from whom the patient had really been estranged, and set up a schedule of home visits with the mobile crisis team to engage the patient in psychotherapy. For reasons that are not clear, the follow-up plan did not work, and the patient reappeared in the emergency room 2 weeks later, tearful, "nervous," and wanting to talk to the emergency room social worker. Another appointment was made for ongoing psychotherapy, which the patient never kept.

AGENT JOHNSON

A tall, well-groomed 30-year-old African American man walked into the emergency room of a large urban hospital, registered under the name Harry Backman, and asked to be admitted to Ward Three of the psychiatric division. He claimed that, despite the fact that all of his identification cards bore the name Harry Backman, his real name was Johnson. "And your first name?" asked the resident psychiatrist. "We're not allowed to divulge our first names," he confided. He went on to explain that in fact he was Agent Johnson, an FBI agent on a mission to find Harry Backman, who had last been seen in Pittsburgh several years earlier. He claimed to have followed Harry from city to city, often posing as a patient in the psychiatric hospitals where Harry had been treated in order to obtain information about him. Harry had a seizure disorder for which he took phenytoin and primidone, and he had also taken trifluoperazine in the past. Agent Johnson did not take any medications. Communicating with his superiors at the FBI via a high-frequency radio stashed in his bag, Agent Johnson had come to this hospital in order to be admitted to the very ward on which Harry Backman had been treated as a 10-year-old boy, in order to seek clues about Harry's whereabouts. The patient confided his fear that the "real" Harry was, in fact, dead, and that an impostor might be posing as Harry in order to collect his welfare checks.

During the interview, the patient was generally cooperative and engaging. His affect ranged from serious to jocular, and when his story was challenged, he became defensive and hostile. There was no evidence of disorganized speech, cognitive impairment, or hallucinations. Results of a physical examination, including a thorough neurological examination, and all laboratory tests were normal.

A call to the shelter where Agent Johnson lived confirmed that his name was Harry Backman, that he carried diagnoses of chronic Schizophrenia and seizure disorder, and that he was maintained on trifluoperazine, phenytoin, and primidone. These medications were subsequently prescribed by the emergency room physician. In addition, a social worker at the shelter said that Harry had been wandering the streets in the past few days, frequently not returning to the shelter at night. She had not witnessed any seizures, and she did not know anything about Agent Johnson.

On the following day, the patient had a generalized tonic-clonic seizure, lasting approximately 2 minutes, during which he hit his head on the floor. He was treated in the medical emergency room; all tests, including a computed tomography scan, were normal. After a brief period of postictal confusion, the patient woke up. He responded to the name Harry and acknowledged that he had had a seizure. The confused resident scratched her head and said, "But I thought Harry had the seizure disorder!" "I AM Harry!" said the patient with a smile. "I've found him!"

Discussion of "Agent Johnson"

The only obvious sign of psychopathology in this case is Harry's belief that he is another person, FBI Agent Johnson. This is clearly a delusion of false identity. Although grandiose delusions of false identity occasionally occur in manic episodes of Bipolar I Disorder, delusions of false identity almost invariably are symptoms of Schizophrenia.

If we try to make a diagnosis on the basis of the very limited information that we have about Harry, the first task is to decide whether his delusion is bizarre. Bizarre delusions involve phenomena that do not occur in real life, such as thought broadcasting or being controlled by an outside force. It is hard to apply the concept of bizarre delusions to Harry's belief that he is Agent Johnson. On the one hand, there are FBI agents who track down other people, and people do deliberately change their identities. On the other hand, people cannot literally stop being themselves and become someone else.

We suspect that Harry's reference to communicating with his superiors via a high-frequency radio indicates that he probably has auditory hallucinations. The combination of delusions (whether bizarre or not) and hallucinations, plus a chronic illness with social and occupational dysfunction, in the absence of a mood disorder or a substance or general medical condition that could account for the disturbance, substantiates a diagnosis of Schizophrenia (DSM-IV-TR, p. 312). We would note the epilepsy only on Axis III, as we doubt that it is etiologically responsible for the disturbance.

ELEPHANT MAN

Chris is a shy, anxious-looking 31-year-old carpenter who has been hospitalized after making a suicide attempt by putting his head in a plastic bag. He asks to meet with the psychiatrist in a darkened room. He is wearing a baseball cap pulled down over his forehead and partially covering his eyes. Looking down at the floor, Chris says he has no friends, has just been fired from his job, and was recently rejected by his girlfriend. When the psychiatrist asks Chris to elaborate, he replies, "It's really hard to talk about this, Doctor. I don't know if I can. It's too embarrassing. Well, I guess I should tell you . . . after all, I'm in the hospital because of it. It's my nose." "Your nose?" the psychiatrist asks. "Yes, these huge pockmarks on my nose. They're grotesque! I look like a monster. I'm as ugly as the Elephant Man! These marks on my nose are all I can think about. I've thought about them every day for the past 15 years. I even have nightmares about them. And I think that everyone can see them and that they laugh at me because of them. That's why I wear this hat all the time. And that's why I couldn't talk to you in a bright room . . . you'd see how ugly I am."

The psychiatrist couldn't see the huge pockmarks that Chris was referring to, even when she later met him in a brightly lit room. Chris is, in fact, a handsome man with normal-appearing facial pores. The psychiatrist says, "I see no ugly pockmarks. Is it possible that your view of your appearance is distorted, that maybe the pockmarks are just normal-looking facial pores?"

"That's a hard question to answer," Chris replies. "I've pretty much kept this preoccupation a secret because it's so embarrassing. I'm afraid people will think I'm vain. But I've told a few people about it, and they've tried to convince me that the pores really aren't visible. Sometimes I sort of believe them. I think I probably am distorting and that they're not so bad. Then I look in the mirror and see that they're huge and ugly, and I'm convinced that people laugh at them. Then no one can talk me out of it. When people try to, I think they just feel sorry for me and that they're trying to make me feel better. This has affected me in a lot of ways, Doctor," Chris adds. "It may be hard for you to believe, but this problem has ruined my life. All I can think about is my face. I spend hours a day looking at the marks in the mirror. But I just can't resist. I started missing more and more work, and I stopped going out with my friends and my girlfriend. I got so anxious when people looked at me that I started staying in the house most of the time. Sometimes when I did go out, I went through red lights so I wouldn't have to sit at the light where people might be staring at me. The hat helped a little, but it didn't cover all the marks. I tried covering them with makeup for a while, but I thought people could see the makeup so that didn't really help. The only time I really felt comfortable was when I wore my nephew's Batman mask on Halloween. Then no one could see the marks. I missed so much work that I was fired. My girlfriend stuck it out with me for a long time, but she finally couldn't take it anymore. One thing that was really hard for her was that I started asking her about 50 times a day whether I looked okay and whether she could see the marks. I think that was the last straw. If I had a choice, I'd rather have cancer. It must be less painful. This is like an arrow through my heart."

Chris went on to discuss the fact that he had seen a dermatologist to request dermabrasion, but was refused the procedure because "the dermatologist said there was nothing there." He finally convinced another dermatologist to do the procedure but thought it did not help. Eventually, he felt so desperate over the supposed marks that he made two suicide attempts. His most recent attempt occurred after he looked in the mirror and was horrified by what he saw. He told the psychiatrist, "I saw how awful I looked, and I thought, I'm not sure it's worth it to go on living if I have to look like this and think about this all the time." His first suicide attempt had also led to hospitalization; but, because Chris was so ashamed of his concern and thought it wouldn't be taken seriously, he had kept it a secret and told the staff only that he was depressed.

Discussion of "Elephant Man"

Chris looks normal but is preoccupied with a supposed defect in his appearance. This preoccupation has clearly caused him much distress and has significantly interfered with his functioning. Although this is a fairly severe case of Body Dysmorphic Disorder (DSM-IV-TR, p. 510), it is not atypical; occupational, social, and other important areas of functioning may be severely impaired, and suicide attempts are not uncommon. However, the degree of distress and dysfunction associated with this disorder spans a spectrum of severity; some people with this disorder—although distressed and perhaps not functioning up to their capacity—nevertheless cope relatively well.

Complaints in Body Dysmorphic Disorder commonly involve facial flaws—often supposed defects of the hair, nose, or skin. However, any body part can be involved, and many people with this disorder are preoccupied with several body parts simultaneously. In some cases, like Chris's, no physical anomaly is actually present. In other cases, a slight physical anomaly is present, but the person's concern is markedly excessive.

Certain associated behaviors are commonly present, although not required, for the diagnosis. They include excessive mirror checking, grooming activities, questioning of others about the "defect," skin picking, comparison with others, camouflaging, and ideas or delusions of reference. Because people with Body Dysmorphic Disorder may be ashamed of their concern, they often keep it a secret and may not reveal it unless specifically asked about it.

A controversy that surrounds this disorder is whether Body Dysmorphic Disorder and its delusional counterpart, Delusional Disorder, Somatic Type, are two different disorders or the same disorder. In Body Dysmorphic Disorder, insight into the imagined or distorted nature of the "defect" is presumed to be present, and it is therefore classified separately from its delusional counterpart, Delusional Disorder, Somatic Type, in which insight is absent (i.e., the person is convinced that the abnormality is real and that his or her view of it is undistorted). However, it can be difficult to differentiate the delusional thinking of Delusional Disorder from the nondelusional thinking of Body Dysmorphic Disorder, as people with Body Dysmorphic Disorder often have poor insight into the fact that the "defect" is imagined or distorted. In addition, it appears that the degree of insight may be more appropriately conceptualized as spanning a spectrum that ranges from good insight to delusional thinking, along which the person's belief may move over time. Indeed, at times Chris's insight was fair, which would warrant a diagnosis of Body Dysmorphic Disorder, but he was often delusional, which would technically warrant a diagnosis of Delusional Disorder, Somatic Type. Does Chris have one disorder or two?

Such classification difficulties, as well as preliminary evidence suggesting that the two disorders may be one and the same, varying only in severity, have raised unresolved questions about how Body Dysmorphic Disorder and its delusional variant should be classified. The solution adopted by DSM-IV (and DSM-IV-TR) is as follows: people with nondelusional Body Dysmorphic Disorder will receive that diagnosis only, but those with delusional Body Dysmorphic Disorder will receive two diagnoses—both Body Dysmorphic Disorder and Delusional Disorder, Somatic Type (DSM-IV-TR, p. 329). Coding what is probably one disorder as two diagnoses highlights the need for continued research to determine whether these two presentations are merely a single disorder with variable manifestations.

AN IRON WILL

A 35-year-old African American woman, Sheila Joyner, was brought to the psychiatric emergency room at the request of the pediatrician examining her 14-month-old baby, Rasheed. Ms. Joyner had first brought her child to see a pediatrician 2 weeks earlier, when the baby's grandmother complained that a diet consisting largely of breast milk was not appropriate for a child of that age. The pediatrician prescribed iron and scheduled a follow-up appointment. When Ms. Joyner reported at follow-up that she had not given her son iron, the pediatrician, concerned because the baby had lost an additional 2 pounds, arranged for the baby to be hospitalized, even though the mother objected. Three security guards were required to wrest the baby from his sobbing mother; and when she began to threaten the staff with a lawsuit, saying the doctors were going to "poison" her baby, Ms. Joyner was brought to the adult psychiatric emergency room, where she spent the night.

The following morning, Ms. Joyner appeared calm but guarded throughout the psychiatric interview. She refused to shake the examiner's hand, explaining that she had just washed her hands in preparation for a snack. She denied any compulsion to wash or obsession with cleanliness. Ms. Joyner reported graduating from college and having taught elementary school until her only child was born, fathered by a friend who lived in another city. Her pregnancy was undetected until 5 months of gestation and complicated by severe anemia. She had had anemia 10 years earlier, but had then refused medical care. She reported curing it herself, by learning to live in a more "natural manner," walking in parks rather than near buildings, and eating only natural foods and "purified" water. This lifestyle, she explained, enabled her to produce a perfectly healthy baby even though her obstetrician had told her that she herself had severe anemia.

Ms. Joyner explained that she had refused to feed her baby "non-organic" iron as prescribed by the pediatrician and insisted on giving him only breast milk because she wanted to provide him with the same diet that had been so good for her. She did not have Rasheed vaccinated, as this was "unnatural," and she supported these views by referring to books and pamphlets from organizations promoting "natural" approaches to health, as well as to discussions with friends who shared these views. Her arguments, although based on questionable data, were understandable and internally consistent. At no time did she show evidence of tangential or disorganized speech, and she appeared quite intelligent.

The psychiatrist tried to explain that Rasheed's anemia was serious and that he was at risk for permanent neurological damage. Ms. Joyner responded by saying that the same treatment that had been good for her would protect her baby. When the doctor explained the ways in which an infant's needs were different from an adult's, she stated that, just as the doctors had been wrong about treating her anemia in the past, the psychiatrist was now wrong about her child. Ms. Joyner clung to her position regarding the danger of "nonorganic" iron, citing as evidence the stomach upset she had experienced when she had taken iron. If given the choice between losing her child and being forced to feed him iron, she would rather lose him, as she did not want any part of "poisoning" her baby.

Because Ms. Joyner was not in need of emergent psychiatric treatment, she was allowed to leave the emergency room and went immediately to her baby's room in the children's hospital. She stayed with Rasheed and made it impossible for the staff to feed him, arguing that the food served was poisonous and the medical tests unnecessary. When the psychiatrist who had seen her in the emergency room was again consulted, the pediatric staff described the dire condition of the baby. Not only was he severely anemic, but he also was grossly malnourished and developmentally delayed, performing motor and communicative tasks at the level of a 7- to 9-month-old. Further, a chest X-ray had revealed possible tuberculosis, but Ms. Joyner would not allow him to be treated.

The psychiatrist met with Ms. Joyner once again and explained the severity of her baby's condition. She countered that the standards used to measure her baby were "Western" and not appropriate for a baby with "African genes." As the medical condition of the baby deteriorated, the pediatric staff turned to legal counsel and the Bureau of Child Welfare; both suggested treating the baby against the mother's will.

Discussion of "An Iron Will"

There can be no disagreement that Rasheed needs to receive medical care if he is to survive. However, it is less clear how one should understand his mother's stubborn insistence that he be given no "unnatural" medication. Does her belief that "unnatural" medicines and foods are poisonous constitute a delusion? If so, the diagnosis would be Delusional Disorder, Persecutory Type. In favor of such a diagnosis is the extreme degree to which she acts on her beliefs even in the face of evidence that doing so has terrible consequences for her son. Her statement that she had treated her own anemia by avoiding walking near buildings suggests an idiosyncratic approach to medical treatment that is unlikely to be found in any of her pamphlets. On the other hand, she has been influenced by nontraditional views of medicine and health that are espoused by a vocal minority.

When making a judgment about whether a particular irrational belief is a delusion, one generally excludes those beliefs that are shared by a subculture. Therefore, the issues are to what extent Ms. Joyner's behavior can be accounted for by this identification with a subculture and to what extent her belief that conventional medical treatment represents "poisoning" is a delusion. We believe that a key consideration is the motivation that she ascribes to the doctors who she believes are poisoning her child. We very much doubt that she believes that the doctors are doing so malevolently—as she would likely believe if she had Delusional Disorder.

Whether she has a psychiatric diagnosis or not, the V code of Neglect of Child (DSM-IV-TR, p. 738) certainly applies. If a psychiatric diagnosis is given, we would opt for the residual category of Psychotic Disorder Not Otherwise Specified (DSM-IV-TR, p. 343).

Follow-Up

The child was treated as an inpatient for 6 weeks. His nutritional status became normal, and he approached appropriate developmental milestones. Ms. Joyner was allowed frequent contact, but was not permitted to interfere with his care. After court proceedings, custody of the child was granted to his grandmother, but Ms. Joyner had full visitation rights. She refused any psychiatric treatment, even if it would increase her chances of regaining custody.

A DOG AND A GUN

A 74-year-old African American woman, Ms. Richardson, was brought to a city hospital emergency room by the police. She is unkempt, dirty, and foul smelling. She does not look at the interviewer and is apparently confused and unresponsive to most of his questions. She knows her name and address, but not the day or the month. She is unable to describe the events that led to her admission.

The police reported that they were called by neighbors because Ms. Richardson had been wandering around the neighborhood and not taking care of herself. The medical center mobile crisis unit went to her house twice but could not get in and presumed she was not home. Finally, the police came and broke into the apartment, where they were met by a snarling German shepherd. They shot the dog with a tranquilizing gun and then found Ms. Richardson hiding in the corner, wearing nothing but a bra. The apartment was filthy, the floor littered with dog feces. The police found a gun, which they took into custody.

The following day, while Ms. Richardson was awaiting transfer to a medical unit for treatment of her out-of-control diabetes, the supervising psychiatrist attempted to interview her. Her facial expression was still mostly unresponsive, and she still didn't know the month and couldn't say what hospital she was in. She reported that the neighbors had called the police because she was "sick," and indeed she had felt sick and weak, with pains in her shoulder; in addition, she had not eaten for 3 days. She remembered that the police had shot her dog with a tranquilizer, and said the dog was now in "the shop" and would be returned to her when she got home. She refused to give the name of a neighbor who was a friend, saying, "He's got enough troubles of his own." She denied ever being in a psychiatric hospital or hearing voices but acknowledged that she had at one point seen a psychiatrist "near Lincoln Center" because she couldn't sleep. He had prescribed medication that was too strong, so she didn't take it. She didn't remember the name, so the interviewer asked if it was Thorazine. She said no, it was "allal." "Haldol?" asked the interviewer. She nodded. The interviewer was convinced that was the drug, but other observers thought she might have said yes to anything that sounded remotely like it, such as "Elavil." When asked about the gun, she denied, with some annoyance, that it was real and said it was a toy gun that had been brought to the house by her brother, who had died 8 years ago. She was still feeling weak and sick, complained of pains in her shoulder, and apparently had trouble swallowing. She did manage to smile as the team left her bedside.

Discussion of "A Dog and a Gun"

When this patient was seen initially in the emergency room, her most prominent symptoms were disorientation, inability to focus attention, and a history of disorganized behavior that probably developed over a relatively short period of time. These are the characteristic features of Delirium (DSM-IV-TR, p. 143); that diagnosis is further supported by the information gained on the second day that her diabetes had been out of control, and her improved mental status with treatment of the diabetes.

A valiant attempt was made to obtain follow-up information to determine whether the Delirium was superimposed on a more chronic disorder, such as Schizophrenia or Dementia. Although the staff on the medical unit recalled having seen the patient previously, they could offer no additional information, and both the patient and her chart were nowhere to be found.

SOMETHING OF VALUE

Eli Wolfe came into the emergency room of a New York hospital complaining of malaise, fever, and a cough. An upper respiratory infection was diagnosed. As the doctor was writing out a prescription, Mr. Wolfe tearfully revealed that he had no home to go to, was depressed, and felt that life was not worth living. A psychiatric resident was called to see the patient and obtained the following additional information.

For the past month Mr. Wolfe had been living in the basement of his apartment building, eating in restaurants, and using a health club for showers. He was eating and sleeping poorly. His own apartment was so full of newspapers, magazines, and books that he could no longer get in the door, but he could not bring himself to get rid of any of his "stuff."

When he was 12, Mr. Wolfe began collecting baseball cards and then books and magazines. His parents were poor immigrants from Eastern Europe, and the idea of holding on to things that might someday be valuable was not strange to them. Eventually, however, the apartment became so cluttered that they threw out much of his collection. He retrieved it from the garbage, and from that point on his "collecting" became a focus of conflict with family and employers.

Mr. Wolfe does not go out of his way to obtain things, but once he has a newspaper, book, or magazine, he cannot throw it away because "there might be something of value written in it." The thought of throwing things out makes him extremely anxious, and, in the end, he simply cannot do it.

For many years he worked as a doorman in elegant apartment buildings, but invariably was fired because he brought his "stuff" to store in his workplace and sometimes got into fistfights with the building maintenance people who tried to throw it out. He was married for 10 years and has a 25-year-old son. His wife finally left him, unable to tolerate his behavior. He rarely sees his son.

Mr. Wolfe first entered treatment not because of his collecting but because, at age 20, "my mood took a turn for the worse. I had a breakdown." He stopped doing virtually everything—working, eating, sleeping. "It was an effort even to lift my leg." He began seeing a psychiatrist as an outpatient and over the years has been in therapy much of the time, treated with a variety of antidepressants and anxiolytics.

After his divorce, 10 years ago, he moved some of his collection into his own apartment and rented storage space for the rest. Gradually his new apartment filled up with newspapers, magazines, and books, and it became a struggle just to get in the front door and make his way to his bed. Finally, last month, he injured his shoulder trying to push things aside and then abandoned the apartment for a cot in the basement of the building. He understands that his inability to throw things out is irrational, but the thought of starting to do it makes him intolerably anxious.

Discussion of "Something of Value"

Mr. Wolfe presents with symptoms suggesting depression: depressed mood, difficulty eating and sleeping, and thoughts that life is not worth living. More information about the severity and persistence of these symptoms would rule out a diagnosis of Major Depressive Disorder. However, what is most striking is that there is a long-standing problem with not being able to throw things out—hoarding—that has totally disrupted his life.

How to diagnose Mr. Wolfe's long-standing difficulty is not at all clear. Many people have trouble throwing things away that they think may be of potential value, but, if this trait does not cause significant distress or impairment, a diagnosis of a mental disorder is not appropriate. That is certainly not the case with Mr. Wolfe. One possibility is that the hoarding is part of a larger picture of Obsessive-Compulsive Personality Disorder, as hoarding behavior is actually one of the criteria for that disorder and is present in approximately half of the cases with the disorder. However, none of the other features of that disorder, such as perfectionism or excessive devotion to work, seem to be present.

Hoarding is sometimes seen as part of the disorganized or bizarre behavior of people with Schizophrenia, but in this case none of the characteristic features of Schizophrenia are present. Mr. Wolfe's anxiety, associated with the thought of throwing things away, suggests an obsession. However, in true obsessions such thoughts are ego-dystonic, whereas in Mr. Wolfe's case, they are not. Is the hoarding behavior a compulsion? Compulsions are repetitive behaviors or thoughts that the person engages in and that are done in a stereotyped manner or in response to an obsession. In contrast, Mr. Wolfe's hoarding is actually the failure to engage in an appropriate behavior (i.e., throwing out his junk). Furthermore, he does not follow any stereotyped rules in collecting his books and papers, and his hoarding is not in response to an obsession.

Experts in Obsessive-Compulsive Disorder generally regard extreme hoarding as part of the spectrum of Obsessive-Compulsive Disorder. They point out that many "hoarders" do in fact exhibit checking or other compulsive rituals that meet the criteria for compulsions even when the hoarding behavior is ego-syntonic. They also point to the extreme anxiety that these patients exhibit if the hoarding behavior is thwarted.

Because Mr. Wolfe does not seem to have any strictly defined obsessions or compulsions, we would give the residual category of Anxiety Disorder Not Otherwise Specified (DSM-IV-TR, p. 484). An alternative way of viewing the hoarding is to consider it a maladaptive personality trait and make the diagnosis Personality Disorder Not Otherwise Specified (DSM-IV-TR, p. 729).

Follow-Up

Mr. Wolfe was admitted to the psychiatric hospital, diagnosed as having a Major Depressive Disorder, and prescribed an antidepressant, the dosage of which was gradually raised. After 4 weeks, with considerable pressure from his therapist, he was able to clear the foyer of his apartment, so he could at least get in the door. His mood improved, and he began eating and sleeping better. In the succeeding 6 months, he has slowly and methodically discarded bundles of articles. Although he is now able to live in his apartment, it remains cluttered with junk.

Melancholy or Malarkey?

Mr. Dennis O'Malley is a small, bent, disheveled 63-year-old man with a very faint Irish accent. He was referred for psychiatric evaluation when he attended the medical clinic where he was being followed for diabetes and maintenance of a colostomy that he had had for 5 years as a result of ulcerative colitis. He told his doctor that he was upset because he had been hearing voices, and was promptly sent to the psychiatry clinic for an evaluation.

Mr. O'Malley is interviewed by a psychiatrist, and begins the telling of his chief complaint, in traditional Irish fashion, with a story. A few weeks ago—he's not quite sure when—he took a fellow home from church and, feeling tired, lay down on the fellow's bed to take a nap. He awoke to find the fellow "on top of" him and raced out the door as fast as he could go. At this point, he's not sure whether it really happened or was a dream or a hallucination. In any case, it was followed some time later by an experience on the street in which a strange man called him "an Irish fag." This upset him a great deal, and he has been brooding about it ever since. He remembers that about a year ago, the owners of a new car wash in the neighborhood called him a fag, and he wonders if these things are related. Two weeks ago he began to hear voices calling him a fag and saying other derogatory things about him, and his "whole system dropped down." He knows he is not homosexual and understands at some level that what is happening is "in my mind." Nevertheless, he feels that everyone in the neighborhood believes that he is homosexual. He has been very nervous and shaky and has gone to his priest, who tells him that it is his imagination and he should ignore it. He is apparently still hearing the voices during the interview.

Mr. O'Malley describes his mood as "lousy" and "nervous and shaky." He doesn't volunteer feeling depressed, but says that he has not been interested in seeing friends or doing anything since this began. He also says that he has no appetite and has lost weight, but denies changes in his sleeping. Although he doesn't acknowledge feeling guilty about things he has done, he says he feels guilty about "the blasphemous words" the voices are saying. When asked specifically about suicide, he says that he's Catholic and he would not go to heaven if he committed suicide, so therefore he would not kill himself; however, he has thought that he would be better off if something just happened to him to make his heart stop.

Mr. O'Malley had a similar experience 12 years ago when he heard blaspheming voices and became preoccupied with religious "scruples." He was treated as an outpatient for several months and took some kind of medication, the name of which he does not remember. He went back to work as a cab driver and continued driving until his deteriorating physical condition caused him to go on disability 5 years ago. He lives with his wife and a 25-year-old son and spends a good deal of time in church-related activities and playing the saxophone for various community affairs. He has not had a drink for 30 years.

When questioned about memory problems, he describes making the wrong turn once on a highway and a few other instances of forgetting whether he had turned off the gas stove in his kitchen.

The following day, Mr. O'Malley's wife was interviewed by the psychiatrist on the ward to which he had been admitted. She reported that he had always tended to exaggerate slights and was quick to take offense and to read criticism into the remarks of others. She saw his distress of the past few weeks as simply an exaggeration of his nature. She noticed that he had been "listless" for a few days, and thought maybe he had a "virus." She described the episode 12 years earlier as similar to this one in that he had become increasingly nervous and suspicious and had begun hearing "voices."

Discussion of "Melancholy or Malarkey?"

The first diagnostic question is whether the "voices" that call Mr. O'Malley an "Irish fag" are hallucinations or obsessions. The symptom has several features that suggest an obsession: they are recurrent, intrusive, and stereotyped. However, the patient does not experience them as products of his own mind, but as accusations that come from other people, which he then elaborates to include everyone in the neighborhood. Therefore, the voices appear to be true hallucinations that are delusionally elaborated.

Are the delusions and hallucinations symptomatic of a mood disorder? He does say that he has not been interested in anything since this all began and that he has lost considerable weight and feels guilty about the blasphemous voices. He has recurrent thoughts of death even though he denies suicidal thoughts. We think there probably are enough symptoms to justify a diagnosis of Major Depressive Disorder (DSM-IV-TR, p. 376). We suspect that the prior episode was similar, so we add Recurrent to the diagnosis. Because the hallucinations and delusions are persecutory and the patient does not feel guilty of the things that he is accused of (as in a typical depressive delusion), we add also With Mood-Incongruent Psychotic Features (DSM-IV-TR, p. 413).

Follow-Up

Mr. O'Malley was treated with antipsychotic medication on an inpatient unit. The treating psychiatrists were not impressed with the depressive symptoms and therefore did not include antidepressant medication until some weeks later when the voices diminished and the patient became more obviously depressed. A full neurological examination, including a computed tomography scan, was negative. He left the hospital in 4 weeks, at which time he was much improved.

His outpatient psychiatrist, who began treating him when he left the hospital, was impressed with a new symptom: Mr. O'Malley's obsessive requests for reassurance that he had not disobeyed church rules, such as having thrown the communion wafer into the toilet, although he recognized that he had not done this. The outpatient psychiatrist gradually reduced his antipsychotic medication and began treating him with a new antidepressant that was thought to be useful also in the treatment of Obsessive-Compulsive Disorder. Maintained on this medication, Mr. O'Malley, a year later, was free of his symptoms and had returned to his baseline functioning.

LATE BLOOMER

A single, unemployed, college-educated 35-year-old African American woman, Ms. Fielding, was escorted to the emergency room by the mobile crisis team. The team had been contacted by the patient's sister after she failed to persuade Ms. Fielding to visit an outpatient psychiatrist. Her sister was concerned about the patient's increasingly erratic work patterns and, more recently, her bizarre behavior since the death of their father 2 years ago. The patient's only prior psychiatric contact had been brief psychotherapy in college.

The patient had not worked since losing her job 3 months ago. According to her boyfriend and roommate (both of whom live with her), she had become intensely preoccupied with the upstairs neighbors. A few days earlier she had banged on their front door with an iron for no apparent reason. She told the mobile crisis team that the family upstairs was harassing her by "accessing" her thoughts and then repeating them to her. The crisis team brought her to the emergency room for evaluation of "thought broadcasting." Though she denied having any trouble with her thinking, she conceded that she had been feeling "stressed" since losing her job, and might benefit from more psychotherapy.

After reading the admission note, which described the patient's bizarre symptoms, the emergency room psychiatrists were surprised to encounter a poised, relaxed, and attractive young woman, stylishly dressed and appearing perfectly normal. She greeted them with a courteous, if somewhat superficial, smile. She related to the doctors with nonchalant respectfulness. When asked why she was there, she ventured a timid shrug, and replied, "I was hoping to find out from you!"

Ms. Fielding had been working as a secretary and attributed her job loss to the sluggish economy. She denied having any recent mood disturbance and answered no to questions about psychotic symptoms, punctuating each query with a polite but incredulous laugh. Wondering if perhaps the crisis team's assessment was of a different patient, the interviewer asked, somewhat apologetically, if the patient ever wondered whether people could read her mind. She replied, "Oh yes, it happens all the time," and described how, on one occasion, she was standing in her kitchen planning dinner in silence, only to hear, moments later, voices of people on the street below reciting the entire menu. She was convinced of the reality of the experience, having verified it by looking out the window and observing them speaking her thoughts aloud.

The patient was distressed not so much by people "accessing" her thoughts as by her inability to exercise control over the process. She believed that most people developed telepathic powers in childhood and that she was a "late bloomer" who had just become aware of her abilities and was currently overwhelmed by them. Although she had begun having telepathic experiences 2 years ago, they had become almost constant in the 3 months since losing her job. She was troubled most by her upstairs neighbors, who would not only repeat her thoughts but would bombard her with their own devaluing and critical comments, such as

"You're no good!" and "You have to leave." They had begun to intrude upon her mercilessly, at all hours of the night and day.

She was convinced that the only solution was for the family to move away. When asked if she had contemplated other possibilities, she reluctantly admitted that she had spoken to her boyfriend about hiring a hit man to "threaten" or, if need be, "eliminate" the couple. She hoped she would be able to spare their two children, who she felt were not involved in this invasion of her "mental boundaries." This concern for the children was the only insight she demonstrated into the gravity of her symptoms. She did agree, however, to admit herself voluntarily to the hospital.

Discussion of "Late Bloomer"

It is extremely unusual for patients with bizarre delusions, such as Ms. Fielding's delusion that her thoughts were "accessed" by others, to appear otherwise perfectly normal. Nevertheless, the presence of bizarre delusions, hallucinations, and social and occupational impairment for at least 1 month, but less than 6 months, in the absence of a mood disorder, substance, or general medical condition that could account for the disturbance, justifies a diagnosis of Schizophreniform Disorder (DSM-IV-TR, p. 319). Her good premorbid functioning and the absence of blunted or flat affect indicate the further specification of With Good Prognostic Features. When the diagnosis is made without waiting for recovery, as in this case, it is further qualified as Provisional, because if continuous signs of the disturbance persist for at least 6 months, the diagnosis would change to Schizophrenia.

Follow-Up

Once admitted to the hospital, Ms. Fielding immediately began pressing for discharge and disavowed her previous symptoms. Her behavior, thinking, and affect seemed otherwise normal. After 2 weeks of observation, she was discharged to her treating physician's clinic. Within a month, however, she again admitted having frightening experiences of hearing voices and of reading other people's thoughts, as well as a general inability to plan for finding work. She agreed to try medication.

She was treated with an antipsychotic drug, and her frightening hallucinations, as well as the belief that she was clairvoyant, remitted. Within 3 months following discharge, she had obtained work with a temporary employment agency. Soon afterward, feeling completely well, she stopped attending the clinic and was lost to follow-up.

Although the total duration of the illness approaches 6 months, we would give her the benefit of the doubt and retain the diagnosis of Schizophreniform Disorder.

ROLLER COASTER

When Ernest Eaton's desperate wife finally got him to agree to a comprehensive inpatient evaluation, he was 37, was unemployed, and had been essentially nonfunctional for several years. After a week during which he was partying all night and shopping all day, Mrs. Eaton said that she would leave him if he did not check into a psychiatric hospital. The admitting psychiatrist found him to be a fast-talking, jovial, seductive man with no evidence of delusions or hallucinations.

Mr. Eaton's troubles began 7 years before when he was working as an insurance adjuster and had a few months of mild, intermittent, depressive symptoms, anxiety, fatigue, insomnia, and loss of appetite. At the time, he attributed these symptoms to stress at work, and within a few months was back to his usual self.

A few years later an asymptomatic thyroid mass was noted during a routine physical exam. One month after removal of the mass, a papillary cyst, Mr. Eaton noted dramatic mood changes. Twenty-five days of remarkable energy, hyperactivity, and euphoria were followed by 5 days of depression during which he slept a lot and felt that he could hardly move. This pattern of alternating periods of elation and depression, apparently with few "normal" days, repeated itself continuously over the following years.

During his energetic periods, Mr. Eaton was optimistic and self-confident, but short tempered and easily irritated. His judgment at work was erratic. He spent large sums of money on unnecessary and, for him, uncharacteristic purchases, such as a high-priced stereo system and several Doberman pinschers. He also had several impulsive sexual flings. During his depressed periods, he often stayed in bed all day because of fatigue, lack of motivation, and depressed mood. He felt guilty about the irresponsibilities and excesses of the previous several weeks. He stopped eating, bathing, and shaving. After several days of this withdrawal, Mr. Eaton would rise from bed one morning feeling better and, within 2 days, be back at work, often working feverishly, though ineffectively, to catch up on work he had let slide during his depressed periods.

Although both he and his wife denied any drug use, other than drinking binges during his hyperactive periods, Mr. Eaton had been dismissed from his job 5 years previously because his supervisor was convinced that his overactivity must be due to drug use. His wife had supported him since then.

When he finally agreed to a psychiatric evaluation 2 years ago, Mr. Eaton was minimally cooperative and noncompliant with several medications that were prescribed, including lithium, neuroleptics, and antidepressants. His mood swings had continued with few interruptions up to the current hospitalization.

In the hospital results of his physical examination, blood chemistry, blood counts, computed tomography scan, and cognitive testing were unremarkable. Thyroid function testing revealed some laboratory evidence of thyroid hypofunction, but he was without clinical signs of thyroid disease. After a week he switched to his characteristic depressive state.

Discussion of "Roller Coaster"

The diagnosis of Bipolar I Disorder, Most Recent Episode Manic, is not difficult to make in this case (DSM-IV-TR, p. 389). In his energetic periods, Mr. Eaton had the characteristic symptoms of a manic episode: decreased need for sleep, overactivity, overtalkativeness, and excessive involvement in pleasurable activities without thinking of the consequences. In his depressed periods, he met the symptom, but not the duration, criteria for major depressive episodes. Because he had had more than four episodes of mania in a 1-year period, separated by periods of depression, the Bipolar I Disorder is further qualified as With Rapid Cycling (DSM-IV-TR, p. 428).

Unlike Mr. Eaton, not all persons with Rapid Cycling experience predictable shifts from mania to depression without intervening periods of euthymia. Rapid Cycling usually involves one or more manic or hypomanic episodes, as in this case, but is also diagnosed if all of the episodes are depressed, manic, or hypomanic so long as they are separated by periods of remission (or switches to the opposite pole).

As noted previously, Mr. Eaton's unusual behavior was attributed by his employers to drug use. It is not uncommon for such an erratic mood pattern to be mistakenly identified as evidence of drug abuse, which should also be part of the differential diagnosis when Rapid Cycling is being considered. Mr. Eaton is somewhat atypical among persons with Rapid Cycling in that the condition is much more common in women. The onset of his symptoms closely followed partial thyroidectomy, and he was found to have evidence of mild thyroid hypofunction. Thyroid disease has been reported in some studies to be a risk factor for Rapid Cycling. An additional risk factor, of unclear significance in this case, is the use of antidepressant medication. Because of high rates of nonresponse to lithium, Rapid Cycling is often treated with anticonvulsants.

Follow-Up

After 3 weeks in the hospital, Mr. Eaton's mood was stable on lithium and thyroxine, the latter being added for mood stabilization rather than to treat the laboratory evidence of thyroid hypofunction. He left the hospital, very quickly found a new job, and did well for the following year. Feeling well, he decided that he didn't need the medication and stopped taking the lithium. Within weeks he became extremely manic and had to be hospitalized again.

FATTY

Andrea Simpson weighed 230 pounds when she returned to her former therapist to get help for the eating and weight problems that had caused her grief since she was a child. She was again having uncontrollable eating binges, and had gained over 50 pounds in 6 months.

Andrea recalled being called "fatty" by her schoolmates in early elementary school, and had had frequent arguments with her mother throughout childhood and adolescence about her excessive eating and weight. During high school she nibbled throughout the day. After each bite, she vowed to herself that this would be the last, and she would go on a diet, but always was unable to keep her vow. She felt very ashamed of her weight, but gradually gained more. She did most of her eating in private so as to be unobserved by others. At graduation from high school, with a height of 5 feet, 5 inches, she weighed 203 pounds.

Andrea believes that her binge eating began in college. She lost about 40 pounds by dieting when she began college, and then began to alternate between periods of dieting and overeating, lasting several weeks to several months. During periods of overeating, she often ate a big breakfast (e.g., several eggs with cheese, two or three slices of toast, and two large glasses of orange juice). She would then take large quantities of food to her dorm room (e.g., two or three peanut butter sandwiches, two or three dozen cookies, potato chips, and sometimes cheese), which she ate over the next few hours. She ate until she felt physically uncomfortable and then fell asleep. She felt very depressed and ashamed about her weight during this time. She does not recall feeling out of control during the eating because she always believed that she would stop when she had finished whatever piece of food she was eating, although this seldom happened. She had a number of weight fluctuations in college, her weight ranging from 170 to 230 pounds.

In her last year of college, Andrea got down to a normal weight, and after graduation, got married. She began to overeat again on her honeymoon. Her husband was angry about the eating and weight gain. They argued a great deal about this and about her dishonesty concerning her eating (motivated largely by shame about what she had eaten). She feels that her eating problems contributed significantly to her subsequent divorce.

Over the next several years, Andrea continued to struggle with her weight and eating. She went to Weight Watchers several times, tried numerous diets in magazines, used prescribed and illicit amphetamines, and spoke to internists about her weight and tried diets they gave her. However, she continued to be overweight, with marked weight fluctuations. During periods of dieting, she was preoccupied with food and urges to eat.

Andrea was in psychotherapy in her mid-20s for issues related to her divorce and family. Although she tried to discuss her weight and eating problems, the therapy was ineffective in this area as the therapist's interventions were largely limited to suggesting diets.

She describes the periods of binge eating as "a nightmare" during which she is preoccupied with fighting the urge to eat, planning additional eating, and feeling guilty and ashamed about her eating and the inevitable weight gain that would follow. Her worst period of daily binge eating, lasting about 10 months, occurred approximately 2 years ago. She ate boxes of cookies, ice cream and other sweets, large amounts of peanut butter and bread, and many bowls of cereal when there was nothing else in the house. She felt out of control and desperate about her inability to stop binge eating. She often ate until she had stomach pains, never felt hungry because she was always eating so much, essentially lost all semblance of a meal structure, avoided eating in front of others because she was ashamed of the eating, and constantly felt depressed. She gained 90 pounds during that period of binge eating.

Discussion of "Fatty"

Many people, particularly women, are concerned about their overeating and inability to maintain a normal weight. They may try a variety of diets and weight-maintenance programs. A minority of them have recurrent eating binges during which they eat large amounts of food and feel that their eating is out of control. When a pattern of binge eating more than twice a week for longer than 6 months occurs, as it does with Andrea, the diagnosis is Binge-Eating Disorder (DSM-IV-TR, p. 787; provided in an appendix for diagnoses requiring further study). This diagnosis is not made if the person engages in the inappropriate compensatory behavior that characterizes Bulimia Nervosa, (e.g., self-induced vomiting or excessive exercise [see "A Visit to Food Hell," p. 40]).

Patients with Binge-Eating Disorder differ in several respects from patients with Bulimia Nervosa. In clinical settings, the patient with Bulimia Nervosa is almost invariably in her 20s, whereas the average age of a patient with Binge-Eating Disorder is in the 40s. Bulimia Nervosa in males is extremely uncommon, whereas in Binge-Eating Disorder, the female-to-male ratio is approximately 3:2. The typical patient with Bulimia Nervosa is of normal or near normal weight, but is preoccupied with being thin, whereas most patients with Binge-Eating Disorder are overweight and would be delighted if they could bring their weight down to the normal range. Finally, patients with Binge-Eating Disorder are less likely than patients with Bulimia Nervosa (but more likely than nonpatients) to have a history of mood, anxiety, and substance abuse disorders.

Follow-Up

Andrea's therapist urged her to join Overeaters' Anonymous (OA), a self-help group program similar to Alcoholics Anonymous. She found the combination of OA and psychotherapy helpful. She lost about 80 pounds, without rigid or restrictive dieting, and has regained only 20 of those pounds in 5 years. She is pleased that she does not often feel preoccupied with food or urges to eat between meals, although she continues to have trouble controlling the size of her meals. She feels quite sure that she will never be entirely free of her eating problem and could begin binge eating again at some unpredictable future time. For this reason, she continues to attend OA meetings.

IN SEARCH OF A HOME

Tony Taylor is a separated, 39-year-old African American man who was admitted to a psychiatric day program in the shelter where he lived when he complained of sudden impulses to stab other residents. The staff in the shelter describe him variously as "manipulative" and "charming." He gives a long history of abuse of alcohol, heroin, and cocaine, but says he has been "clean" for 3 weeks. He reports several arrests for felonies, including armed robbery and kidnapping, for which he always seems to have an explanation that minimizes his own responsibility.

Mr. Taylor entered the city shelter system 2 years ago when the woman he was living with threw him out because she couldn't tolerate his temper and substance abuse. During his marriage to another woman 20 years ago, he was able to work briefly in blue-collar jobs in between prison and hospital stays. He has not worked for the past 7 years and has never paid child support to his wife.

Life did not begin easily for Mr. Taylor. His father left home before he was born, leaving behind a family scandal. The family story is that his father impregnated his wife's sister, causing Tony to be treated like an outcast by the family. His mother had nine children, each with a different father. She had chronic depression and had received extensive psychiatric treatment. All of her children have psychiatric or substance abuse problems.

When Mr. Taylor was 3, his mother turned him over to a succession of reluctant caretakers on both sides of the family. He was physically abused by some of his mother's boyfriends, being whipped with belts and electrical cords. He dropped out of school in seventh grade because "a teacher embarrassed me." He began drinking when he entered the Job Corps at age 16. In his late teens and early 20s, he used nasal cocaine and heroin, then intravenous heroin for about a year. He stopped using drugs in his mid-20s, but continued to binge on alcohol every few weeks.

At age 19, after an argument with his wife, he cut his wrists and was hospitalized for 6 months. He was given an antidepressant, an unknown tranquilizer, and psychotherapy following his discharge, but stopped treatment when he felt better. Over the ensuing 20 years there have been multiple hospitalizations when he was suicidal or had violent impulses. At one point he jumped off a bridge, sustaining multiple fractures. He has never exhibited manic symptoms, nor has he ever had delusions or hallucinations.

The one psychiatric chart that is available outlines an extensive criminal record and gives the patient the diagnosis of Antisocial Personality Disorder. His criminal history includes charges for multiple armed robberies, desertion and neglect of a minor, and kidnapping of a 20-year-old man. With reference to this last crime, he says that he held the man at bay with a machete while friends stole the man's car.

Discussion of "In Search of a Home"

Like many single men who find themselves in shelters for the homeless, Mr. Taylor has a long history of contacts with the criminal justice system and problems with alcohol and drugs. Also typical is a history of an unstable family and childhood abuse. Mr. Taylor, like most shelter residents, has never had a psychotic disorder.

We have no trouble making past diagnoses of Alcohol (DSM-IV-TR, p. 214), Cocaine (DSM-IV-TR, p. 243), and Heroin (DSM-IV-TR, p. 271) Abuse; if more information were available, it is likely that, at some point, he was dependent on each of these substances. His history of violent behavior, lack of remorse, failure to sustain employment, illegal acts, and irresponsible behavior toward his spouse and child all suggest a provisional diagnosis of Antisocial Personality Disorder (DSM-IV-TR, p. 706). (This diagnosis is provisional because the criteria require a history of childhood Conduct Disorder, which was probably present, but could not be confirmed in this case.)

This case demonstrates that some of the same behaviors that indicate a diagnosis of Antisocial Personality Disorder can be viewed as evidence for Borderline Personality Disorder (DSM-IV-TR, p. 710)—for example, his unstable interpersonal relationships, impulsivity, and uncontrolled anger. Other symptoms of Borderline Personality Disorder are his history of suicidal behavior and affective instability. Because not all patients with Antisocial Personality Disorder also have these Borderline features, we would diagnose both conditions.

Symptoms of depression, including suicide attempts, have been present in Mr. Taylor, as they often are in shelter residents whose lives are so bleak; but it is unclear in this case whether a full Major Depressive Episode was ever present.

Follow-Up

Over a 10-month treatment period, Mr. Taylor exhibited an intense attachment to his female caseworker. He often demanded immediate attention. When frustrated, he would occasionally become intoxicated and verbally abusive. This was especially the case when his caseworker left the program for another job. However, he did refrain from violent behavior and enrolled in a group for drug abusers who also have other psychiatric problems. An anticonvulsant drug helped him control his aggressive impulses. He also received individual and group counseling and social skills training and took part in a work and money-management program.

Mr. Taylor was accepted into a community residence and has been able to maintain his housing and his outpatient treatment in a day program during a 9-month period. He is monitored closely by his shelter caseworker, who intervenes when problems arise.

JUNKIE

Joe Havel, a 54-year-old administrator in a Midwestern university, was asked to tell the story of his struggle to give up cigarettes. He has not smoked at all for 2 years, following a 6-week treatment with a nicotine patch that was prescribed by a colleague who runs a smoking cessation research program.

Mr. Havel began smoking when he was age 18, usually smoking one or two packs a day. Beginning in his late 30s, he vowed to stop every morning, but says that by 9:30 A.M., "It was over and I was lighting my first cigarette of the day." When he was age 45, under a lot of pressure from family, friends, and his cardiologist, he asked his colleague to prescribe an antidepressant that has been used to help smokers break the habit. Over 4 days the dosage was gradually increased, and he did not smoke. On the fourth day he began to feel like he "was on an LSD trip." His surroundings seemed unreal, and "people opened and closed their mouths, but no words came out." Frightened about what was happening to him, he stopped the drug abruptly. For the next few weeks he still felt drugged, but did not smoke. Back to normal, he began smoking again and was soon up to a pack or two a day.

Over the next 5 years there was more social pressure for him to stop smoking. Smoking was outlawed in his office building, and his wife and doctor were relentless in their badgering. He also began to notice that he was short of breath when he walked up a few flights of steps. Again he asked his colleague for help and this time was given a nicotine patch. "I had always thought that I smoked because it was a part of my life, but then I got the patch and didn't need to smoke, and in that moment I realized I was a junkie."

For the 6 weeks that he wore the patch, life was "beautiful." He was happy, productive, and focused, and did not crave cigarettes. He gave up the patch after 6 weeks, as prescribed, and for months thereafter felt "cranky" and without his usual *joie de vivre*. "One day I was reading an ad for an antidepressant, and I had all the symptoms!" In addition, he began to have frequent, mild viral infections, which he had never experienced before.

Two years later he is still not smoking and no longer has symptoms of depression yet feels that something is missing: "The period, the comma, and the exclamation point are missing from my life."

Discussion of "Junkie"

Because the acute effects of nicotine do not include the maladaptive behavior that is characteristic of intoxication from other drugs commonly abused, such as alcohol or cocaine, it is only recently that the similarity between dependence on nicotine and other abused drugs has been recognized. Mr. Havel referred to himself as a "junkie" because he recognized that he was as dependent on nicotine as any heroin user might be on heroin. He was repeatedly unable to cut down or control his smoking, he smoked all day, and he smoked despite the knowledge that it was causing him physical problems. Therefore, for many years, Mr. Havel had Nicotine Dependence (DSM-IV-TR, p. 264).

Periodically, as Mr. Havel sought to cut down on his smoking, he tried to avoid withdrawal symptoms by using an antidepressant or by using a nicotine patch that slowly administers a low dose of nicotine into the bloodstream.

Although Mr. Havel is glad that he has been able to kick his nicotine habit, like many other successful former addicts, he misses the pleasure that the drug once gave him. Mr. Havel has apparently never had a Major Depressive Disorder. Research has indicated that tobacco users with such a history find it much harder to give up the drug.

LOW LIFE LEVEL

Louise Larkin is a pale, stooped woman of 39 years, whose childlike face is surrounded by scraggly blond braids tied with pink ribbons. She was referred for a psychiatric evaluation for possible hospitalization by her family doctor, who was concerned about her low level of functioning. Her only complaint to him was, "I have a decline in self-care and a low life level." Her mother reports that there has indeed been a decline, but that it has been over many years. In the last few months Louise has remained in her room, mute and still.

Twelve years ago Louise was a supervisor in the occupational therapy department of a large hospital, living in her own apartment, and engaged to a young man. He broke the engagement, and she became increasingly disorganized, wandering aimlessly in the street, wearing mismatched clothing. She was fired from her job, and eventually the police were called to hospitalize her. They broke into her apartment, which was in shambles, filled with papers, food, and broken objects. No information is available from this hospitalization, which lasted 3 months, and from which she was discharged to her mother's house with a prescription for an unknown medication that she never had filled.

After her discharge, her family hoped that Louise would gather herself together and embark again on a real life, but over the years, she became more withdrawn and less functional. Most of her time was spent watching TV and cooking. Her cooking consisted of mixing bizarre combinations of ingredients, such as broccoli and cake mix, cooking them, and then eating them alone because no one else in the family would eat her meals. She collected cookbooks and recipes, cluttering her room with stacks of them. Often when her mother entered her room, she would quickly grab a magazine and pretend to be reading, when in fact she had apparently just been sitting and staring into space. She stopped bathing and brushing her hair or teeth. She ate less and less, although she denied loss of appetite, and over a period of several years lost 20 pounds. She would sleep at odd hours. Eventually she became enuretic, wetting her bed frequently and filling the room with the pungent odor of urine.

On admission to the psychiatric hospital, Louise sat with her hands tightly clasped in her lap and avoided looking at the doctor who interviewed her. She answered questions readily and did not appear suspicious or guarded, but her affect was shallow. She denied depressed mood, delusions, or hallucinations. However, her answers became increasingly idiosyncratic and irrelevant as the interview progressed. In response to a question about her strange cooking habits, she replied that she did not wish to discuss recent events in Russia. When discussing her decline in functioning, she said, "There's more of a take-off mechanism when you're younger." Asked about ideas of reference, she said, "I doubt it's true, but if one knows the writers involved, it could be an element that would be directed in a comical way." Her answers were interspersed with the mantra, "I'm safe. I'm safe."

Discussion of "Low Life Level"

Several features of this case suggest the diagnosis of Schizophrenia. There are Louise's extreme decline in functioning over a period of several years and her many oddities of behavior and speech. In addition, there is no evidence of a mood disorder or of a general medical condition or substance that could account for this disturbance. What makes the diagnosis more problematic is the apparent absence of delusions or hallucinations, which are usually present during the active phase of Schizophrenia.

DSM-III and DSM-III-R did permit the diagnosis of Schizophrenia, even in the absence of delusions and hallucinations, if there were two of the following three symptoms: incoherence or marked loosening of association, catatonic behavior, or flat or grossly inappropriate affect. It would have been difficult to diagnose this as a case of Schizophrenia without stretching these criteria. Louise's speech is at times incoherent, but her affect, although described as shallow, is not flat or grossly inappropriate, and she has no catatonic symptoms. The criterion describing the characteristic symptoms of Schizophrenia in DSM-IV (and DSM-IV-TR) includes additional negative symptoms: alogia (poverty of amount or content of speech) and avolition (pervasive inability to persist in goal-directed activities). Because her speech is at times incoherent and she is unable to work or cope with more than minimal self-care (avolition), the DSM-IV-TR diagnosis would be Schizophrenia (DSM-IV-TR, p. 312).

Follow-Up

Louise was treated with an antipsychotic medication in the hospital and was also given an antidepressant that is thought to be effective in Obsessive-Compulsive Disorder (some of the staff thought that her strange cooking and eating behaviors might be symptoms of Obsessive-Compulsive Disorder). She improved significantly over a 3-month hospitalization and then returned to her mother's home, enrolled in a day program, and continued in outpatient treatment with her hospital psychiatrist. Her psychiatrist discontinued the antidepressant because she believed that Louise's "obsessive-compulsive behavior" was actually a symptom of Schizophrenia. Louise worked in a cooking group and became so proficient that there were plans to get her a work-study job in a bakery. However, after a few months she stopped taking her medication, and she began to be preoccupied with irrelevant details in the cooking group. Her speech became tangential, and eventually she dropped out of the program and stayed at home, ruminating and eating very little. Her self-care deteriorated; and when she lost 30 pounds, she was rehospitalized.

She was treated with a different antipsychotic drug and was discharged after 6 weeks. Two years after her first admission, Louise attends a less-demanding day program, takes good care of her physical appearance, and demonstrates only very slight tangentiality in her speech.

EYEWITNESS

A 39-year-old television reporter, Karen Davis, saw a psychiatrist at her network employee assistance program a few weeks after witnessing the execution of a murderer. For several years she had been following the story of the inmate as he approached execution. The execution itself was remarkably protracted and gruesome; along with colleagues, she maintained a deathwatch for several hours while various last-minute reprieves were gained and then set aside by judicial bodies. At one point the inmate was actually strapped into the chair when a phone call from a federal judge, literally at the last minute, reprieved him, and the inmate was removed from the gas chamber alive. When execution finally occurred, Karen and her colleagues watched from a distance of about 10 feet through the windows of the gas chamber. The inmate's eyes rolled back in his head, and he began to convulse involuntarily, eventually gasping and drooling as his body was racked by convulsions. After approximately 5 minutes, his body was still, and he was declared dead by prison authorities.

Karen told the psychiatrist, "Once you see someone die, you don't forget what it looks like." She felt that her professional role as an objective recorder was helpful to her initially in that it separated her from her emotional response. She recalled, for example, the sensation of her mouth going dry just at the moment of execution, but this was unaccompanied by any emotional response. A feeling of detachment, which she described as "surreal and macabre," persisted for some days after the event. For a week after the execution, she continued to be detached from her feelings and was "in a daze and not like my usual self."

For the last few weeks, since the execution, she has felt unexcited about her work. She was surprised, for example, at her unwillingness to cover a riot that occurred shortly after the execution, a story about which she normally would have been very enthusiastic. Moreover, she described becoming irritable, with angry outbursts at her husband, which prompted him to suggest that they see a marriage counselor. Karen has had trouble staying asleep and often has nightmares. She says that she thinks of the event at least daily, having vivid "snapshot" images of the moment of execution.

Discussion of "Eyewitness"

Karen is experiencing the aftereffects of watching a gruesome execution. Her reexperiencing the trauma in intrusive recollections, the irritability that threatens her marriage, and her refusal to take a job assignment that ordinarily would cause her no difficulty all suggest the diagnosis of Posttraumatic Stress Disorder (PTSD). However, that diagnosis is reserved for cases that persist beyond a month, because transient, acute PTSD-like symptoms are so common following traumatic events, and most people with such symptoms recover in a few days or weeks. DSM-IV added a diagnosis, Acute Stress Disorder (DSM-IV-TR, p. 471), for those cases with PTSD-like symptoms that are sufficiently severe to require treatment and persist for more than 2 days, but less than 1 month. Whereas dissociative symptoms are common in PTSD but are not required for making the diagnosis, in Acute Stress Disorder the person must have three dissociative symptoms, such as, in this case, detachment either during or after experiencing the trauma, derealization ("surreal and macabre"), and a reduction in awareness of one's surroundings ("in a daze").

DISCO DI

Diana Miller, age 25, entered a long-term treatment unit of a psychiatric hospital after a serious suicide attempt. Alone in her enormous suburban house, with her parents away on vacation, depressed and desperately lonely, she made herself a Valium and Scotch cocktail, drank it, and then called her psychiatrist.

Diana had been a tractable child with a mediocre school record until she turned age 12. Then her disposition, which had been cheerful and outgoing, changed drastically: she became demanding, sullen, and rebellious, shifting precipitously from a giddy euphoria to tearfulness and depression. She took up with a "fast" crowd, became promiscuous, abused marijuana and hallucinogens, and ran away from home at 15 with a 17-year-old boy. Two weeks later, having eluded the private investigators her parents had hired, they both returned. She reentered school, but dropped out for good in her junior year of high school. Her relationships with men were stormy, full of passion, unbearable longing, and violent arguments. She craved excitement and would get drunk, dance wildly on table tops in discos, leave with strange men, and perhaps have sex in their cars. If she refused their sexual advances, she was sometimes put out onto the street. After one such incident, at 17, she made her first suicide attempt, cutting her wrist severely, which led to her first hospitalization.

After her first hospitalization, Diana was referred to a therapist for intensive, twice-weekly dynamic psychotherapy, for which she had little aptitude. She filled up most of her sessions with a litany of complaints against her family, from whom she expected "100% attention." She called her therapist several times a day about one "crisis" or another.

During her long period of unsuccessful outpatient treatment, punctuated by several brief hospitalizations, she had many symptoms. She was afraid to travel even to her doctor's office without one of her parents. She was depressed, with suicidal preoccupations and feelings of hopelessness. She drank excessively and used up to 40 mg/day of Valium. She had eating binges, followed by crash diets to get back to her normal weight. She was obsessed with calories and with the need to have her food cut into particular shapes and arranged on her plate in a particular manner. If her mother failed to comply with these rules, she had tantrums, sometimes so extreme that she broke dishes and had to be physically restrained by her father.

Diana has never worked, except for a few months as a receptionist in her father's company. She has never had an idea of what she wants to do with her life, apart from being with a "romantic man." She has never had female friends, and her only source of solace is her dog. She has often been "eaten alive" with boredom.

Efforts by her therapist to set limits have had little effect. She refused to join Alcoholics Anonymous or attend a day program or vocational rehabilitation center, regarding these as "beneath" her. Instead, she languished at home, grew more depressed and agoraphobic, and escalated her Valium use to 80 mg/day. It was a serious suicide attempt this time that led to her current (seventh) psychiatric hospitalization.

Discussion of "Disco Di"

Diana's history of many different symptoms over many years suggests several Axis I disorders. The depression and suicide attempt that prompted the last hospitalization suggest a diagnosis of Major Depressive Disorder or Dysthymic Disorder or both. Because this case was presented to us several years after the hospitalization, we have insufficient information to make these diagnoses.

Her escalating dosage of Valium (with the resulting development of tolerance) and continued use despite its negative effect on her life suggest a diagnosis of Valium Dependence (DSM-IV-TR, p. 285). Her binge eating may have been frequent enough to warrant the additional diagnosis of Binge-Eating Disorder (DSM-IV-TR, p. 787).

What is most striking is her chronically chaotic life, her pervasive pattern of instability in mood and relationships, and her impulsivity. These suggest an Axis II personality disorder as the primary disturbance, specifically, Borderline Personality Disorder (DSM-IV-TR, p. 710). Diana demonstrates at least five of the characteristic symptoms of this disorder. She certainly has unstable and intense interpersonal relationships, and the "violent arguments" suggest an alternation between extremes of idealization and devaluation. She has an identity disturbance (no goals in life), impulsive behavior in many areas (sex, substance abuse, eating), recurrent suicidal behavior, affective instability (sudden shifts of mood), and inappropriate and intense anger, and we suspect that her being "eaten alive" with boredom is evidence of chronic feelings of emptiness.

As is commonly the case in people with severe personality disorders, features of several other personality disorders are also present: Narcissistic (Alcoholics Anonymous was "beneath her"), Histrionic (craving excitement), Obsessive-Compulsive (rigidity about food), and Dependent (inability to manage without her family).

Follow-Up

In the hospital Diana complained that the nurses were "cruel" to her and that other patients "hated" her. Many sessions were spent with the parents, counseling them to resist her pleas to return home. She was exquisitely sensitive to the slightest decrement in her Valium level, so that she could be weaned only a milligram at a time. It took 3 months before she was "off" the drug. Afterward, her progress was unexpectedly good. Her disposition became cheerful. She grew cooperative toward the staff and friendly toward other patients. She learned secretarial skills in a hospital rehabilitation program and became less fearful of going outside and less fussy about food. By the end of her 10-month stay, she had developed a friendship with another convalescing patient, and the two arranged to share an apartment. Both found part-time work, and Diana continued therapy once a week as an outpatient.

Diana responded primarily to a supportive mode of psychotherapy, one that emphasized education, exhortation, encouragement, and limit setting. She was too anxious and too action prone to benefit from a psychodynamic approach that required introspection and reflection. Brief hospitalizations could not stem the tide of her multiple and intense symptoms, of which her substance abuse was the most threatening. For Diana, what seemed to work best was a long-term hospitalization, in which the substance abuse could be properly dealt with and vocational rehabilitation could take hold. The enforced separation from her parents helped her and her mother realize that each could survive without the other.

During 7 years of follow-up, Diana has held her ground, continues to work and live with the same roommate, and is able to visit her parents with regularity without falling back into the old pattern of mother–daughter interdependence. Sensation-seeking remains a noticeable part of her adaptation—she likes flashy clothes, discos, rock concerts—but she is less impulsive, abstains from alcohol, and no longer places herself in jeopardy with strange men.

A VISIT TO FOOD HELL

Abby Thurmond, age 42, had not had a food binge for over 2 years when she flew from Miami to Chicago to attend the wedding of her friend's daughter. Single, independent, and devoted to her work, Abby had just sold her first screenplay. She was pleased, but she was also experiencing the "postpartum" letdown that always occurred when she finished a major project.

Despite knowing, from 2 years in Overeaters Anonymous (OA), that she needed to keep a safe distance from food, especially in emotionally hard times, Abby spent the entire day of the wedding rehearsal party in the company of food. She stood in her friend's kitchen for hours—cutting, chopping, sorting, arranging, and, eventually, picking at the food.

When night and the guests came, the flurry of activity made it easy for Abby to disappear—physically and emotionally—into a binge. She started with a plate of what would have been an "abstinent" meal (an OA concept for whatever is included on one's meal plan): pasta salad, green salad, cold cuts, and a roll. Although the portions were generous, Abby wanted more. She spent the next 5 hours eating, at first trying to graze among the guests, but then, when shame set in, retreating to dark corners of the room to take frantic, stolen bites.

Abby stuffed herself with crackers, cheeses, breads, chicken, turkey, pasta, and salads, but all that was a prelude to what she really wanted—sugar. She'd been waiting for the guests to leave the dining room, where the desserts were. When they finally did, she cut herself two pieces of cake, then two more, then ate directly from the serving tray, shoveling the food into her mouth. She reached for cookies, more cake, and cookies again. Heart racing, terrified of being discovered, Abby finally tore herself away and slipped out onto the terrace.

By now, in what she thought of as a "food trance," Abby piled her plate with bread, onto which she smeared some unidentifiable spread. Though the food tasted like mud, Abby kept eating. Soon, other guests came out to the terrace, leaving Abby feeling she had to move again, which she did, stepping into the kitchen—and the light. When Abby glanced down at her plate, she was horrified; ants were crawling all over it. Instead of reflexively spitting out the food, Abby, overcome by shame, could only swallow. Then her eyes began to search the debris on her plate for uncontaminated morsels. Witnessing her own madness, Abby began to cry. She flung the plate into the trash and ran to her room.

That event marked the beginning of a 6-month relapse into binge eating—Abby's worst experience with bingeing since the problem began 15 years earlier. During the relapse, she binged on sugar foods and refined carbohydrates, returned to cigarette smoking to control the bingeing, and once again was driven to "get rid" of the calories by incessant exercise after each binge, walking 4 or 5 hours at a time, dragging her bicycle up and down six flights of stairs, and biking miles after dark in a dangerous city park.

Discussion of "A Visit to Food Hell"

The term *eating binge* is often used by people to describe occasions on which they eat more food than they should. However, Abby's description of her eating episode at the wedding rehearsal leaves little doubt that her episodes of binge eating, during which she has no control over how much she eats, represent a serious symptom. In diagnosing a person with recurrent eating binges, the first question is whether or not that person regularly compensates for the overeating by some drastic inappropriate behavior. If the answer is no, the diagnosis is probably Binge-Eating Disorder, a nonofficial diagnosis that is included in a DSM-IV-TR appendix of diagnoses requiring further study (see "Fatty," p. 25). If the answer is yes and, as is usually the case, self-evaluation is unduly influenced by body shape and weight, the diagnosis is Bulimia Nervosa. Most patients with Bulimia Nervosa compensate for the binge eating by some method of purging—either self-induced vomiting (most common) or the use of diuretics or laxatives. Abby's disorder is an example of the relatively unusual diagnosis of Bulimia Nervosa, Nonpurging Type (DSM-IV-TR, p. 594), in which the patient uses methods such as excessive exercise (Abby's method) or fasting.

Follow-Up

Throughout the relapse, Abby went to therapy and to OA. But the bingeing worsened, as did the accompanying isolation and depression, which kept her awake, often crying uncontrollably, until the early morning hours. Finally, her therapist, a social worker, referred her to a psychiatrist, who put her on an antidepressant that has been used to control binge eating and on a structured food plan that excluded refined sugars, breads, crackers, and similar carbohydrates. Within a few weeks, Abby was able to stop bingeing, come out of the depression, and resume her life. After 2 years on the medication, no binges, and the gradual reintroduction of breads and related carbohydrates into her diet, Abby was able to stop taking the antidepressant, without depression or a return to binge eating. She continues to be active in OA.

COFFEE MACHINE

Eric Evans is a 41-year-old attorney whose internist has referred him for a psychiatric consultation. He has been complaining of fatigue, loss of motivation, sleepiness, headaches, nausea, feeling unsociable, and difficulty concentrating. His symptoms occur mostly on weekends, and as a result he often begs off of weekend social activities, which causes his wife to be very annoyed with him. She complains that he's fine during the week, but never feels like going out with friends or playing with the children on weekends. He is in good health, with no recent history of medical disorders.

Mr. Evans works a 60-hour week in a busy law practice and barely sees his family during the week. At work he is often anxious, restless, and constantly busy. He frequently has trouble sleeping on weeknights because he worries about his job. He denies marital or family problems, other than those caused by his not wanting to do anything on the weekends.

He has a history of alcohol problems, but has not had a drink for 5 years. He used to smoke 20 cigarettes a day, but stopped 2 months ago, hoping this would improve his condition. (It did not.) At work he drinks four cups of coffee a day. He has stopped using coffee on the weekends

because he suspects that it may be contributing to his anxiety and sleeplessness.

Discussion of "Coffee Machine"

Many people recognize that they need a cup of coffee to get going
in the morning. What they do not recognize is that often what they
are doing by taking one or more cups of coffee is avoiding the development of caffeine withdrawal symptoms. Typically, withdrawal
symptoms begin approximately 12 hours after the last cup of coffee.
What often happens is that the heavy coffee drinker who has coffee
with dinner starts to develop withdrawal symptoms the next morning if he or she, for some reason, does not have coffee at breakfast.

Although caffeine withdrawal is rarely severe enough to cause
a person to seek clinical attention, surveys of the general popula-
tion indicate that 25% of people who regularly drink coffee report
developing headaches, fatigue, or drowsiness if they miss their
usual dose. Interestingly, when actually tested in the laboratory,
approximately 50% of regular coffee drinkers develop headaches.
Even some who regularly take as little as one cup of coffee a day
(100 mg of caffeine) can develop withdrawal symptoms.

It is clear that Mr. Evans, on weekends, had the characteristic
symptoms of Caffeine Withdrawal (DSM-IV-TR, p. 765), a nonofficial diagnosis that is included in an appendix to DSM-IV-TR.

Follow-Up

The psychiatrist was impressed with the relationship between the
onset of the symptoms of headache, fatigue, difficulty concentrating, sleepiness, and loss of motivation and Mr. Evans's cessation of
coffee drinking on weekends. Mr. Evans was advised to decrease
his consumption of coffee during the week, but he found that he
couldn't function well without his usual dose of coffee. Instead, he
decided to resume drinking coffee on the weekends as there was
no medical contraindication to his regular use of caffeine. He decided to live with the anxiety and difficulty sleeping that had originally prompted his giving up his weekend coffee.

SLIME

A psychiatrist with a special interest in the long-term effects of childhood traumatic experiences first saw Linda Darby when she was 26. She was a paralegal who had many physical complaints for which no clear etiology could be found; she was also chronically depressed and anxious. Her family doctor, who made the referral, had been unsuccessful in treating her with medication. He noted that she was exquisitely sensitive to medications (e.g., she would go into a daylong sleep after taking 5 mg of an antianxiety medication, diazepam; she would develop severe side effects on 25 mg of an antidepressant, amitriptyline.)

The psychiatrist noted that at age 26 Linda lives with her parents and brother and feels that she needs to stay around in order to minimize the constant threat of family violence. She frequently thinks of suicide and has engaged in self-mutilation, using a razor blade on her breasts and thighs, which she claims helps her feel "like myself" and restores a sense of calm after an upsetting experience. At work her performance is exemplary. She is assigned the most complex cases and often stays late doing library research. She also volunteers as a fund-raiser for a charitable organization on weekends. Even though she seems to possess adequate social skills, she has no real friends and no social life.

She began treatment with the psychiatrist and gradually revealed a history of chronic family violence and incest. Her father was only occasionally employed, often in illegal activities. He had recurrent alcoholic binges and used to beat up his two sons regularly, to the point that they both had been hospitalized with broken bones.

Linda remembered first having sex with her father at age 8, when she and her father and two brothers were snowed in while her mother was in the hospital. She was terrified by her father's breaking open a locked door and forcing her to have intercourse with him, but also remembers feeling that she now had become "special" to her father. These episodes of sexual abuse continued until she moved out of the house to go to college when she was age 18. She recalled her relationship with her father with much self-loathing, convinced for many years that she was to blame for the incest, which made her feel like "slime" and "a bag of shit."

Throughout her childhood, Linda's mother was often ill and Linda took care of many of the routine household duties. She always suspected that her mother was aware of the incestuous relationship.

She did not remember much of her childhood, and described episodes of "spacing out" during which she found herself in places without knowing how she got there. Despite the fact that she had a lot of attention from men, she avoided dating. She felt terrified when a man showed any interest in her. Any sexual feelings appeared to be associated in her mind with thoughts of violence. Probably her greatest source of shame was the fact that she was sexually aroused by thoughts of sexual violence.

After 2 years of supportive psychotherapy, Linda gained enough courage to move into an apartment of her own. At once expressing fear of intimacy (for fear that people might find out what a despicable person she is) and a longing for care, she adopted four stray cats and two dogs, which she considered her family. The presence of her animals, she claimed, help her deal with her frequent nightmares about being sexually assaulted. She entered a women's psychotherapy group in which she proved to be extremely insightful about other people's problems, astounding them with her insights and her capacity to put her finger on the crucial issues. When it was pointed out that she only helped others and avoided talking about herself, she became angry and threatened to leave the group.

Two years later she was raped in her apartment in the inner city. She lived on the ground floor, and the rapist entered through a window without a grate. She had talked to her therapist about the lack of safety in her apartment, but had been unable to confront her landlord about it. After the rape, she moved back home, forfeiting 2 months' security deposit. Although shaken by the assault, she claimed that it just compounded her sense of living "in hell already—the hell of my memories."

Through judicious use of small amounts of medications, Linda's symptoms gradually subsided. She is now able to sleep through the night and has lost her pervasive sense of psychic numbing. At work she sometimes feels so enraged about real and imagined slights that she thinks expressing her rage would have cataclysmic results. On the other hand, she has become Big Sister to an abused 10-year-old girl and has some social contacts with cousins. In dealings with her family, she continues to feel that she has no rights and is still financially exploited by them. She continues to avoid all contacts with sexual implications. She still has no sense of having a future that she can influence and that has personal meaning. Her medical bills, aggravated by three fender-benders during the past year, the result of "spacing out" while driving, continue to mount. Her work performance is still exemplary, and she does not mutilate herself anymore.

Discussion of "Slime"

In recent years there has been increasing recognition of the long-term effects of chronic interpersonal trauma, such as sexual and physical abuse during childhood. The consequences of such trauma on personality and functioning may be pervasive. Recent research indicates that the diagnostic criteria for Posttraumatic Stress Disorder (PTSD) capture only a limited aspect of the posttraumatic psychopathology seen in these people. This case was presented to illustrate many of the characteristic features of a syndrome seen in people who have been exposed as children to long-term interpersonal trauma. The syndrome is usually observed in those who also have PTSD. Many researchers in the area of chronic stress have used the unofficial acronym DESNOS (Disorders of Extreme Stress Not Otherwise Specified) to indicate that the syndrome is not fully captured by any of the stress-induced disorders recognized in the official classification.

Linda reexperiences her trauma in the form of recurrent nightmares. She tries to avoid feelings associated with the trauma (avoids sex), is detached from others (avoids intimate relationships), and has no sense of a future for her life. These symptoms suggest the diagnosis of Posttraumatic Stress Disorder, but additional symptoms of increased arousal (e.g., difficulty falling asleep or irritability) are required for the diagnosis, and we are unsure whether such symptoms are present. Therefore, we would note, rule out Posttraumatic Stress Disorder (DSM-IV-TR, p. 467).

However, Linda's main difficulties are with the characteristic symptoms of DESNOS. She is chronically depressed and self-destructive and has brief dissociative episodes. She has chronic guilt and shame and is unable to trust or maintain close relationships. She has a tendency to be revictimized (returning to her abusive family), and she has many physical complaints that are without an adequate medical explanation. Other symptoms of DESNOS that she does not show include extreme risk-taking behavior, victimizing others, minimizing the importance of the trauma, and idealizing the perpetrator.

Many patients who have had similar childhood experiences go on to develop Borderline Personality Disorder or a Dissociative Disorder. Linda certainly has some of the features of Borderline Personality Disorder (e.g., self-destructive behavior and distorted self-image). Because she does not have enough features to warrant the diagnosis, we are left with the diagnosis of Personality Disorder Not Otherwise Specified (DSM-IV-TR, p. 729). Although she has brief dissociative periods (lost time), they are not sufficiently severe to warrant a diagnosis of Dissociative Amnesia, and certainly there is no evidence of two or more distinct identities, as would be seen in Dissociative Identity Disorder (Multiple Personality Disorder).

SIXTY-SEVEN-POUND WEAKLING

When Peggy was first evaluated for admission to an inpatient eating disorder program, she was a 20-year-old woman who had difficulty supporting her 5-foot, 3-inch body with a weight of only 67 pounds. She had begun to lose weight 4 years earlier, initially dieting to lose an unwanted 6 pounds. Encouraged by compliments on her new body, she proceeded to lose 8 more pounds. Over the next 2 years she continued to lose weight, increased her physical activity until her weight reached a low of 64 pounds, and stopped menstruating. She was admitted to a medical unit, treated for peptic ulcer disease, and discharged, only to be admitted 3 months later to the psychiatric unit of a general hospital. During that 8-week hospitalization, she went from 84 pounds to 100 pounds. She did well until she went off to college, where, with increased academic and social demands, she again began to diet until she weighed only 67 pounds. Her eating habits were ritualized: she cut food into very small pieces, moved them around on the plate, and ate very slowly. She resisted eating foods with high fat and carbohydrate content. She was troubled by the changes in her body and became increasingly anxious as her figure developed. She was forced to drop out of school and to accept another hospitalization.

Peggy was motivated to comply with treatment, but her fears of gaining weight and becoming obese affected her progress. She was expected to gain a minimum of 2 pounds every week, and she was restricted to bed rest if she failed to gain sufficient weight. In psychotherapy Peggy was gradually guided to discuss her feelings and to actually look at herself in the mirror. She was initially instructed to look at one part of her body for a minimum of 10 seconds, and the time was progressively increased until she could look at her whole body without any anxiety. Her menses returned at a weight of 93 pounds. After 7 months of individual and family treatment, she was discharged at a weight of 100 pounds. Peggy returned to college, worked part time, and lived with her parents.

Discussion of "Sixty-Seven-Pound Weakling"

As is usually the case with Anorexia Nervosa (DSM-IV-TR, p. 589), the characteristic signs and symptoms leave little doubt concerning the correct diagnosis. Peggy has all of the salient features, including refusal to maintain body weight at or above a minimally normal weight for age and height; intense fear of gaining weight or of becoming fat, even though underweight; disturbance in the way in which her body weight or shape is experienced (anxiety when viewing her body); and in postmenarchal females, amenorrhea. Because her method of losing weight has never involved purging (self-induced vomiting or use of laxatives or diuretics) or binge eating (consumption of large amounts of food with a sense of loss of control), the subtype is specified as Restricting Type.

Peggy exhibited compulsive ritualistic behavior with regard to food (e.g., cutting her food into very small pieces and moving it around on her plate before eating it), a feature commonly seen in patients with Anorexia Nervosa. Although her compulsive eating behavior might suggest the possible additional diagnosis of Obsessive-Compulsive Disorder, a separate diagnosis is not given, as the compulsive behavior is accounted for by the diagnosis of Anorexia Nervosa.

During the course of the Anorexia Nervosa, Peggy experienced depression and panic attacks. There is insufficient information about these symptoms to make a definitive diagnosis of a Mood or an Anxiety Disorder. However, the occurrence of these comorbid disorders is common in patients with Anorexia Nervosa.

Anorexia Nervosa is a serious and often life-threatening disorder. This case illustrates that with expert treatment, a good outcome is possible.

> ## Follow-Up
>
> Over the next 10 years, Peggy graduated from college with a degree in nutrition and was selected to do an internship with a major corporation. She has excelled in her work, receiving several promotions. She married, but the relationship deteriorated as her husband became physically abusive. She moved out and obtained a court order of protection and eventually a divorce. Her most recent correspondence told of her return to graduate school (all expenses paid and full salary), a new romance, and success in a marathon (third place in a 26-mile race). She has maintained her weight at around 116 pounds and menstruates normally. She did seek counseling to sort out issues related to her broken marriage and her estrangement from her sister, which has since been resolved. She describes her life now as full and satisfying.

POL POT'S LEGACY

Mrs. Chan is a 38-year-old Cambodian widow who was referred by her family physician for evaluation of several years' history of headaches and neck pains for which no medical cause could be found. She says she has had headaches since she arrived in the United States, about 4 years before. She also describes many other pains and psychiatric symptoms. These include poor sleep, sadness, poor concentration, poor memory, low energy, loss of interest in her environment, and a weight loss of 20 pounds in the last 3 months. She often feels dizzy and sometimes sees her mother's ghost at night, usually in a dream. She has nightmares almost nightly, visions of being killed, and intrusive thoughts of the disasters she experienced during the war. Sometimes these thoughts seem so real that she feels she is reexperiencing the events. She has tried to avoid memories of the past, but cannot stop thinking about these things. In the past few months she has become increasingly irritable and angry toward her children and has felt hopeless.

Mrs. Chan was born in a rural area of Cambodia where her family were farmers. She had no formal education. When the Pol Pot regime came to power, the family members were separated. She heard that one brother was executed. She was reunited briefly with her mother, who died of starvation several hours after their reunion. Mrs. Chan cried intensely, but was threatened with death for "being attached to the old ways." She was forced to marry, but did not stay with her husband long because she was assigned to a forced labor group. She had very little food and saw many people starve to death or be killed. By the time the Vietnamese invaded in 1979, she felt that she, too, was destined to die.

She was reunited with her husband and escaped to Thailand, but 3 years later her husband died from multiple medical problems. Since coming to the United States, she has been involved with several Cambodian men and has had two children with two different fathers. She now lives with her children in a Cambodian community, but has few friends. In addition to her numerous physical complaints, it is her irritability with the children that is now very distressing to her.

Discussion of "Pol Pot's Legacy"

This patient's symptom picture is typical of that seen in many Southeast Asian refugees. She has multiple somatic symptoms that apparently do not result from a general medical condition. In addition, she has a specifically Cambodian cultural experience of seeing visions of her dead mother. This is a common way of experiencing grief in this culture and is not regarded as abnormal.

Mrs. Chan exhibits the characteristic symptom picture of Posttraumatic Stress Disorder (PTSD) (DSM-IV-TR, p. 467). She reexperiences overwhelming traumas in nightmares and waking images. These include watching her mother die of starvation and seeing her neighbors killed. She tries to avoid memories of the traumas. She has little interest in activities; her social isolation is probably a manifestation of detachment or estrangement from others. She has symptoms of increased arousal, including difficulty concentrating and sleeping and irritability. All of these symptoms have persisted for more than 1 month and clearly cause her significant distress.

The patient also has symptoms of a Major Depressive Episode. In the last 3 months she has had persistent depressed mood, poor sleep, poor concentration, low energy, loss of interest in her environment, and a weight loss of 20 pounds. Although the depression occurred after the deaths of loved ones, this would not be considered Bereavement because the symptoms have persisted far beyond the 2-month period noted in the DSM-IV-TR description of the V code for

Bereavement (DSM-IV-TR, p. 740). In the absence of a history of a previous episode or symptoms of a Manic Episode, we would also diagnose Major Depressive Disorder, Single Episode, Moderate (DSM-IV-TR, p. 375).

The physical symptoms suggest Undifferentiated Somatoform Disorder, but this diagnosis is not made if the symptoms occur exclusively during the course of another mental disorder, such as a mood or anxiety disorder.

A FAMILY AFFAIR

Paula Perot brought her 9-year-old daughter, Cynthia, to the emergency room three times in 3 weeks. Cynthia had a fever and rash that were not responding to treatment for viral and bacterial illnesses. By the third visit, Cynthia was irritable and lethargic and was admitted to the hospital for evaluation of her unusual syndrome. Soon after admission she was found to be in renal failure and was transferred to a large hospital center for dialysis. Ms. Perot suggested that Cynthia might have mercury poisoning because her maternal grandmother had once had mercury poisoning. An extensive laboratory search was undertaken to explain Cynthia's renal failure, and several consultations were obtained to diagnose and manage Cynthia's illness and its complications. A diagnosis of acute interstitial nephritis secondary to mercury toxicity was eventually made, based on drastically elevated mercury levels.

When questioned, Ms. Perot explained that she felt Cynthia's school had a vendetta against her family, beginning with her own mother who had been poisoned by the same teacher there. In fact, she wouldn't let Cynthia have friends over to visit because she was afraid they might be part of the evil conspiracy and would try to poison the food with mercury. Cynthia also believed she had been poisoned with mercury by her teacher. Ms. Perot believed that other students had also been poisoned. The school, the Department of Social Service for Children, the police, and the district attorney were contacted, but Ms. Perot's claims could not be substantiated.

In further discussion, Ms. Perot alleged other incidents that she felt were related to the vendetta. Cynthia had reportedly been sexually abused in the past at two different day-care centers, and Ms. Perot had herself been sexually abused as a child in one of these same centers. In one instance involving her daughter, Ms. Perot reported the allegation; but no basis for it was found. In the other instance, she did not report it, thinking she would not be believed.

Cynthia had developed normally, had briefly had some behavioral problems in school, but was in a gifted class before her illness. Cynthia's father was in prison intermittently and rarely saw his child. Ms. Perot's sister had been hospitalized in a state hospital and was treated with neuroleptics. She was said to be mentally retarded, violent, and self-mutilating. Ms. Perot had been healthy, had completed a general equivalency diploma, and had trained as a nurse's aide. She had no psychiatric history, did not feel depressed, denied hallucinations, and did not use alcohol or drugs.

During Cynthia's hospitalization, Ms. Perot remained attentive and devoted, and the staff found her very personable. However, she became agitated about the plan to treat her daughter with prednisone, which she believed was evil and had made her mother ill in the past. Because the staff had by now become convinced that Ms. Perot had somehow been poisoning her daughter, she was restricted to supervised visits only and was not permitted to bring her daughter any food. After 2 months, Cynthia became well enough to leave the hospital and was placed in foster care. Her mother was mandated by the court to enter psychiatric treatment. In treatment she continued to insist that various evil people were responsible for her daughter's illness.

Discussion of "A Family Affair"

For many years doctors have recognized that there are rare cases in which a person will intentionally produce or feign symptoms of a physical or mental illness when there is no apparent external incentive. This has been called Munchausen syndrome (see "Misery," p. 391). More recently, an even rarer syndrome, called Munchausen by proxy, has been described, in which a person, almost always a mother, produces symptoms in her child. At first glance, this diagnosis might seem to apply in this case, given that it is clear that the mother is the perpetrator of the mercury poisoning of her daughter. (In the prior edition of the Casebook, this case was diagnosed as Factitious Disorder by proxy [DSM-IV-TR, p. 783]). On closer examination, the criteria are not met for Factitious Disorder by proxy because the diagnosis depends on a consideration of the motivation for the mother's behavior. In Factitious Disorder, the motivation for the feigned symptoms is to assume the sick role; in Factitious Disorder by proxy, the perpetrator assumes the sick role by proxy (i.e., through the attention and care directed toward the dependent child). In this case, there is no evidence that the mother is motivated by the need for her child (and by extention, herself) to be taken care of. Instead, the motivation appears related to the delusion that there is an "evil conspiracy" to poison her and her daughter. Even though the case material does not elucidate the precise reason why the mother ended up administering the poison herself, perhaps she felt she was under the control of those outsiders who were attempting to harm the family.

Given that the mother's delusional system does not appear to involve any bizarre beliefs, the most appropriate diagnosis for her case would be Delusional Disorder, Persecutory Type (DSM-IV-TR, p. 329). The child, of course, has no psychiatric diagnosis but instead would be identified with the V code Physical Abuse of Child (DSM-IV-TR, p. 738).

HAIR

Celeste, now age 25, had always thought she was unique. When she was a teenager, her parents made her feel as though nobody else had ever pulled out her eyebrows until there were none left. This had been going on since she was age 12. And her eyebrows had not been the worst of it: over the years there had been quarter-size bald patches on her head. There was a 1-year period (about 5 years ago, when she was a sophomore at college) when she was practically bald.

It always amazed her how "together" everyone thought her to be. She got good grades; she got into law school. "If they only knew," she often said to herself. But through careful brushing of whatever hair she still had, artful use of scarves and, at one time, a hair "piece," and avoiding all gym classes, not a soul ever found out. The eyebrows were easy; she just drew in new ones.

It was a merciless habit. It went on every day. Usually she would be sitting in front of the TV, distractedly watching reruns, and then she would notice her fingers were in her hair, rummaging about, looking for a hair with a nice thick shaft. Then she would rapidly tug with an expertise gained from long experience. Out would come the hair, root and all. She would then notice the little pile of hairs accumulating on the arm of the sofa and realize she must have been doing this for many minutes already. She would try to stop, but the nervousness would escalate, and the hair-pulling would recommence and go on until the urge just wore itself out. On good days this would be 10 minutes. On bad days, it could last for an hour.

She might never have known that other people had this habit until a month ago when a sudden rainstorm messed up her strategically coiffed hair, exposing the large ratty patch just above her left ear. Horrified that she was now revealed to her co-worker, Sylvia, she was surprised when she heard, "You're a hair-puller too?" Three days later Sylvia took Celeste to a self-help group where she met seven other "pullers," five women and two men. She thought she was hearing her own life in other people's words:

> I felt like I must be an awful person, with no self-control. That's what my parents said.
>
> High school gym terrified me. I was constantly afraid of my wig coming off.
>
> I figured, who could ever want to marry me? First of all, I'm scared to have any real sex. I know my hair will come undone. And what if someone does fall in love with me? How would he react when he realized I did this thing? I had one boyfriend whom I told that I got messed up by a chemical reaction to a bad permanent. But I wouldn't be able to say that forever.
>
> I thought I was the only one in the world.

Discussion of "Hair"

Celeste has an unusual habit. She cannot resist the impulse to pull out her hair. This has resulted in extensive hair loss, both on her head and from her eyebrows. When she tries to resist, she becomes increasingly anxious and inevitably gives in. She apparently derives some pleasure and relief of tension from the activity. These are the

characteristic features of the impulse control disorder Trichotillomania (DSM-IV-TR, p. 677). This case is typical in that the patient is
a woman and the onset was in adolescence.

The absence of intense pleasure associated with the activity (as
contrasted to the pleasure associated with other disorders of impulse
control, such as Pathological Gambling or drug abuse) and the intrusive quality of the impulses suggest Obsessive-Compulsive Disorder.
However, in Obsessive-Compulsive Disorder, the compulsions are
in response to an obsession or are performed in a stereotyped way
and are often aimed at preventing some dreaded event. Furthermore, in Obsessive-Compulsive Disorder the obsessions and compulsions usually are not limited to a single behavior, as is the case
in Trichotillomania.

Follow-Up

In the self-help group, Celeste learned the name of a doctor who
specialized in the treatment of Trichotillomania. This doctor prescribed an antidepressant, which seemed to help substantially for
about 3 months. Then the symptoms worsened again, and Celeste
was switched to another antidepressant. It took a while for the sleepiness caused by the medication to remit, but her symptoms improved considerably, and the improvement persisted. Six months
later Celeste went to see a hypnotist, which helped reduce the
hair-pulling urge further. She now has days and even weeks when
she doesn't pull her hair at all, and the symptom is never as bad as
it used to be. Surprisingly, the use of the two medications had an
unexpected benefit. Even though she felt herself demoralized by her
hair-pulling, Celeste had never thought of herself as "depressed." But
on medication her mood became much brighter. She was more enthusiastic about work and felt better about herself when she went
out on dates—even before the hair-pulling got better. She continues to attend the self-help group and credits it for some of her improvement, particularly in her self-esteem.

MARY QUITE CONTRARY

Mary Kendall is a 35-year-old social worker who was referred to a psychiatrist for treatment of chronic pain caused by a reflex sympathetic dystrophy in her right forearm and hand. She had a complex medical history that included asthma, migraine headaches, diabetes mellitus, and obesity. She was found to be highly hypnotizable and quickly learned to control her pain with self-hypnosis.

Mary was quite competent in her work, but had a rather arid personal life. She had been married briefly and divorced 10 years earlier, and she had little interest in remarrying. She spent most of her free time volunteering in a hospice.

As a thorough psychiatric evaluation continued, she reported the strange observation that on many occasions, when she returned home from work the gas tank of the car was nearly full, yet when she got into car to go to work the next day, it was half empty. She began to keep track of the odometer, and discovered that on many nights 50 to 100 miles would be put on the car overnight, although she had no memory of driving it anywhere. Further questioning revealed that she had gaps in her memory for large parts of her childhood.

Because of the gaps in her memory, the physician suspected a dissociative disorder, but it was only after several months of hypnotic treatment for pain control that the explanation for the lost time emerged. During a hypnotic induction, the physician again asked about the lost time. Suddenly a different voice responded, "It's about time you knew about me." The (alter) personality with a slightly different name, Marian, now spoke and described the drives that she took at night, which were retreats to the nearby hills and seashore to "work out problems." As the psychiatrist got to know Marian over time, it was apparent that she was as abrupt and hostile as Mary was compliant and concerned about others. Marian considered Mary to be rather pathetic and far too interested in pleasing and said that "worrying about anyone but yourself is a waste of time."

In the course of therapy, some six other personalities emerged, roughly organized along the lines of a dependent/aggressive continuum. Considerable tension and disagreement emerged among these personalities, each of which was rather two-dimensional. Competition for control of time "out" was frequent, and Marian would provoke situations that frightened the others, including one who identified herself as a 6-year-old child. The subjective experience of distinctness among some of the personality states was underscored when one rather hostile alter personality made a suicide threat. The therapist insisted on discussing this with other personalities, and she objected that to do so would be a "violation of doctor–patient confidentiality."

The memories that emerged with these dissociated personalities included recollections of physical and sexual abuse at the hands of her father and others and considerable guilt about not having protected other children in the family from such abuse. Mary recalled her mother as being infrequently abusive, but quite dependent, and forcing Mary to cook and clean from a very early age.

After 4 years of psychotherapy, Mary gradually integrated portions of these personality states. Two similar personalities merged, although she remained partially dissociated. The personality states were aware of one another and continued to "fight" with each other periodically.

Discussion of "Mary Quite Contrary"

It does not take much training in psychopathology to recognize this as a case of Multiple Personality Disorder, which in DSM-IV was renamed Dissociative Identity Disorder (DSM-IV-TR, p. 529). Mary apparently has several distinct personality states, each with its own relatively enduring pattern of perceiving, relating to, and thinking about the environment and self. At various times, one or another of these identities takes control of her behavior. As is often the case, the clue to the presence of the disorder is gaps in the patient's memory—in this case substantiated by unexplained mileage on her car's odometer. Almost invariably, as became apparent in this case, there is a history of childhood sexual or physical abuse.

There is considerable controversy regarding the validity of this disorder. On the one hand, those clinicians who specialize in its treatment claim that the condition is much more common than is generally recognized. They point out that the diagnosis is almost always first made several years after the patient has had the symptoms, often having accumulated many different diagnoses because of the shifting nature of the symptoms. On the other hand, there are some critics of the diagnosis who claim that most or all cases are either the result of the therapist's suggesting the symptoms or the patient assuming the characteristics of the patient in a famous case of the disorder, such as *The Three Faces of Eve*.

There may well be patients who are incorrectly diagnosed as having this newly fashionable disorder. However, when one has observed in a patient the emergence of an alter with a completely different speech pattern and body language, one becomes convinced of the validity of the diagnosis.

MUTE

Cathy Jarvis, a 25-year-old mother with a 3-year history of systemic lupus erythematosus, was admitted to a university hospital in an acute confusional state with inability to maintain attention or to carry on a coherent conversation and with marked disorientation to time and place. Before her hospitalization, she had become progressively more confused over a number of days and started to believe that the neighbors were watching her. On the day of admission, she had run out of her house and into the street in a state of uncontrollable agitation.

On admission to the hospital emergency room, Cathy was given intramuscular haloperidol, an antipsychotic; but by the next morning, her clinical picture had changed dramatically for the worse. She was now rigid, mute, uncommunicative, and unresponsive to all questions; and she exhibited facial grimacing. Her course fluctuated so that at times she became excited, screamed continuously, and seemed to be responding to auditory and visual hallucinations. At other times she was mute and rigid. She required total nursing care, with intravenous feeding, catheterization, and four-point restraint. She received frequent sedation with lorazepam, a short-acting benzodiazepine. Because she was thought to have lupus cerebritis, intravenous methylprednisolone, a steroid, was begun, but there was no improvement in her clinical condition.

During the next 3 weeks, Cathy's condition deteriorated. She lost considerable weight, was unable to stand, and continued to require total nursing care. On day 28 she was referred for electroconvulsive therapy (ECT). After seven treatments she gradually responded, sought to feed herself and to stand, was more alert, and recognized her family. Rigidity was now only occasionally present. A lumbar puncture demonstrated the presence of IgG antineuronal antibodies in high titer, consistent with a diagnosis of central nervous system involvement with lupus.

Over the next few weeks, periods of lucidity alternated with rigidity, mutism, negativism, and staring. By day 90 of Cathy's hospitalization, a second course of ECT was begun. After 10 treatments, she was verbal, euthymic, and cooperative.

Discussion of "Mute"

Before admission Ms. Jarvis exhibited a number of features of a delirium: problems with attention, disorientation, agitation, incoherence, and delusional thinking. Upon admission this quickly evolved into the clinical syndrome of catatonia. She alternated between periods of catatonic negativism and stupor (body rigidity, mutism) and periods of catatonic excitement (agitation and psychotic symptoms).

Catatonic symptoms are associated with a number of different conditions. First, they are seen in the catatonic type of Schizophrenia. Although this form is now relatively rare in patients with Schizophrenia in the United States and Europe, in other parts of the world it is far more common. The most frequent condition associated with catatonic symptoms is a Mood Disorder, particularly Manic Episodes. Far less often, catatonic symptoms result from a general medical condition, or are related to medications (e.g., neuroleptics) or substance use (e.g., cannabis, phencyclidine).

Given the history of lupus and the initial presentation with a delirium, the most likely etiology for the catatonia in this case is the lupus, which was supported by the presence of antibodies in the cerebrospinal fluid. Because of the clinical significance of both the delirium and the catatonic symptoms, the diagnosis would be Delirium Due to Systemic Lupus Erythematosus (DSM-IV-TR, p. 143) and Catatonic Disorder Due to Systemic Lupus Erythematosus (DSM-IV-TR, p. 187).

Although this patient received a neuroleptic, which sometimes can cause catatonic symptoms, the persistence of the catatonia long after the administration of the neuroleptic makes it unlikely that it was responsible for the catatonic symptoms. The initial agitation and delusions suggest the possibility that a mood disorder was present (e.g, Bipolar I Disorder, Single Manic Episode With Catatonic Features) that might have accounted for the catatonic symptoms. However, the absence of other features suggesting a manic episode, as well as the presence of marked cognitive impairment and a fluctuating course, makes it unlikely that the catatonic symptoms result from a mood disorder.

It has been reported that catatonic symptoms may be present in as many as 8% of hospitalized psychiatric patients. Many instances of catatonia resolve spontaneously. Intravenous administration of a short-acting sedative often eliminates the symptoms, although usually only transiently. For some patients, like Ms. Jarvis, the definitive treatment is ECT; in fact, regardless of the etiology, catatonic symptoms generally respond to ECT.

Follow-Up

Seen a year later, Ms. Jarvis was without evidence of psychiatric disturbance. She was alert, oriented, cooperative, and fully capable of managing her home and taking care of her children. A repeat lumbar puncture revealed the absence of antineuronal antibodies in the cerebrospinal fluid.

BAD VOICES

Carmen Galvez is an attractive, divorced, 25-year-old Dominican mother of two children. A redhead with a pouty and seductive demeanor, Ms. Galvez was referred to the psychiatric emergency room by a psychiatrist who was treating her in an anxiety disorders clinic. After telling her doctor that she heard voices telling her to kill herself, and then assuring him that she would not act on the voices, Ms. Galvez skipped her next appointment. Her doctor called her to say that if she did not voluntarily come to the emergency room for an evaluation, he would send the police for her.

Interviewed in the emergency room by a senior psychiatrist with a group of emergency room psychiatric residents, Ms. Galvez was at times angry and insistent that she did not like to talk about her problems, saying that the psychiatrists would not believe her or help her anyway. This attitude alternated with flirtatious and seductive behavior.

Ms. Galvez had first seen a psychiatrist 7 years previously, after the birth of her first child, when she began to hear a voice commenting on her behavior and telling her to kill herself. She would not say exactly what it told her to do, but she reportedly drank nail polish remover in a suicide attempt. At that time she remained in the emergency room for 2 days and received an unknown medication that reportedly helped quiet the voices. She did not return for an outpatient appointment after discharge and continued having intermittent auditory hallucinations at various intervals over the next 7 years. For example, often when she was near a window, a voice would tell her to jump out; and when she walked near traffic, it would tell her to walk in front of a car.

She reports that she continued to function well after that first episode, finishing high school and rearing her children. She was divorced a year ago but refused to discuss her marital problems. About 2 months ago, she began to have trouble sleeping and felt "nervous." It was at this time that she responded to an ad for the anxiety clinic. She was evaluated and given an antipsychotic drug. She claims that there was no change in the voices at the time she applied to the anxiety clinic, and only the insomnia and anxiety were new. She specifically denied at that time depressed mood or anhedonia, or any change in her appetite, but did report that she was more tearful and lonely and sometimes ruminated about "bad things," such as her father's attempted rape of her at age 14. Despite these symptoms, she continued working more than full time as a salesperson in a department store.

Ms. Galvez says she did not keep her follow-up appointment at the anxiety clinic because the medication was making her stiff and nauseated, and was not helping her symptoms. She denies wanting to kill herself, and cites how hard she was working to rear her children as evidence that she would not "leave them that way." She did not understand why her behavior had alarmed her psychiatrist.

Ms. Galvez denies alcohol or drug use, and a toxicology screen for various drugs was negative. Findings of a physical examination and routine laboratory tests were normal. She had stopped taking the medication on her own 2 days before the interview.

Following the interview, there was disagreement among the staff about whether to let the patient leave. It was finally decided to keep her overnight, until her mother could be seen the following day. When told she was to stay in the emergency room, she replied angrily, yet somewhat coyly: "Go ahead. You'll have to let me out sooner or later, but I don't have to talk to you if I don't want to." During the night, nursing staff noticed that she was tearful, but she said she didn't know why she was crying.

When the mother was interviewed the following morning, she said she did not see a recent change in her daughter. She did not feel that Ms. Galvez would hurt herself, but agreed to stay with her for a few days and make sure she kept follow-up appointments. In the family meeting, Ms. Galvez complained that her mother was unresponsive and did not help her enough. However, she again denied depression and said she enjoyed her job and her children. About the voices, she said that over time she had learned how to ignore them, and that they did not bother her as much as they had at first. She agreed to outpatient treatment provided the therapist was a woman.

Discussion of "Bad Voices"

This is a puzzling case. Ms. Galvez applied to the anxiety disorder clinic because of symptoms of increasing anxiety. The anxiety clinic doctor, however, was more concerned with Ms. Galvez's most malignant symptom—the voices that she has heard repeatedly over many years. Chronic and prominent hallucinations certainly suggest Schizophrenia. However, there is no evidence of the disorganization of personality, delusions, and deterioration in level of functioning that are usually seen in Schizophrenia. One wonders whether her voices are true hallucinations or represent a histrionic description of thoughts that trouble her. Could the voices even be of dissociated personalities, as in Dissociative Identity Disorder (Multiple Personality Disorder)? Patients with Borderline Personality Disorder may also have brief psychotic episodes, but Ms. Galvez's voices do not appear to be limited to brief episodes.

In the absence of any other data, we would be forced to diagnose Psychotic Disorder Not Otherwise Specified (DSM-IV-TR, p. 343), but we would probably suspect that Ms. Galvez has a benign form of Schizophrenia that is not frequently seen in clinical settings.

LOBSTERMAN

Harold Robbins was stopped as he was leaving a grocery store with three cans of lobster hidden in his pockets. He was charged with shoplifting, but the court asked for a psychiatric evaluation after determining that he had no prior criminal record and no particular need for the food he had stolen.

Mr. Robbins is a young-looking, well-groomed 42-year-old man who is married and has two teenage sons. He has worked for 15 years in an insurance company and has never been arrested before. He admits to the psychiatrist that he has been shoplifting for years, following a pattern that only this time resulted in his arrest. He describes how he entered the store impulsively, without any specific purpose. While walking around in the store, he experienced an increasing sense of tension, which grew in intensity the longer he remained in the store. Then he had a desire to take the cans of lobster. He had no particular need for the food and actually does not like seafood. He had not been asked by anyone to buy canned lobster, and it is not something that he or his family would usually eat. He had more than enough money in his wallet to buy the lobster had he wanted it. The tension increased until he could no longer resist it. He took the cans and stuffed them in his pockets, after which he experienced a sense of relief. He went on to explain that he knew nothing about this particular grocery store or about its owners. The choice of a store was apparently random.

For the previous few years he had been having similar urges to steal, which he could not resist. They usually came on suddenly and for no apparent reason. Typically, he would be in a store and would experience an increasing sense of tension and feel that he needed to pick up something and leave the store without paying for it. The items he shoplifted were never expensive and usually were nothing that he particularly needed or wanted. For reasons that he did not understand, he most commonly stole canned seafood. A few moments after the shoplifting, he would have strong feelings of guilt and resolve never to do it again, but would be able to resist the urge for only 2 or 3 weeks before again succumbing to the impulse.

He and his wife have excellent jobs and no financial problems. He can think of no particular stresses either in his family or at work that might be related to the impulse to steal. He doesn't know why he takes these "useless little things" and wishes he were able to control the urge to steal.

Mr. Robbins has not had other serious problems with impulse control. He does, however, reveal that over the last 10 years, while walking at night, he often has an increasing sense of tension and an urge to look at women in the windows of ground-floor apartments, which he does perhaps every 2 or 3 months. During these times he has a feeling of tension and excitement, but claims it is nonsexual. He does not masturbate or fantasize about the woman observed. Once the incident is over, he feels guilty, whether or not the woman he observed was naked.

Mr. Robbins says that for the past 2 years, he has had a growing sense of futility about his life. His children are approaching the point when they will be leaving home, and he has no interests or hobbies that do not revolve specifically around the children. He occasionally feels that "life is not worth living," but denies active suicidal thoughts or other persistent symptoms of depression. His feelings of shame and guilt are limited to his shoplifting and peeping. Otherwise, he considers himself to be a hard-working, law-abiding person who contributes to his community by coaching sports.

Mr. Robbins is the only child of an alcoholic father who physically abused his wife. There were many periods during which he and his mother lived away from his father, and he has always felt very close to her. As an adult he has been a dutiful and supportive son.

He describes himself as an adolescent as being irritable and quite aggressive. He was often in fights, usually with boys larger than himself who had made some kind of derogatory remark about his size. Generally, his response was grossly out of proportion to the remark.

Discussion of "Lobsterman"

Although superficially Mr. Robbins acts like an ordinary shoplifter, he is not motivated simply by the desire to have what he takes without paying for it. He has no particular need or desire for the things that he takes and does not understand why he often takes seafood. He knows only that he has recurrent impulses to steal objects that he does not need and that, with an increasing sense of tension, he inevitably gives in to the impulse and steals, after which he feels relief, guilt, and remorse. He does not plan to steal, but succumbs to the impulse once he is in a store. These are the characteristic features of Kleptomania, an Impulse-Control Disorder Not Elsewhere Classified (DSM-IV-TR, p. 669).

Kleptomania is probably more common in females than males. It is a rare condition; even among arrested shoplifters, only about 5% give a history that is consistent with the disorder. It is assumed that in some of these cases, the history is fabricated in order to conform to the stereotype of the disorder, thereby allowing the person to avoid criminal prosecution. The onset may be as early as childhood, and it usually waxes and wanes and tends to become chronic.

In Kleptomania, as in other Impulse-Control Disorders, such as Pathological Gambling and Pyromania, the person usually has impulses to engage in a single inappropriate activity. Mr. Robbins seems to be an exception to this, and it is hard to know what to make of his peeping Tom impulses. He denies the sexual arousal that one would expect in Voyeurism (a Paraphilia). If one wanted to give a separate diagnosis for that behavior, the appropriate diagnosis would be Impulse-Control Disorder Not Elsewhere Specified (DSM-IV-TR, p. 677).

STILL A STUDENT

Ellen Waters's psychotherapist referred her for a medication consultation because of her continuing depressed mood and panic attacks. She is a 37-year-old part-time graduate student who lives alone and supports herself by working as a home health aide. She completed the course work for a Ph.D. in sociology 3 years ago, but has not yet begun her thesis.

Ellen is indeed an unhappy-looking woman and describes being unhappy through much of her life, with no long periods of feeling really good. Her father had a history of alcohol problems, and there was always a great deal of strife in her parents' marriage. She denies sexual or physical abuse, but feels that her parents were "emotionally abusive" to her. She was first referred for treatment after she made a suicide attempt at age 14, and there have been many times over the years during which her usual low-level depression has become considerably worse, but she has not sought treatment.

Two years ago, when she had been seeing her current boyfriend for about 4 years, it finally became clear that he was unwilling to marry her or live with her. She began to get more depressed and to experience acute panic attacks, and it was at that time that she entered psychotherapy.

In the month before the consultation, she says she was depressed most of the time. She had gained about 10 pounds because she was constantly nibbling on chips or cookies or making herself peanut butter sandwiches. She often awakened in the middle of the night, was unable to go back to sleep for hours, and then overslept the following day, often sleeping up to 18 hours. She says she feels like dead weight, her legs and arms are heavy, and she is always tired. She ruminates about her own failures and cannot concentrate on any serious reading. Although she often wishes to be dead, she has not made any recent suicide attempts.

Ellen's mood is clearly reactive to favorable events. Small attentions from her therapist or her boyfriend can cause her to feel really good for hours at a time. She has an equally extreme reaction to any sort of rejection. If a friend does not return a call, or if someone appears romantically interested and then withdraws, she feels devastated to the point where she cannot work. She then stays at home, overeats, and avoids people.

Ellen's academic and vocational history have been erratic. She has a master's degree in psychology and worked as a counselor for a while, but found this too upsetting. She then began a Ph.D. program in sociology, completed her course work, but interrupted this to train in physical therapy. She has never worked in one job for more than a few years and has spent much of her adult life as a student. Her current romance is the longest she has sustained. She lived with a man once previously, but this was a brief and tumultuous relationship. Boyfriends have described her as "needy and clinging," and it appears her current boyfriend fears her neediness.

Although Ellen reports chronic depression, when she is asked about "high" periods, she describes many episodes of abnormally elevated mood that have lasted for several months. During these times she would function on 4 or 5 hours of sleep a night, run up huge telephone bills, and feel that her thoughts were racing. She was able to get a lot done, but her friends were obviously concerned about the change in her behavior, urging her to "slow down" and "calm down." She has never gotten into any real trouble during these episodes.

Discussion of "Still a Student"

Ellen's long history of mild depressive symptoms suggests the diagnosis of Dysthymic Disorder. However, her many episodes of elevated mood, decreased sleep, increased activity, and racing thoughts clearly indicate Hypomanic Episodes (DSM-IV-TR, p. 368), which rule out a diagnosis of Dysthymic Disorder in favor of a diagnosis of Bipolar II Disorder (DSM-IV-TR, p. 397). Because she currently has a Major Depressive Episode (weight gain, insomnia, trouble concentrating, self-deprecation, suicidal ideation), it would be further specified as Current Episode Depressed.

Whereas most patients with a Major Depressive Episode have trouble sleeping and loss of appetite, Ellen often sleeps 18 hours and has had an increase in appetite. These features, often referred to as "reverse vegetative symptoms," in the presence of depressed mood that brightens in response to positive events and rejection sensitivity, warrant the additional specification of With Atypical Features. This clinical picture has been demonstrated to be associated with good response to monoamine oxidase inhibitors and poorer response to traditional tricyclic antidepressant medications.

Ellen also complains of "panic attacks." We suspect that she has the characteristic symptoms of panic attacks and concern about their recurrence, but does not have agoraphobic symptoms. If this is the case, we would add the diagnosis of Panic Disorder Without Agoraphobia (DSM-IV-TR, p. 440).

YOU MAY KEEP THE YACHT

Eddie Stover was escorted from jail to a forensic psychiatry inpatient unit by sheriff's deputies. They brought with them involuntary detention papers citing him as "gravely disabled because of a psychiatric disorder." He was in a jail uniform and ambulatory restraints, chatting cheerfully, incoherently, and rapidly to himself. The accompanying deputy explained to the admitting nurse: "He won't shut up. He's been keeping the inmates awake for the last 2 nights talking nonsense. The charges are for rape in another state; we don't have any details. He won't talk to us, won't eat any food, refuses to take medicine, and stays naked under the blankets on his cot. He says he's plucking his pubic hair because it increases his virility."

An attending psychiatrist arrived to examine the patient and noted that he was a tall, thin, black male who appeared his stated age of 35 years. He had "unruly" hair that was matted and apparently neglected. He was noted to have "intense affect" that was "menacing." His speech was articulate, but rambling, loud, and pressured. His responses were judged to be "guarded" and "questionably reliable." He gave bizarre responses with loose associations, such as when he was asked to spell the word "world" and responded, "w-zero-r-l-d. I used the number, but I know it's a letter . . . it's part of the metric system, world system, you know." He denied hallucinations, violent impulses, and any previous psychiatric treatment.

The psychiatrist thought the most likely diagnosis was Schizophrenia, Chronic, Undifferentiated Type, with a need to rule out drug intoxication. Antipsychotic medication was prescribed, but Mr. Stover refused it. He also refused the physical exam and laboratory tests, except for urinalysis and VDRL. He did later agree to a physical examination and reported to the examining nurse practitioner a history of intravenous heroin use, syphilis infection treated 8 years prior to admission, and a gunshot wound to the heart. The examination revealed no evidence of old scars of gunshot wounds or track marks. Syphilis serology tests were within normal limits, and his urine toxicology screen at approximately 72 hours after admission was negative. On the afternoon of his transfer, the patient was released from criminal custody when the rape charges were dropped. He remained involuntarily detained for psychiatric treatment, however, and was transferred to a locked general ward that evening.

On the locked ward, Mr. Stover was cooperative, but agitated and unable to sleep. After a few hours he began to complain of homosexual activity by "others" in his room, though he had no roommates. The staff feared he would lose control; and because he continued to refuse medication, they placed him in open seclusion. This did not alleviate his agitation, and he began to yell. When the seclusion door was locked, he became calmer, thanked the staff for ensuring his safety, and slept briefly.

The following day Mr. Stover was kept in seclusion, where he remained lying on the floor, pacing, or in a corner vocalizing to himself. He displayed bizarre, ritualistic movements and was increasingly withdrawn. He refused medication and solid food, but did take fluids. A nurse described him as having a "playful and aloof attitude." He responded to questions by repeating, "I refuse, I refuse. I'm in a meeting conducting business." On day four of his hospitalization, the female psychiatrist examining him observed "menacing and sexually inappropriate behaviors." Upon being questioned regarding his refusal of medication, he shouted, "You're not listening," and began making kissing gestures and thrusting his pelvis.

Because of his persistent symptoms and refusal of medicines, Mr. Stover was presented for court-ordered treatment. At the hearing, he continued to behave inappropriately, passing flatus and referring to the woman court commissioner as "Carol Channing." He lost the hearing because of his "lack of rational refusal." He was offered oral medication, but preferred to be restrained and therefore received his first dose of antidepressant medication parenterally. Within 8 hours he agreed to oral medication.

On day four of medication, Mr. Stover was dramatically improved. He was weaned from seclusion and began to groom himself and attend group therapy. Although his conduct was mostly appropriate, occasional bizarre behaviors were still observed, such as during one grooming group when he shaved his head of his long dreadlocks, stating he was "allowing his head to cool down." On mental status examination he no longer exhibited loose associations, but he continued to be "suspicious" and declined to supply information regarding his past. He actively lobbied for discharge and requested that the doctor contact his former physician in a midwestern state. His only revelations were that his parents were alive, he had four female siblings, and he had been a construction company employee, but now received disability payments because of an industrial accident.

Because the rape charge had been dropped and his mental condition no longer warranted involuntary treatment, the staff attempted to convince him to stay voluntarily. He refused, and the hospital was forced to discharge him. He indicated that he planned to remain in town only long enough to purchase some "superior leather goods," and then he planned to return to the Midwest. As he left the unit, Mr. Stover turned to his primary nurse and said: "You've been the best servant I've ever had; you may keep the yacht!"

Discussion of "You May Keep the Yacht"

When African American patients present in ways that are unfamiliar to the clinicians evaluating them, the target symptoms may be overlooked. It is apparent that the admitting psychiatrist here, having noted a history of violence and perceiving a "menacing," agitated, incoherent, large, dark male, was most impressed by these features, which led to a diagnosis of Schizophrenia. The doctor apparently did not recognize that what he perceived as "unruly" hair was actually a popular Caribbean hairstyle. Had it not been for Mr. Stover's frightening presentation, the doctor might have viewed him as flamboyant rather than as wild and disorganized. He might also have noticed that his speech was pressured, he was not sleeping, and he was irritable and hypersexual—all symptoms suggesting a possible Manic Episode (DSM-IV-TR, p. 362). The subsequent course, in which Mr. Stover demonstrated grandiosity and an expansive mood, further supports this diagnosis. In the absence of any information about prior Manic or Major Depressive Episodes, the diagnosis would be Bipolar I Disorder, Single Manic Episode, Severe With Psychotic Features (DSM-IV-TR, p. 388).

Studies have demonstrated that clinicians often misdiagnose African American patients as having Schizophrenia rather than Bipolar Disorder. In this case the preliminary suspicion of Schizophrenia or of a substance intoxication was reasonable, but the differential diagnosis should have included Bipolar I Disorder With Psychotic Features.

CERTIFIED PUBLIC ACCOUNTANT

Maurice Rosen was 69 when he made an appointment for a neurological evaluation. He had recently noticed that his memory was slipping and he had problems with concentration that were beginning to interfere with his work as a self-employed tax accountant. He complained of slowness and losing his train of thought. Recent changes in the tax laws were hard for him to learn, and his wife said he was becoming more withdrawn and reluctant to initiate activities. However, he was still able to take care of his personal finances and accompany his wife on visits to friends. Although mildly depressed about his disabilities, he denied other symptoms of depression, such as disturbed sleep or appetite, feelings of guilt, or suicidal ideation.

Mr. Rosen has a long history of treatment for episodes of depression, beginning in his 20s. He has taken a number of different antidepressants and once had a course of electroconvulsive therapy. As recently as 6 months before this evaluation, he had been taking an antidepressant.

Two years ago he developed an intermittent resting tremor in his left hand and a shuffling gait. Although the diagnosis of Parkinson's disease was considered by his psychiatrist, it was not confirmed by a neurologist, and therefore no additional treatment was given.

The neurologist who was now evaluating him found that his spontaneous speech was hesitant and unclear (dysarthric). Cranial nerve examination was normal. Motor tone was increased slightly in the neck and all limbs. Alternating movements of his hands were performed slowly. He had a slight intermittent tremor of the left arm at rest. Reflexes were symmetrical. A diagnosis of idiopathic Parkinson's disease was made, and he was placed on a low dose of carbidopa, a medication that alleviates the symptoms of Parkinson's disease.

A neuropsychological examination performed three weeks later revealed average performance on the Wechsler Adult Intelligence Scale—Revised (full scale IQ = 104), but a verbal IQ of 118 and a performance IQ of 84. Memory as assessed by a 12-item, 10-trial, selective reminding task was poor, with no more than 7 items recalled on any trial, and only 3 words recalled after a 15-minute delay, though the patient could recognize the remaining words. He showed marked difficulty in drawings of overlapping figures and parallel lines. He was unable to draw three-dimensional figures. In language testing he demonstrated impaired naming. In summary, Mr. Rosen displayed evidence of impairment in memory, naming, and constructional abilities. These may have been secondary to slowness, poor planning, and perseveration. The deficits were believed to result from Parkinson's disease. Additional evaluation included a magnetic resonance imaging scan, which revealed only generalized atrophy, and an electroencephalogram, which was significant for background generalized slowing.

Discussion of "Certified Public Accountant"

Although the first neurologist who saw Mr. Rosen did not make a diagnosis of Parkinson's disease, the subsequent development of an intentional tremor at rest and abnormalities in speech and other motor functions confirmed the diagnosis. The second neurological evaluation was prompted primarily by cognitive symptoms, including failing memory, problems with concentration, and difficulties in initiating goal-directed activities. On neuropsychological examination, Mr. Rosen showed impairment in memory, naming, and constructional abilities. All of these symptoms, when they are sufficiently severe to cause significant impairment in functioning, indicate the presence of a dementia. Thus, the diagnosis is Dementia Due to Parkinson's Disease, Without Behavioral Disturbance (DSM-IV-TR, p. 168).

Most patients with Parkinson's disease eventually develop some cognitive impairment. If the onset of the Parkinson's disease is late in life or if there is a history of depression (both of which were true in this case), the development of dementia is more likely.

Follow-Up

Mr. Rosen's motor function improved on carbidopa, but his memory worsened. He now noted occasional difficulty telling time and writing checks. His wife said he would immediately forget conversations or movie plots. He was again treated with fluoxetine, but without improvement in his cognitive status. He then had a small stroke that temporarily affected his motor function. With all of these new difficulties, he decided to retire. The following year he reported increasing difficulty in decision making and memory impairment and more word-finding problems. His Parkinson's disease also worsened. In the second year after his evaluation, his speech became more difficult to understand, and he had "freezing" episodes (his foot sticking to the floor), resulting in falls. He frequently used the wrong words in conversation. His memory continued to worsen, and he was unable to care for himself without a great deal of assistance from his wife.

A WANDERING MIND

Noreen Hamilton, a 35-year-old clerk and mother of three small children, applied for treatment at a Montana mental health clinic with the complaint that "My mind wanders. It's hard for me to keep my attention on one task, and I get distracted so easily." She also described herself as disorganized, restless, irritable, and bad tempered. She tended to overreact emotionally and was often depressed for days at a time. Her relationship with her long-time lover had begun to unravel. The couple had frequent arguments, exacerbated by Noreen's temper. Her lover complained that "problems just never get solved." She also found it difficult to handle her two boys, whom she described as "hyperactive."

The psychiatrist asked the patient's mother to complete a questionnaire in which she was asked to recall Noreen's behavior as a child. The results placed Noreen in the 95th percentile of childhood "hyperactivity." Although Noreen's memories of her own childhood were sketchy, she recalled being a disciplinary problem and often being sent to the principal's office in elementary school. She had no treatment as a child, but at age 20 and again at age 23 saw a counselor because she had difficulty "coping." Her marriage, which had been very stormy, terminated after the birth of her third child, at age 25, and she was again briefly in treatment. Finally, 2 years ago she went to the community mental health clinic and was given antidepressant medication, which she took for several months without any noticeable improvement.

Discussion of "A Wandering Mind"

The long-term symptoms of mood lability, problems with interpersonal relationships, and difficulty controlling anger suggest a possible diagnosis of Borderline Personality Disorder. However, Noreen does not have any of the other characteristic features of the disorder, such as identity problems, intense and unstable relationships, suicidal behavior, or chronic feelings of emptiness. The clue to what is probably the correct diagnosis is in her chief complaint: "My mind wanders. It is hard for me to keep my attention on one task, and I get distracted so easily." This problem with attention and focusing is one of the cardinal symptoms of Attention-Deficit/Hyperactivity Disorder; and her mother confirms that as a child, Noreen had hyperactivity, the other characteristic feature.

Currently Noreen has the following typical features of attention deficit: difficulty sustaining attention and organizing tasks, and distractibility. We assume that as a child she probably had other symptoms, such as failing to attend to details and follow through on instructions. Because she has some symptoms of the disorder but not the full syndrome, as is usually the case when the disorder persists into adulthood, the diagnosis is Attention-Deficit/Hyperactivity Disorder, In Partial Remission (DSM-IV-TR, p. 92).

When an adult complains of inattentiveness, distractibility, affective lability, problems controlling temper, and impulsivity, the clinician should be alert to the possibility of the persistence of the childhood disorder. Such patients frequently also have an unusually high energy level, but this was apparently not true of Noreen.

Follow-Up

Noreen was entered into a placebo-controlled trial of methylphenidate, a drug that is frequently given to children with Attention-Deficit/Hyperactivity Disorder. She showed no response to placebo, but experienced a clear-cut and substantial response to the drug, characterized by marked improvement in her concentration, organization, restlessness, affective lability and "the blues," temper, and handling of stress. She has been maintained on this medication, and during 7 years has developed no tolerance to the drug's effects. She reentered school and received her general equivalency diploma, and then completed 2 years of community college. She became a legal secretary and married her live-in lover. Her work performance, relationship with her children, and relationship with her partner are greatly improved.

ATAQUES DE NERVIOS*

Belinda Otero, agitated and screaming, was brought to the emergency room of a city hospital by her family, complaining of severe left-sided facial pain. The previous week, after she heard that her former husband had remarried in the Dominican Republic, she had become increasingly agitated and developed insomnia and anorexia. She moved into her mother's home with her two children, and that day developed the facial pain.

By the time she was seen by the attending psychiatrist, Ms. Otero was alternately mute and mumbling unintelligibly in Spanish and English. She was given small doses of an antipsychotic medication with no

---

*From Oquendo H, Horwath E, Martinez A: "Ataques de Nervios: Proposed Diagnostic Criteria for a Culture Specific Syndrome." *Culture, Medicine and Psychiatry* 16:367–376, 1992.

response. Because of her behavior, she was admitted to the psychiatric ward for further evaluation.

On the ward Ms. Otero was agitated and had outbursts of bizarre behavior. For example, she would suddenly snatch another patient's purse or grab at gold chains around a male patient's neck. Once she ate plastic flowers from a vase. She appeared sad, frightened, and disheveled. She reported ideas of reference and command auditory hallucinations of her daughter's voice telling her to kill herself. She received larger doses of antipsychotic medication. Though there was some decrease in her agitation, she continued intermittently to display bizarre behavior.

On the following day, a family meeting was held with Ms. Otero, her mother, daughter, and son. It now became clear that when Ms. Otero heard that her ex-husband had remarried, she became terrified that he would no longer support her and their children. A meeting was scheduled with the ex-husband the next day to discuss these issues, at which he indicated his intention to continue to pay child support. After this meeting, there was a pronounced change in Ms. Otero. Her psychotic symptoms resolved, and her intermittent episodes of agitation stopped. Her medication was tapered and discontinued without recurrence of symptoms. Having returned to her previous level of functioning, she was discharged after 1 week of hospitalization.

Discussion of "Ataques de Nervios"

This case is presented as an example of a culture-specific syndrome that is not recognized in the official classification of mental disorders. *Ataques de nervios* is a sudden, dramatic, but transient change in behavior observed in people from Spanish-speaking countries following the occurrence of major stress. It is sometimes attributed to malevolent spirits. It generally involves dissociative symptoms and frequently symptoms that suggest a panic attack, such as palpitations, chest tightness, shortness of breath, and dizziness. There may also be, as in this case, bizarre behavior and frankly psychotic symptoms, such as hallucinations. The disturbance usually begins in the presence of family members, and the family often mobilizes to provide support and even removal of the stressor.

Although in this case the hallucinations and incoherence, lasting only a few days, support an official diagnosis of Brief Psychotic Disorder (DSM-IV-TR, p. 332), it would be a serious mistake to ignore the fundamental difference between this seemingly psychotic disorder and other psychotic disorders in which stress and dissociation do not play a major role. In retrospect, the failure to recognize that this was not the usual psychotic disorder and that complete recovery was to be expected was undoubtedly responsible for the inappropriate administration of the antipsychotic medication.

Cases of this syndrome raise the interesting question of whether it is appropriate to give a pathological diagnosis to a condition like *ataques de nervios,* because it can be considered a culture-specific expression of distress, analogous to normal bereavement. One could argue that had this woman received the necessary social support from her family, she would have recovered quickly and never would have required medical care.

Ms. Otero experienced the remarriage of her ex-husband as very stressful, though it is not clear whether this would be markedly stressful to almost anyone in similar circumstances in the person's culture. However, because it is clearly the stress of her ex-husband's remarriage that has precipitated this episode, if one were to make the DSM-IV-TR diagnosis of Brief Psychotic Disorder, one would add With Marked Stressor.

BUSTED NERVES

A 49-year-old housewife, Norma Jean Luby, was seen in a central Appalachian clinic on referral from her primary care physician for evaluation of depression. She was a pale, neatly and plainly dressed woman, with hair combed straight back and no makeup. Her eyes were filled with tears during most of the interview, although she did not weep openly. She spoke slowly and so softly that at times she was inaudible. She appeared timid, abject, dependent, helpless, and hopeless, claiming she had been ill all of her life, and summed up her situation by stating, "My nerves are busted. I can't do anything."

There were multiple complaints of pain, including "black ankles," painful "knots" in her neck, "busted discs" in her back, headaches that radiated all over her body, and pelvic and abdominal pain. She described a variety of gastrointestinal and respiratory complaints. It became apparent upon conducting a routine review by systems that she would respond positively to every query. She said she had been depressed all her life, and it was getting worse. She was sad, helpless, hopeless, and fearful. She had no energy and did little but "sit around the house." She had no interest in anything, and nothing gave her pleasure. She was able to fall asleep, but would awaken repeatedly during the night and be awake for good before daylight. She had no appetite and had lost 10 pounds over the preceding 2 months. She had had many episodes of weight loss and gain in the past. She said she was inattentive and disinterested. "People are talking to me and I forget what they are saying right in the middle of things." From time to time she heard voices calling her name. She would look about, but no one was present. Frequent episodes of "smothering" occurred. At these times she felt that she might choke to death. She would become dizzy, her heart would pound, and her hands would tingle.

Ms. Luby had never had a formal psychiatric evaluation or treatment; however, detailed observations made by her physician in her chart 25 years earlier revealed a picture similar in almost every respect to her current presentation. She has taken multiple minor tranquilizers over the years, with no benefit. Aside from mild, self-limited episodes of physical illness, usually infections, results of physical exams and laboratory studies have always been within normal limits, as they were at the time of this referral.

The patient was born and lived all of her life in the central Appalachian mountains. She attended school through the eighth grade, but "could not learn." She was unable to say how old she was when she stopped going to school and "stayed at home" with her mother and father. All of her siblings left home, but she "stayed home and helped her mother." This was the state of affairs until she met and married her husband, at age 23. They have three grown daughters. Her husband, a former coal miner, is drawing disability pay because of black lung disease.

Discussion of "Busted Nerves"

This case is an example of a syndrome frequently seen in people living in rural Appalachia. The syndrome is characterized by a pattern of somatic and emotional complaints that are attributed to "nerves" rather than to specific physical causes or illnesses. Common symptoms include fainting, partial paralysis, forgetfulness and amnesia, inertia and weakness, and inability to engage in any strenuous physical activity without getting faint, shaky, or "going to pieces." The people with this syndrome are often described as fearful and nonassertive, showing surprisingly little resentment over their lot in life. In previous times, similar cases were given the diagnosis of Hysteria.

Using the official classification, we need to consider Somatization Disorder when we hear that Ms. Luby responds positively to every query about physical symptoms. However, we do not know whether she has been actively complaining and seeking help for all of these symptoms, a requirement for the diagnosis of Somatization Disorder.

Clearly, the patient's chronic mild depressed mood and associated symptoms indicate a diagnosis of Dysthymic Disorder (DSM-IV-TR, p. 380). It is unclear whether she also has had superimposed Major Depressive Episodes. The episodes of smothering and dizziness suggest a probable additional diagnosis of Panic Disorder Without Agoraphobia (DSM-IV-TR, p. 440).

Should one also diagnose a Personality Disorder because of her pattern of timidity, social isolation, and general ineffectiveness, or are these symptoms of her underlying mood disorder? Because her personality problems are not aptly described by any specific DSM-IV-TR Personality Disorder, we see little advantage to adding a diagnosis of Personality Disorder Not Otherwise Specified. Furthermore, most patients with longstanding Dysthymic Disorder also display some nonspecific personality disturbance.

Follow-Up

Ms. Luby was seen for individual supportive psychotherapy and medication management biweekly for 5 months. The chronicity, fixity, and recalcitrant nature of her symptoms were remarkable. She appeared regularly for sessions, was always on time, but displayed little insight into her condition. She had trials of various medications. Finally, on trazodone, she reported that her sleep was improved and, consequently, she seemed to feel " a little better" during the day. According to a review of her medical records for the past 25 years, this is the first time she has reported even a faintly positive response to any psychotropic medication.

MEMORIES

Zelda Podlevner, a married, 67-year-old Orthodox Jewish woman, is referred to a psychiatrist for an evaluation in preparation for an appeal to the board that had previously denied her claim for Workers' Compensation. Zelda's problems began 6 months earlier, following a fire in the dress factory where she had been employed as a seamstress for 15 years. The fire was minor and easily contained, but the synthetic fabrics that burned had produced an extremely acrid smell. After the fire, Zelda developed abdominal pains, nausea, and heart palpitations. She was hospitalized in an intensive care unit for a week because her doctor suspected asthma or a heart condition. A thorough medical evaluation revealed no evidence of physical illness.

Zelda went home, but felt depressed and so frightened about leaving her apartment that she was unable to go to work. Her symptoms persisted and intensified when her compensation claim was rejected 2 months ago. She has been staying at home, cooking and cleaning, and has no interest in doing anything else.

In the psychiatric interview she appears mildly depressed and says that whatever the decision of the appeal board, she cannot bring herself to go back to work. She feels comfortable and safe at home; but whenever she has to go out, she becomes apprehensive, although she cannot say exactly what she fears. She feels more comfortable when her husband accompanies her to stores in the neighborhood; but when she has to travel to a different neighborhood (e.g., to go to a doctor's office), she feels uncomfortable despite his presence, afraid that his long sideburns and ethnic garments will attract hostile attention from non-Jews. She has trouble sleeping because of recurrent nightmares of her experiences in a concentration camp over 40 years ago and finds herself dwelling on these memories during the day and unable to concentrate on reading.

Zelda has always been an active and competent person, and she does not understand why she has developed all of these problems since the fire and why she now feels that she is a "dead person." Although she would not describe herself as a particularly "happy" person before the fire, she believes that she was "content." She has always thought about how she would have been a very different person were it not for the war, but she claims this was not a thought that preoccupied her.

The psychiatrist asks her to talk about her experiences in the concentration camp and learns that she was in Auschwitz in 1943, at age 17.

Having been young and healthy, she was selected by Dr. Mengele, the sadistic camp doctor, to be part of the work force. After the selection, she and hundreds of other women were told to undress and wait for instructions. As the camp was extremely overcrowded, they were shoved into a strange-looking, empty, windowless hall. The place had a peculiar odor. When they were transferred a few hours later, she found out that she and the other women had been temporarily kept in a gas chamber. She began to cry as she realized that the smell in the factory fire had brought back the memory of the gas chamber.

Discussion of "Memories"

This is an example of Posttraumatic Stress Disorder, Chronic, With Delayed Onset (DSM-IV-TR, p. 467). The fire in the factory in which Zelda worked had triggered a reliving of her experience in Auschwitz, even though she was not aware of the connection until she spoke with the psychiatrist. Why such a relatively minor event could trigger such an extreme response after so many years is a mystery.

The characteristic symptoms of Posttraumatic Stress Disorder are apparent: the traumatic experience of being in a concentration camp is certainly one that involves actual or threatened death of oneself or others and produces intense fear, helplessness, or horror. In Zelda's case the trauma is reexperienced in the form of nightmares and distressing recollections. She avoids situations that remind her of the trauma (going back to work). She has lost interest in her usual activities, has a restricted range of affect (feels "dead"), and has symptoms of increased arousal, including difficulty sleeping and concentrating.

Follow-Up

The psychiatrist sent his report to the Workers' Compensation Board. At the hearing, the presiding officer said that he did not want to hear the story again and agreed to full compensation. Zelda has now been in treatment for 6 months. She is still afraid to go to work, but is less depressed. Her therapist says she is dealing with the feeling that her life stopped when she was age 17.

TWISTED SISTER

A 19-year-old youth sporting a punk-style haircut and T-shirt with "Twisted Sister" written across the front is brought, by ambulance, at midnight to a hospital emergency room in Baltimore. He is accompanied by a 23-year-old male friend who called the ambulance because he was afraid his companion "was going to die like that basketball player" (a reference to a famous basketball player who died from a cocaine overdose).

The patient is agitated and argumentative, his breathing is irregular and rapid, his pulse is rapid, and his pupils are dilated. Reluctantly, the patient's friend admits they used a lot of cocaine that evening.

In addition to attending to the patient, the medical staff attempts to contact the patient's parents. As often happens at this inner-city hospital, the patient is not carrying any identifying information. The friend is hesitant to say anything, but he finally provides the patient's name and home phone number. The patient's mother, sounding groggy and confused on the phone, has difficulty understanding the seriousness of her son's predicament, and only after a lengthy discussion does she finally agree to come to the hospital. Worried about her state of mind, the hospital sends a police car to pick her up.

By the time the mother arrives, the patient's condition has improved somewhat, although he creates a commotion in the emergency room with his loud singing and gesticulations. The mother, looking disheveled and smelling of alcohol, is distraught and tearful. She tells a disorganized story about her son's problems at home: he is disobedient and resentful of authority, unwilling to take part in family activities, and violently argumentative when confronted about his carrying on and partying at all hours of the night. She reports that he has been arrested twice for shoplifting and once for driving while intoxicated and that he spends almost all of his time with an older crowd. "They drag race a lot and hang out in the streets," she says.

Divorced for almost 15 years, the mother admits that not having a stable father figure in the household makes disciplining quite difficult.

She suspects that her son uses drugs because she has heard him talk to his friends about drugs, but she does not have any direct evidence. She claims that her son is not all bad, that he is a fairly good student and even a star member of the basketball team. (In fact, the son is quite successful in deceiving his nonvigilant mother into believing that he is a good student and star basketball player. Actually, the patient never completed high school, had poor or failing grades, and never played on the school's basketball team.) When asked about her own drinking habits, the mother becomes defensive and claims she drinks only occasionally and in small amounts.

Within 24 hours the patient is physically well and quite willing to talk. He states, almost boastfully, that he has been using alcohol and other drugs regularly since age 13. Initially, his drug use was limited to alcohol and marijuana, particularly because alcohol was readily available in his home and marijuana was commonly sold in the neighborhood. Once he reached high school, however, he began to associate with an older and more experienced drug-using group. Choice and level of drug use were largely a function of availability and price. By the time the patient had reached age 17, he was regularly using various combinations of alcohol, marijuana, speed pills, and cocaine, with no one drug predominating. After about 1 year of this pattern of mixing several drugs, he settled on a preference for cocaine.

He tells of repeated instances in which he and his friends have each consumed an entire case of beer in a day ("I can drink a lot before I feel anything. We call ourselves the 'Andre the Giant Club.'") in addition to using other drugs. These drug orgies have often included a dangerous game called "hurricane drag racing," in which intoxicated contestants engage in drag racing on side roads until somebody "chickens out" to avoid an oncoming car. During this heavy drug use, it is common for him to skip school because of the drug activity; when he has to be in school, he typically is intoxicated. To help support his drug involvement, he has devised various schemes for acquiring money, such as "borrowing" money from friends that will never be repaid or stealing car radios from the student parking lot, plus blatant stealing of money from his mother. This behavior is justified by a "Robin Hood" attitude: "I take from people who have a lot of money anyway."

Despite the patient's admission of heavy drug involvement, he stops short of admitting that he has a real problem. In response to a question about his ability to control drug use, he replies, hostilely, "Of course I could. No problem. I just don't see any damn good reason to stop."

Somewhat fidgety and restless, the patient says he is finished with the interview. Before the interviewer has an opportunity to press him further about seeking treatment, the patient begins to roam around the hospital unit, looking for someone who has an extra cigarette.

Discussion of "Twisted Sister"

This young man comes into the hospital experiencing the acute effects of Cocaine Intoxication (DSM-IV-TR, p. 245). He is agitated and argumentative (maladaptive behavior) and has a rapid pulse and dilated pupils. From what we know of his recent use of cocaine, we can say only that it causes serious social problems (he steals money and lies to his mother). Although we suspect that he probably has other symptoms of loss of control of his cocaine use that would justify the diagnosis of Cocaine Dependence, we give him the benefit of the doubt and diagnose only Cocaine Abuse (DSM-IV-TR, p. 243).

The patient's indiscriminate use of many drugs when he was younger follows the pattern of a polydrug user. During this period he spent a great deal of time "doing drugs," used drugs when it was dangerous to do so ("drag racing"), and skipped school to use drugs. All of these symptoms of loss of control over his drug use and the pattern of indiscriminate use of many drugs indicate a past diagnosis of Polysubstance Dependence (DSM-IV-TR, p. 293).

In addition to his problems with drugs, this young man exhibits considerable antisocial behavior, not all of which is directly associated with his dependence on drugs (e.g., he is disobedient and resentful of all authority). He fulfills the adult criteria for Antisocial Personality Disorder in that he exhibits consistent irresponsibility (does not go to school regularly or hold a job, fails to honor financial obligations), fails to conform to social norms with respect to lawful behavior, and has no regard for the truth. Although we do not know at what age he began to lie, steal, and skip school, we suspect that this behavior began before he was 15. Therefore, we make a provisional diagnosis of Antisocial Personality Disorder (DSM-IV-TR, p. 706).

MY FAN CLUB

During the course of a routine physical examination, Nick, a single, 25-year-old African American man, suddenly started crying and blurted out that he was very depressed and was thinking about a suicide attempt he had made when he felt this way as a teenager. His doctor referred him for a psychiatric evaluation.

Nick is tall, bearded, muscular, and handsome. He is meticulously dressed in a white suit and has a rose in his lapel. He enters the psychiatrist's office, pauses dramatically, and exclaims, "Aren't roses wonderful this time of year?" When asked why he has come for an evaluation, he replies laughingly that he has done it to appease his family doctor, "who seemed worried about" him. He has also read a book on psychotherapy and hopes that "maybe there is someone very special who can understand me. I'd make the most incredible patient." He then takes control of the interview and begins to talk about himself, after first remarking, half jokingly, "I was hoping you would be as attractive as my family doctor."

Nick pulls out of his attaché, case a series of newspaper clippings, his resumé, photographs of himself, including some of him with famous people, and a photostatted dollar bill with his face replacing George Washington's. Using these as cues, he begins to tell his story.

He explains that in the last few years he has "discovered" some now-famous actors, one of whom he describes as a "physically perfect teenage heartthrob." He volunteered to coordinate publicity for the actor, and as part of that, posed in a bathing suit in a scene that resembled a famous scene from the actor's hit movie. Nick, imitating the actor's voice, laughingly, and then seriously, describes how he and the actor had similar pasts. Both were rejected by their parents and peers, but overcame this to become popular. When the actor came to town, Nick rented a limousine and showed up at the gala "as a joke," as though he were the star himself. The actor's agent expressed annoyance at what he had done, causing Nick to fly into a rage. When Nick cooled down, he realized that he was "wasting my time promoting others, and that it was time for me to start promoting myself." "Someday," he said, pointing to the picture of the actor, "he will want to be president of my fan club."

Nick has had little previous acting experience of a professional nature, but he is sure that success is "only a question of time." He pulls out some promotional material he has written for his actors and says, "I should write letters to God—He'd love them!" When the psychiatrist is surprised that some materials are signed by a different name than the one Nick has given the receptionist, Nick pulls out a legal document explaining the name change. He has dropped his family name and taken as his new second name his own middle name.

When asked about his love life, Nick says he has no lover, and this is because people are just "superficial." He then displays a newspaper clipping in which he had letterset his and his ex-lover's names in headlines that read: "The relationship is over." More recently he has dated and adored a man with the same first name as his own; but as he became disenchanted, he realized that the man was ugly and was an embarrassment because he dressed so poorly. Nick then explains that he owns more than 100 neckties and about 30 suits and is proud of how much he spends on "putting myself together." He has no relationships with other homosexual men now, describing them as "only interested in sex." He considers heterosexual men "mindless and without aesthetic sense." The only people who have understood him are older men who have suffered as much as he has. "One day, the mindless, happy people who have ignored me will be lining up to see my movies."

Nick's alcoholic father was very critical of him, was rarely around, and had many affairs. His mother was "like a friend." She was chronically depressed about her husband's affairs and turned to her son, often kissing him on the lips, until he was 18, when she started an affair of her own. Nick then felt abandoned and made his suicide gesture. He described a tortured childhood, being picked on by his peers for looking odd, until he began body building.

At the end of the interview, Nick is referred to an experienced clinician associated with the clinic, who charges a minimal fee (10 dollars), which he can afford. However, Nick requests a referral to someone who would offer him free treatment, seeing no reason for paying anyone as the therapist "would be getting as much out of it" as he would.

Discussion of "My Fan Club"

What is remarkable about Nick is his unabashed grandiosity and preoccupation with unrealistic fantasies of success. His behavior and attitude are arrogant and haughty. He believes that he is so special that he is entitled to be treated gratis. He is preoccupied with envy of the stars that he emulates and presumes that others are envious of him. He seems to require constant attention and admiration, and we strongly suspect that he is unable to recognize and experience how others feel (lack of empathy). He can adore and flatter others if they are of use to him, but he quickly changes his mind if they are not, coldly devaluing them and pointing out their flaws. This pervasive pattern of grandiosity and need for admiration indicates Narcissistic Personality Disorder (DSM-IV-TR, p. 717).

Nick also has many of the features of Histrionic Personality Disorder (DSM-IV-TR, p. 714). He uses physical appearance to draw attention to himself, expresses emotions with inappropriate exaggeration and theatricality, is probably uncomfortable in situations in which he is not the center of attention, and undoubtedly displays rapidly shifting and shallow expressions of emotions. Therefore, we would note histrionic traits on Axis II.

In addition, there are many suggestions of the pervasive pattern of instability of interpersonal relationships, self-image, and affects that is characteristic of Borderline Personality Disorder (DSM-IV-TR, p. 710), and we would also note these traits on Axis II.

No Joke[*]

A woman heard a man shouting for help and went to his apartment door. Calling through the door, she asked the man inside if he needed help.

"Yes," he said. "Break the door down."

"Is this a joke?"

"No."

The woman returned with her two sons, who broke into the apartment. They found the man lying on the floor, his hands tied behind him, his legs bent back, and his ankles secured to his hands. A mop handle had been placed behind his knees. He was visibly distraught, sweating, and short of breath, and his hands were turning blue. He had defecated

[*] From Dietz PE, Burgess AW, Hazelwood RR: "Autoerotic Asphyxia, the Paraphilias, and Mental Disorder," in *Autoerotic Fatalities*. Edited by Hazelwood RR, Dietz PE, Burgess AW. Lexington, MA, Lexington Books, 1983, pp 83–85.

and urinated in his trousers. In his kitchen the woman found a knife and freed him.

When police officers arrived and questioned the man, he stated that he had returned home that afternoon, fallen asleep on his couch, and awakened an hour later only to find himself hopelessly bound. The officers noted that the apartment door had been locked when the neighbors broke in. The man continued his story. As far as he knew, he had no enemies, and certainly no friends capable of this kind of practical joke. The officers questioned him about the rope. The man explained that, because he had considered moving in the near future, he kept a bag of rope in his bedroom. Near the couch lay a torn bag, numerous short lengths of thin rope, and a steak knife.

When the officers filed their report, they noted that "this could possibly be a sexual deviation act." Interviewed the next day, the man confessed to binding himself in the position in which he was found.

A month later, the police were called back to the same man's apartment. A building manager had discovered him face down on the floor in his apartment. A paper bag covered his head like a hood. When the police arrived, the man was breathing rapidly with a satin cloth stuffed in his mouth. Rope was stretched around his head and mouth and wrapped his chest and waist. Several lengths ran from his back to his crotch, and ropes at his ankles had left deep marks. A broom handle locked his elbows behind his back. Once freed, the man explained, "While doing isometric exercises, I got tangled up in the rope."

Police interviewed the man's employer, and the employer subsequently advised him to seek counseling. When the man agreed to follow through on a referral to a private psychiatrist, his boss supported his assertion that the incident, although unfortunate, had been unique and would not recur.

Two years passed and the man moved on to another job. He failed to appear for work one Monday morning. A fellow employee found him dead in his apartment.

During their investigation, police were able to reconstruct the man's final minutes. On the preceding Friday, he had bound himself in the following manner: sitting on his bed and crossing his ankles, left over right, he had bound them together with twine. Fastening a tie around his neck, he then secured the tie to an 86-inch pole behind his back. Aligning the pole with his left side, the upper end crossing the front of his left shoulder, he placed his hands behind his bent legs and there, leaving his wrists 4 inches apart, secured them with a length of rope. He then tied the rope that secured his wrists to the pole and to an electric cord girdling his waist. Thus bound, he lay on his bed on his back and stretched his legs. By thus applying pressure to the pole, still secured to the tie around his neck, he strangled himself. In order to save himself, he might have rolled over onto his side and drawn up his legs; but the upper end of the pole pressed against the wall. He was locked into place.

Discussion of "No Joke"

This man aroused himself sexually by depriving himself of oxygen while masturbating, thereby risking death. Such bizarre sexual behavior has to be regarded as a paraphilia, a sexual disorder in which the person is aroused by stimuli that are not part of normative arousal-activity patterns and that in varying degrees may interfere with the capacity for reciprocal, affectionate sexual activity.

This particular paraphilia, Hypoxyphilia (hypoxy = lack of oxygen), is not common enough to be included as a specific paraphilia in DSM-IV and therefore is coded as a Paraphilia Not Otherwise Specified (DSM-IV-TR, p. 576). This case was chosen because it is one of the few that have come to psychiatric attention before the death of the patient. When people with the disorder seek treatment, it is usually for depression, and they are unlikely to reveal their sexual practices unless a therapist takes a very careful sexual history. The most commonly associated paraphilias are Sexual Masochism and Transvestic Fetishism.

An estimated 500–1,000 people die annually in the United States from autoerotic asphyxiation; almost all (96%) are male. Deaths occur among persons from adolescence through the 70s, the greatest frequency being in the 20s. A complication of Hypoxyphilia, other than death, is anoxic brain damage.

THE RADIOLOGIST

A 38-year-old radiologist is evaluated after returning from a 10-day stay at a famous out-of-state diagnostic center to which he had been referred by a local gastroenterologist after "he reached the end of the line" with the radiologist. The patient reports that he underwent extensive physical and laboratory examinations, X-ray examinations of the entire gastrointestinal tract, esophagoscopy, gastroscopy, and colonoscopy at the center. Although he was told that the results of the examinations were negative for significant physical disease, he appears resentful and disappointed rather than relieved at the findings. He was seen briefly for a "routine" evaluation by a psychiatrist at the diagnostic center, but had difficulty relating to the psychiatrist on more than a superficial level.

On further inquiry concerning the patient's physical symptoms, he describes occasional twinges of mild abdominal pain, sensations of "fullness," "bowel rumblings," and a "firm abdominal mass" that he can sometimes feel in his left lower quadrant. Over the last few months he has gradually become more aware of these sensations and convinced that they may be the result of a carcinoma of the colon. He tests his stool for occult blood weekly and spends 15–20 minutes every 2–3 days carefully palpating his abdomen as he lies in bed at home. He has secretly performed several X-ray studies on himself in his own office after hours.

Although he is successful in his work, has an excellent attendance record, and is active in community life, the patient spends much of his leisure time at home alone in bed. His wife, an instructor at a local school of nursing, is angry and bitter about this behavior, which she describes as "robbing us of what we've worked so hard and postponed so much for." Although she and the patient share many values and genuinely love each other, his behavior causes a real strain on their marriage.

When the patient was 13, a heart murmur was detected on a school physical exam. Because a younger brother had died in early childhood of congenital heart disease, the patient was removed from gym class until the murmur could be evaluated. The evaluation proved the murmur to be benign, but the patient began to worry that the evaluation might have "missed something" and considered the occasional sensations of "skipping a beat" as evidence that this was so. He kept his fears to himself; they subsided over the next 2 years, but never entirely left him.

As a second-year medical student he was relieved to share some of his health concerns with his classmates, who also worried about having the diseases they were learning about in pathology. He realized, however, that he was much more preoccupied with and worried about his health than they were. Since graduating from medical school, he has repeatedly experienced a series of concerns, each following the same pattern: noticing a symptom, becoming increasingly preoccupied with what it might mean, and having a negative physical evaluation. At times he returns to an "old" concern, but is too embarrassed to pursue it with physicians he knows, as when he discovered a "suspicious" nevus only 1 week after he had persuaded a dermatologist to biopsy one that proved to be entirely benign.

The patient tells his story with a sincere, discouraged tone, brightened only by a note of genuine pleasure and enthusiasm as he provides a detailed account of the discovery of a genuine, but clinically insignificant, urethral anomaly as the result of an intravenous pyelogram he had ordered himself. Near the end of the interview, he explains that his coming in for evaluation now is largely at his own insistence, precipitated by an encounter with his 9-year-old son. The boy had accidentally walked in while he was palpating his own abdomen for "masses" and asked, "What do you think it is this time, Dad?" As he describes his shame and anger (mostly at himself) about this incident, his eyes fill with tears.

Discussion of "The Radiologist"

It is apparent that this doctor's symptoms are not caused by any general medical disorder. Preoccupation with physical symptoms can be seen in disorders such as Schizophrenia, Major Depressive Disorder, or Anxiety Disorders, but there is no evidence for any of these disorders in this case. This suggests, therefore, a Somatoform Disorder—a mental disorder with physical symptoms suggesting a general medical disorder, but for which there is positive evidence, or a strong presumption, that the symptoms are linked to psychological factors.

A variety of physical symptoms not adequately explained by general medical conditions is seen in Somatization Disorder. In this case the symptoms are few, whereas in Somatization Disorder typically there are a large number of different symptoms that appear in many different organ systems. Furthermore, in Somatization Disorder the preoccupation is generally with the symptoms themselves. In this case the disturbance is preoccupation with the fear of having a serious disease resulting from an unrealistic interpretation of physical signs or sensations. The persistence of this irrational fear for more than 6 months, despite medical reassurance, indicates Hypochondriasis (DSM-IV-TR, p. 507).

RX FLORIDA

In the winter of 1982, John Redland, a 42-year-old physician, married with two children, applied to a special depression treatment program of the National Institute of Mental Health (NIMH). He stated that over the last few weeks, he felt he was again slipping into a depression.

John says his first depression occurred at age 21 after he had moved to the Washington, D.C., metropolitan area from Florida, where he had lived until that time. Depressions recurred the next four winters, while he was in college and early in medical school. During the last of these episodes, John was hospitalized and was told that, because of his recurrent depressions, he was unlikely ever to succeed in becoming a physician, which had been his lifelong goal. He remained depressed and in the hospital for the next year, during which time he was treated with psychotherapy alone. His depression remitted in the spring and he remained free of depressions for several years, during which he completed medical school and his internship. However, the winter depressions had returned each year for the 9 years before he applied to the NIMH treatment program.

John now realizes that all of his depressive episodes seem to follow the same pattern. They start around the first of December (plus or minus 3 weeks) and begin to lift by April. In most years the onset of depression is gradual, but sometimes it occurs more precipitously, apparently in response to some environmental stress. When depressed, John is lethargic, apathetic, irritable, and pessimistic. His mood is worse in the morning. He cannot sleep through the night. He craves carbohydrates (bread, cake, cookies) and gains weight. He has noticed that his winter clothes are often two sizes larger than his summer ones. He recalls feeling much better during a winter vacation in Bermuda, the mood improvement occurring a few days after he arrived there. However, he relapsed a few days after returning home. He also recalls one particularly difficult winter when he worked in Syracuse, New York. These associations between latitude, the weather, and his mood make him wonder whether the climate might actually be influencing his mood changes.

John has been treated for several years with psychotherapy and a tricyclic antidepressant, both of which he has found to be "quite helpful."

Discussion of "Rx Florida"

There can be little doubt that John has a Major Depressive Disorder, Recurrent (DSM-IV-TR, p. 376). He has had numerous episodes of persistent depressed mood, disturbed sleep, increased appetite and weight gain, decreased energy, and loss of interest in usual activities. As he is once again "slipping into a depression," we note the current severity as Mild, although in the past his depressions have been severe.

What is unusual about John's depressions is that they apparently all began in the winter and remitted in the spring. Recurrent mood disorders that regularly begin and end during a particular period of the year have been called Seasonal Affective Disorders. John's case illustrates the most common pattern, in which depression begins in fall or winter and ends in spring. Less common patterns involve recurrent depressions or Manic Episodes that begin in the summer and remit in the fall or winter. In DSM-IV-TR, the concept of Seasonal Affective Disorder is expressed with the specification With Seasonal Pattern (DSM-IV-TR, p. 427). The seasonal pattern should have been present, as in this case, during at least each of the past 2 years, with no nonseasonal episodes during the same period. Seasonal episodes should substantially outnumber nonseasonal episodes over the patient's lifetime.

John's weight gain and craving for carbohydrates are typical of patients with Seasonal Affective Disorder. In other ways John's case is atypical; most patients with Seasonal Affective Disorder are women, and most complain of increased sleeping (hypersomnia) rather than of disturbed sleep (insomnia).

Follow-Up

When John entered the NIMH treatment program, he was maintained on an antidepressant and entered a light treatment research protocol involving exposure for 3 hours, twice a day, morning and evening, to 2,500 lux of full-spectrum light. The light treatments involved his sitting 3 feet in front of a standard 2-foot by 4-foot metal light fixture containing six 40-watt Powertwist Vitalite™ tubes and glancing at the light for a few seconds every 1 or 2 minutes. After 1 week of treatment, he became much less depressed, and his Hamilton Rating Scale for Depression (Hamilton 1960) score fell from 21 to 8.

After the formal light treatment study was over, John's anti-depressant was increased. He was maintained on light treatment during the day and in the evening hours and remained free of depression on the combination of light and medication. John has used lights each winter since then and remains on the antidepressant during the winter months. He has been virtually free of depression and is not currently in psychotherapy.

Like many patients with Seasonal Affective Disorder, during the summer John is able to reduce the dose of antidepressant medication and discontinue the light treatment; however, in the winter he is unable to stop the light treatment for more than a few days without experiencing a return of his depressive symptoms.

SAM SCHAEFER

A psychiatrist was asked by the court to evaluate a 21-year-old man arrested in a robbery because his lawyer raised the issue of his competence to stand trial. During the course of a 2½-hour evaluation, the patient acknowledged frequent encounters with the law since he was age 11 and incarceration in various institutions for criminal offenses, but was reluctant to provide details about them.

During the interview the man appeared calm and in control, sat slouched in the chair, and had good eye contact. His affect showed a good range. His thought processes were logical, sequential, and spontaneous even when he was describing many difficulties with his thinking. He seemed guarded in his answers, particularly to questions about his psychological symptoms. He gave the impression of thoughtfully considering his answers before responding and seemed to be pretending a reluctance to talk about symptoms suggesting psychosis when, in fact, he apparently enjoyed elaborating the details of presumably psychotic experiences.

He claimed to have precognition on occasion, knowing, for instance, what is going to be served for lunch in the jail; that people hear his thoughts, as if broadcast on the radio; and that he does not like narcotics because Jean Dixon doesn't like narcotics either, and she is in control of his thoughts. He stated that he has seen a vision of General Lee in his cell and that his current incarceration is a mission in which he is attempting to be an undercover agent for the police, although none of the local police realize this. He said that Sam Schaefer is his "case name." He felt that the Communists were taking over and were locking up those who would defend the country. Despite the overtly psychotic nature of these thoughts as described, the patient did not seem to be really engaged in the ideas; he seemed to be simply reciting a list of what appeared crazy rather than recounting actual experiences and beliefs.

He was asked about the processes and procedures of a trial and stated that there was a jury, which he thought consisted of 8–10 friends. He also thought there was a judge present, who asked for money and made decisions about the procedure. He described the prosecuting attorney as someone who pointed out all your faults and tried to make the jury think that you were bad, and the defense attorney as someone who tried to point out your good points. He saw no particular reason why he could not cooperate with his attorney. When asked the date, he said that it was June 28, either 1970 or 1985. He then saw the inconsistency in the dates he gave for the year and said that this therefore must be 1978, as he was 20 and was born in 1958. When asked where he was, he said it was a Communist control center in Austin, Texas. He reported that he graduated from high school in 1976. When asked to do serial 7 subtractions from 100, his responses were 88, 76. Asked to do additions, he responded: $4 + 6 = 10$, $4 + 3 = 7$, $4 + 8 = 14$. Asked to recall Presidents, he mentioned Ford and said that Agnew was President before him.

When asked the color of the red rug in the room, he said it was orange; his blue and white striped shirt he said was white on white. When presented with some questions from an aphasia screening test, he copied a square faithfully except for rounding the corners; a cross was copied as a capital "I." When shown a picture of a clock, he said he did not know what it was, but it looked familiar. A dinner fork was identified as a "pitchfork."

When asked whether he thought he was competent to stand trial, he replied, "Yes," and said he did not think there was anything wrong with him mentally. When told that the examiner agreed with his assessment, he thought for several seconds and then, somewhat angered, protested that he probably couldn't cooperate with his attorney because he couldn't remember things very well, and therefore was incompetent to stand trial.

Discussion of "Sam Schaefer"

This gentleman is in trouble, and apparently he has concluded that his best chance of avoiding prosecution is to prove that he is crazy and therefore not competent to stand trial. He goes about trying to prove this by claiming to have a variety of unrelated bizarre beliefs and by giving responses to questions that would suggest severe cognitive impairment. However, he presents the responses in a manner that is inconsistent with the disorganization of psychological functioning that would be expected if the symptoms were genuine. Furthermore, some of his responses to the questions testing cognitive functioning, although clearly wrong, indicate that he knows the correct response (e.g., rounding the corners of a square indicates appreciation that a square has four sides). If there is any doubt about his motivation, it is eliminated when he becomes angry with the examiner for agreeing that he is sane and competent to stand trial.

There is little question that in this case the "psychotic" symptoms are under voluntary control. The differential diagnosis is therefore between a Factitious Disorder and Malingering. Because the goal this fellow hopes to achieve is obviously motivated by external incentives (avoiding prosecution) and there is no evidence of an intrapsychic need to maintain the sick role, what is involved is an act of malingering, which in DSM-IV-TR is given a V code as a Condition That May Be a Focus of Clinical Attention.

This clinical picture has some of the features of what has been referred to as Ganser's syndrome—the giving of "approximate" answers to questions, commonly associated with other symptoms such as amnesia, disorientation, perceptual disturbances, fugue, and conversion symptoms. The full picture of Ganser's syndrome is classified in DSM-IV-TR as a Dissociative Disorder Not Otherwise Specified. Because there is no evidence of dissociative symptoms in this case, a diagnosis of a Dissociative Disorder is not made.

From the history there is a strong suggestion of Antisocial Personality Disorder—a diagnosis that needs to be ruled out, but that will be of no help to this man in avoiding prosecution. Even if there were sufficient evidence to warrant a diagnosis of Antisocial Personality Disorder, it would still be appropriate to note Malingering on Axis I. Lying is a common symptom of Antisocial Personality

> Disorder; but when it is elaborated to create the impression of a mental disorder, then it should be identified in its own right as the V code Malingering (DSM-IV-TR, p. 739).

CLOSE TO THE BONE[*]

A 23-year-old woman from Arkansas wrote a letter to the head of a New York research group after seeing a television program in which he described his work with patients with unusual eating patterns. In the letter, which requested that she be accepted into his program, the woman described her problems as follows:

> Several years ago, in college, I started using laxatives to lose weight. I started with a few and increased the number as they became ineffective. After 2 years I was taking 250–300 Ex-Lax pills at one time with a glass of water, 20 per gulp. I would lose as much as 20 pounds in a 24-hour period, mostly water and some food, [and would be] dehydrated so that I couldn't stand, and could barely talk. I ended up in the university infirmary several times with diagnoses of food poisoning, severe gastrointestinal flu, etc., with bland diets and medications. I was released within a day or two. A small duodenal ulcer appeared and disappeared on X-rays in 1975.
>
> I would not eat for days, then would eat something, and, overcome by guilt at eating, and *hunger,* would eat, eat, eat. A girl on my dorm floor told me that she occasionally forced herself to vomit so that she wouldn't gain weight. I did this every once in a while and discovered that I could consume large amounts of food, vomit, and still lose weight. This was spring of 1975. I lost nearly 50 pounds over a few months, to 90 pounds. My hair started coming out in handfuls, and my teeth were loose.
>
> I never felt lovelier or more confident about my appearance: physically liberated, streamlined, close-to-the-bone. I was flat everywhere except my stomach when I binged, when I would be full-blown and distended. When I bent over, each rib and back vertebra was outlined. After vomiting, my stomach was once more flat, empty. The more I lost, the more I was afraid of getting fat. I was afraid to drink water for days at a time because it would add pounds on the scale and make me miserable. Yet

---

[*]From Spitzer RL, Skodol AE, Gibbon M, et al.: *Psychopathology: A Case Book.* New York, McGraw-Hill, 1983.

I drank (or drink; perhaps I should be writing this all in the *present* tense) easily a half-gallon of milk and other liquids at once when bingeing. I didn't need the laxatives as much to get rid of food and eventually stopped using them altogether (although I am still chronically constipated, I become nauseous whenever I see them in the drugstore).

I exercised for hours each day to tone my figure from the weight fluctuations, and joined the university track team. I wore track shoes all the time and ran to classes and around town, stick-legs pumping. I went to track practice daily after being sick, until I was forced to quit; a single lap would make me dizzy, with cramps in my stomach and legs.

At some point during my last semester before dropping out I came across an article on anorexia nervosa. It frightened me; my own personal obsession with food and body weight was shared by other people. I had not menstruated in 2 years. So, I forced myself to eat and digest healthy food. Hated it. I studied nutrition and gradually forced myself to accept a new attitude toward food—vitalizing—something needed for life. I gained weight, fighting panic. In a rigid, controlled way I have maintained myself nutritionally ever since: 105–115 pounds at 5'6". I know what I need to survive and I eat it—a balanced diet with the fewest possible calories, mostly vegetables, fruits, fish, fowl, whole grain products, and so on. In 5 years I have not eaten anything like pizza, pastas or pork, sweets, or anything fattening, fried or rich without being very sick. Once I allowed myself an ice cream cone. But I am usually sick if I deviate as much as one bite.

It was difficult for me to face people at school, and I dropped courses each semester, collecting incompletes but finishing well in the few classes I stayed with. The absurdity of my reclusiveness was even evident to me during my last semester when I signed up for correspondence courses, while living only two blocks from the correspondence university building on campus. I felt I would only be able to face people when I lost "just a few more pounds."

Fat. I cannot stand it. This feeling is stronger and more desperate than any horror at what I am doing to myself. If I gain a few pounds I hate to leave the house and let people see me. Yet I am sad to see how I have pushed aside the friends, activities, and state of energized health that once rounded my life.

For all of this hiding, it will surprise you to know that I am by profession a model. Last year when I was more in control of my eating-vomiting I enjoyed working in front of a camera, and I was doing well. Lately I've been sick too much and feel out-of-shape and physically unself-confident for the discipline involved. I keep myself supported during this time with part-time secretarial work, and whatever unsolicited photo bookings my past clients give me. For the most part I do the secretarial work. And I can't seem to stop being sick all of the time.

The more I threw up when I was in college, the longer it took, and the harder it became. I needed to use different instruments to induce vomiting. Now I double two electrical cords and shove them several feet down into my throat. This is preceded by 6–10 doses of ipecac [an emetic]. My knees are calloused from the time spent kneeling sick. The eating-vomiting process takes usually 2–3 hours, sometimes as long as 8. I dread the gagging and pain and sometimes my throat is very sore and I procrastinate using the ipecac and cords. I sit on the floor, biting my nails, and pulling the skin off around my nails with tweezers. Usually I wear rubber gloves to prevent this somewhat.

After emptying my stomach completely I wash thoroughly. In a little while I will hydrate myself with a bottle of diet pop, and take a handful of Lasix [furosemide; a diuretic] 40 mg (which I have numerous prescriptions for). Sometimes I am faint, very cold. I splash cool water on my face, smooth my hair, but my hands are shaking some. I will take aspirin if my hands hurt sharply . . . so I can sleep later. My lips, fingers are bluish and cold. I see in the mirror that blood vessels are broken. There are red spots over my eyes. They always fade in a day or two. There is a certain relief when it is over, that the food is gone, and I am not horribly fat from it. And I cry often . . . for some rest, some calm. It is foolish for me to cry for someone, someone to help me; when it is only me who is hiding and hurting myself.

Now there is a funny new split in my behavior, this honesty about my illness. Hopefully it will bring me more help than humiliation. Sometimes I feel a hypocrisy in my actions, and in the frightened, well-ordered attempts to seek out help. All the while I am still sick, night after night after night. And often days as well.

Two sets of logic seem to be operating against each other, each determined, each half-canceling the effects of the other. It is the part of me which forced me to eat that I'm talking about . . . which cools my throat with water after hours of heaving, which takes potassium supplements to counteract diuretics, and aspirin for torn hands. It is this part of me, which walks into a psychiatrist's office twice weekly and sees the liability of hurting myself seriously, which makes constant small efforts to repair the tearing-down.

It almost sounds as if I am being brutalized by some unrelenting force. Ridiculous to feel this way, or to stand and cry, because the hands that cool my throat and try to make small repairs only just punched lengths of cord into my stomach. No demons, only me.

For your consideration, I am

Gratefully yours,
Nancy Lee Duval

Ms. Duval was admitted to the research ward for study. Additional history revealed that her eating problems began gradually during her adolescence and had been severe for the past 3–4 years. At age 14 she weighed 128 pounds and had reached her adult height of 5 feet, 6 inches. She felt "terribly fat" and began to diet without great success. At age 17 she weighed 165 pounds and began to diet more seriously for fear that she would be ridiculed and went down to 130 pounds over the next year. She recalled feeling very depressed, overwhelmed, and insignificant. She began to avoid difficult classes so that she would never get less than straight A's and began to lie about her school and grade performance for fear of being humiliated. She had great social anxiety in dealing with boys, which culminated in her transferring to a girls' school for the last year of high school.

When she left for college, her difficulties increased. She had trouble deciding how to organize her time—whether to study, to date, or to see friends. She became more desperate to lose weight and began to use laxatives, as she describes in her letter. At age 20, in her sophomore year of college, she reached her lowest weight of 88 pounds (70% of ideal body weight) and stopped menstruating.

As Ms. Duval describes in her letter, she recognized that there was a problem and eventually forced herself to gain weight. Nonetheless, the overeating and vomiting she had begun the previous year worsened. As she was preoccupied with her weight and her eating, her school performance suffered, and she dropped out of school midway through college at age 21.

Ms. Duval is the second of four children and the only girl. She comes from an upper-middle-class professional family. From the patient's description, it sounds as though the father has a history of alcoholism. There are clear indications of difficulties between the mother and the father, and between the boys and the parents; but no other family member has ever had psychiatric treatment.

Discussion of "Close to the Bone"

Ms. Duval has Anorexia Nervosa (DSM-IV-TR, p. 589), a disorder that was first described 300 years ago and given its current name in 1868. Although theories about the cause of the disorder have come and gone, the essential features have remained unchanged. Ms. Duval poignantly describes these features.

She had an intense and irrational fear of becoming obese, even when she was emaciated. Her body image was disturbed in that she perceived herself as fat when her weight was average and "never lovelier" when, to others, she must have appeared grotesquely thin. She lost about 30% of her body weight by relentless dieting and exercising, self-induced vomiting, and use of cathartics and diuretics. She had not menstruated for the past 3 years.

Significantly, Ms. Duval's dieting takes place despite persistent hunger; thus, the anorexia (loss of appetite) in the name of the disorder is a misnomer. In fact, she also has recurrent episodes of binge eating—rapid, uncontrolled consumption of high-calorie foods. These binges are followed by vomiting and remorse. This pattern of recurrent binge eating and purging, if it occurred by itself, would warrant the diagnosis of Bulimia Nervosa, Purging Type. However, when it occurs during the course of Anorexia Nervosa, only the diagnosis of Anorexia Nervosa is made, but it is qualified as Binge-Eating/Purging Type.

When an emaciated patient with Anorexia Nervosa insists that she is fat, this suggests the presence of a somatic delusion, as might be seen in Schizophrenia or Major Depression. However, such a patient is generally not considered to have a delusion because she is describing how she experiences herself rather than disputing the facts of her weight.

Follow-Up

Ms. Duval remained in the research ward for several weeks, during which time she participated in research studies and, under the structure of the hospital setting, was able to give up her abuse of laxatives and diuretics. After her return home, she continued in treatment with a psychiatrist in psychoanalytically oriented psychotherapy two times a week, which she had begun 6 months previously. That therapy continued for approximately another 6 months, when her family refused to support it. The patient also felt that, although she had gained some insight into her difficulties, she had been unable to change her behavior.

Two years after leaving the hospital, she wrote that she was "doing much better." She had reenrolled in college and was completing her course work satisfactorily. She had seen a nutritionist and felt that form of treatment was useful for her in learning what a normal diet was and how to maintain a normal weight. She was also receiving counseling from the school guidance counselors, but she did not directly relate that to her eating difficulties. Her weight was normal and she was menstruating regularly. She continued to have intermittent difficulty with binge eating and vomiting, but the frequency and severity of these problems were much reduced. She no longer abused diuretics or laxatives.

UNDER SURVEILLANCE

Mr. Simpson is a single, unemployed, 44-year-old white man brought to the emergency room by the police for striking an elderly woman in his apartment building. His chief complaint is, "That damn bitch. She and the rest of them deserved more than that for what they put me through."

The patient has been continuously ill since age 22. During his first year of law school, he gradually became more and more convinced that his classmates were making fun of him. He noticed that they would snort and sneeze whenever he entered the classroom. When a girl he was dating broke off the relationship with him, he believed that she had been "replaced" by a look-alike. He called the police and asked for their help to solve the "kidnapping." His academic performance in school declined dramatically, and he was asked to leave and seek psychiatric care.

Mr. Simpson got a job as an investment counselor at a bank, which he held for 7 months. However, he was getting an increasing number of distracting "signals" from co-workers, and he became more and more suspicious and withdrawn. It was at this time that he first reported hearing voices. He was eventually fired and soon thereafter was hospitalized for the first time, at age 24. He has not worked since.

Mr. Simpson has been hospitalized 12 times, the longest stay being 8 months. However, in the last 5 years he has been hospitalized only once, for 3 weeks. During the hospitalizations he has received various antipsychotic drugs. Although outpatient medication has been prescribed, he usually stops taking it shortly after leaving the hospital. Aside from twice-yearly lunch meetings with his uncle and his contacts with mental health workers, he is totally isolated socially. He lives on his own and manages his own financial affairs, including a modest inheritance. He reads the *Wall Street Journal* daily. He cooks and cleans for himself.

Mr. Simpson maintains that his apartment is the center of a large communication system that involves all three major television networks, his neighbors, and apparently hundreds of "actors" in his neighborhood. There are secret cameras in his apartment that carefully monitor all his activities. When he is watching TV, many of his minor actions (e.g., going to the bathroom) are soon directly commented on by the announcer. Whenever he goes outside, the "actors" have all been warned to keep him under surveillance. Everyone on the street watches him. His neighbors operate two different "machines"; one is responsible for all of his voices, except the "joker." He is not certain who controls this voice, which "visits" him only occasionally and is very funny. The other voices, which he hears many times each day, are generated by this machine, which he sometimes thinks is directly run by the neighbor whom he attacked. For example, when he is going over his investments, these "harassing" voices constantly tell him which stocks to buy. The other machine he calls "the dream machine." This machine puts erotic dreams into his head, usually of "black women."

Mr. Simpson describes other unusual experiences. For example, he recently went to a shoe store 30 miles from his house in the hope of getting some shoes that wouldn't be "altered." However, he soon found out that, like the rest of the shoes he buys, special nails had been put into the bottom of the shoes to annoy him. He was amazed that his decision concerning which shoe store to go to must have been known to his "harassers" before he himself knew it, so that they had time to get the altered shoes made up especially for him. He realizes that great effort and "millions of dollars" are involved in keeping him under surveillance. He sometimes thinks this is all part of a large experiment to discover the secret of his "superior intelligence."

At the interview, Mr. Simpson is well-groomed, and his speech is coherent and goal-directed. His affect is, at most, only mildly blunted. He was initially very angry at being brought in by the police. After several weeks of treatment with an antipsychotic drug failed to control his psychotic symptoms, he was transferred to a long-stay facility with a plan to arrange a structured living situation for him.

Discussion of "Under Surveillance"

Mr. Simpson's long illness apparently began with delusions of reference (his classmates making fun of him by snorting and sneezing when he entered the classroom). Over the years his delusions have become increasingly complex and bizarre (his neighbors are actually actors, his thoughts are monitored, a machine puts erotic dreams in his head). In addition, he has prominent hallucinations of different voices that harass him.

Bizarre delusions and prominent hallucinations are the characteristic psychotic symptoms of Schizophrenia (DSM-IV-TR, p. 312). The diagnosis is confirmed by the marked disturbance in his work and social functioning and the absence of a sustained mood disturbance or a general medical condition or use of a substance that can account for the disturbance.

All of Mr. Simpson's delusions and hallucinations seem to involve the single theme of a conspiracy to harass him. This preoccupation with a delusion, in the absence of disorganized speech, flat or inappropriate affect, or catatonic or grossly disorganized behavior, indicates the Paranoid Type (DSM-IV-TR, p. 314), further specified as Continuous, as he has not been free of psychotic symptoms for many years. The prognosis for someone like Mr. Simpson with the paranoid type of schizophrenia is expected to be better than the prognosis for disorganized and undifferentiated types. Mr. Simpson has, in fact, done remarkably well despite a chronic psychotic illness, in that over the past 5 years he has been able to take care of himself.

DEAR DOCTOR

Myrna Field, a 55-year-old woman, was a cashier in a hospital coffee shop 3 years ago when she suddenly developed the belief that a physician who dropped in regularly was intensely in love with her. She fell passionately in love with him, but said nothing to him and became increasingly distressed each time she saw him. Casual remarks that he made were interpreted as cues to his feelings, and she believed he gave her significant glances and made suggestive movements, though he never declared his feelings openly. She was sure this was because he was married.

After more than 2 two years of this, she became so agitated that she had to give up her job; she remained at home, thinking about the physician incessantly. She had frequent, intense abdominal sensations, which greatly frightened her. (These turned out to be sexual feelings, which she did not recognize as she had never been orgasmic before.) Eventually she went to her family doctor, who found her so upset he referred her to a male psychiatrist. She was too embarrassed to confide in him, and it was only when she was transferred to a female psychiatrist that she poured forth her story.

Myrna was an illegitimate child whose stepfather was excessively strict. She was a slow learner and was always in trouble at home and at school. She grew up anxious and afraid, and during her adult life consulted many doctors because of hypochondriacal concerns. She was always insecure in company.

Myrna married, but the marriage was asexual, and there were no children. Although her husband appeared long-suffering, she perceived him as overly critical and demanding. Throughout their married life she had periodically abused alcohol and, during the past 3 years, had been drinking more heavily and steadily to try to cope with her distress. She could not confide in her husband about her "love" affair.

When she was interviewed, Myrna was very distressed and talked under great pressure. Her intelligence was limited and many of her ideas appeared simple; but the only clear abnormality was the unshakable belief that her physician "lover" was passionately devoted to her. She could not be persuaded otherwise.

Discussion of "Dear Doctor"

Myrna's only symptom is a delusion that she is loved by a doctor whom she barely knows. Although her belief seems false, it is certainly possible that a doctor could fall in love with her; thus, it is a nonbizarre delusion. This kind of delusion, in the absence of prominent hallucinations, bizarre behavior, a mood syndrome, or a general medical condition or use of a substance that could account for it, indicates a diagnosis of Delusional Disorder (DSM-IV-TR, p. 329). The content of the delusion, that the person is loved by someone (usually of higher status), makes it the Erotomanic Type.

Because we think that Alcohol Abuse (DSM-IV-TR, p. 214) is very likely, we would note it as a provisional diagnosis.

Follow-Up

Myrna readily accepted medication, and an antipsychotic drug was prescribed. Over a period of 3–4 weeks she became much calmer, the delusion became less insistent, and she reduced her alcohol consumption considerably. She developed an episode of depression, which responded to a tricyclic antidepressant that was temporarily added to her antipsychotic medication.

Three years later, Myrna remains well and rarely drinks. She and her husband appear content with their marriage, which remains platonic. She occasionally thinks of the physician with some nostalgia and still believes he loves her, but is no longer distressed about this. She continues to take her antipsychotic medication.

MR. MACHO[*]

Hank Allen was charged with the murder of 10 women. His wife, Jody, who eventually testified against him, had worked as his partner, luring victims to their deaths.

Wanting to further her husband's fantasy of finding the "perfect lover," Jody had accompanied him to shopping centers or county fairs and talked young girls into climbing into their customized van. Once inside, the victims were confronted by her husband, who held a handgun and bound them with adhesive tape. Most were teenagers, though two of the final victims were adults; the youngest was 13. The oldest victim, age 34, was a bartender who closed up late one night, went out to her car, then rolled down her window to talk to the couple, who had been inside drinking and who now approached her. The Allens kidnapped her and drove her back to their own residence. While Jody sat inside watching an old movie on television, Hank assaulted his victim in the back of the van, scripting her to play the role of his teenage daughter. When he was

---

[*] From Dietz PE, Harry B, Hazelwood RR: "Detective Magazines: Pornography for the Sexual Sadist?" *Journal of Forensic Sciences* 31:197–211, 1986.

through, Jody rejoined him and drove away in the early morning hours, the radio blaring to drown out the sounds of her husband in the back of the van, strangling his victim to death. That evening they celebrated Hank's birthday at a restaurant.

Most of Hank's victims were petite blonds like Jody and Hank's own daughter. All were sexually abused, then shot or strangled to death; several were buried in shallow graves. One, a pregnant 21-year-old hitchhiker (Jody was also pregnant at the time), was raped, strangled, and buried alive in sand.

Hank rated the sexual performance of each of his victims and always made sure that Jody knew she was never number one. Jody tried to redeem herself in the eyes of her difficult husband by submitting to his every demand. Even when she finally separated from him, she was unable to say no. They had been apart for several months when Hank called her, asking that they get together one more time. She agreed, and that day they claimed their ninth and tenth victims.

Hank's violence was a legacy from his father. When he was born, his 19-year-old father was serving a prison sentence for auto theft and passing bad checks. A later conviction earned him a term for second-degree robbery, but he escaped. In an ensuing saga of recapture, escape, recapture, and escape, he killed a police officer and a prison guard, blinding the latter by tossing acid into his face before beating him to death. A short time before he was executed, his father wrote: "When I killed this cop, it made me feel good inside. I can't get over how good it did make me feel, for the sensation was something that made me feel elated to the point of happiness. . . . "

Often told that he was going to be just like his father when he grew up, Hank was 16 when he learned that his father had been captured and executed in a gas chamber after his mother betrayed his hiding place. Hank later confessed to the police: "Sometimes I [think] about blowing her head off. . . . Sometimes I wanta put a shotgun in her mouth and blow the back of her head off. . . . "

In a forensic psychiatric evaluation, Hank revealed that his mother was the object of his most intense sexual fantasy:

> I was gonna string her up by her feet, strip her, hang her up by her feet, spin her, take a razor blade, make little cuts, just little ones, watch the blood run out, just drip off her head. Hang her up in the closet, put airplane glue on her, light her up. Tattoo "bitch" on her forehead. . . .

Hank's mother had beaten and mocked her son, a bed wetter until age 13, calling him "pissy pants" in front of guests. One of her husbands punished him mercilessly, forcing him to drink urine and burning a cigar coal into his wrist. When his mother tried to intervene, his stepfather smashed her head into a plaster wall. From that point on, she joined in the active abuse of her children. As far back as he could remember, Hank had nightmares of being smothered by nylon stocking material and being strapped to a chair in a gas chamber as green gas floated into the room.

Hank began to burglarize with an older brother at 7, and at 12 was put on probation. A year later he was sent to the California Youth Authority for committing "lewd and lascivious acts" with a 6-year-old girl. As a teenager he faced charges of armed robbery and auto theft. A habitual truant, he was suspended from high school at 17 with F's in five academic subjects and F's in five categories of "citizenship." That same year he married for the first time.

Often knocked unconscious in fights, he was comatose twice, briefly at 16 and for over a week at 20. A computed tomography brain scan revealed "abnormally enlarged sulci and slightly enlarged ventricles." A neuropsychological battery showed "damage to the right frontal lobe."

Hank married seven times. He beat each of his wives, sometimes badly. Most of the marriages lasted no more than a few months. One wife described him as "dominant" and said "he's got to be in control." Another, who had had clumps of hair yanked from her head, called him "a Jekyll and Hyde." Yet another said he was "vicious." When she told him she wanted out, he took revenge by beating her parents. His first marriage ended when he beat his wife with a hammer. When she left him, she replaced his mother in his central fantasy. They had married 5 days after the birth of a baby daughter and a custody battle ensued. In spite of his lengthy record of assaults, thefts, and parole violations, Hank won.

When he was 23, Hank went on a crime spree that eventually covered five states. Stealing license plates and cars, holding up bars and drugstores, he eluded capture until caught and convicted for the armed robbery of a motel. Sent to prison for 5 years to life, he molested his 6-year-old daughter for the first time during a conjugal visit.

Upon release, Hank went to live with his mother, who had not visited him during his 3½ years in prison. While there, he got involved with a woman whom he impregnated and whom he once kicked out of bed, literally, when she refused him anal intercourse. He chose not to marry her, she later recalled, as "he didn't want the responsibility." Thirteen days after she gave birth, he married another woman, his fifth wife. He was 28.

Hank and his fifth wife separated when he was released from parole. He took up residence with his 13-year-old daughter, whom he soon impregnated. She had an abortion. His daughter had, by this time, replaced his first wife in his favorite fantasy, and he often raped her in the back of the van to which he and Jody would later lure victims. He had first raped her when she was in the fourth grade and, for the next 6 years, assaulted her at least once a week. When a friend of hers arrived for a 2-week visit, he also raped her.

He was 30, and his divorce from his fifth wife had not been finalized when he moved in with Jody. By the time they met, Hank had been arrested on 23 separate occasions. The following summer Hank was fired from his job as a driver. He had been fired often, and it was an event that usually left him sexually impotent. An employer at the time termed him "inadequate." A week earlier he had celebrated his birthday by sodomizing his 14-year-old daughter. When his daughter finally informed authorities of the 6 years of abuse, felony charges were filed against Hank for incest, unlawful sexual acts, sodomy, and oral copulation. Hank responded by changing his name. Using the stolen driver's license of a state police officer, he obtained a new birth certificate and Social Security number, and he and Jody moved to another town.

Shortly before his final arrest, Hank, a gun enthusiast, owned a semiautomatic assault rifle, an automatic pistol, two revolvers, and a derringer. He was working as a bartender. A co-worker described him as a ladies' man and said that women called him at work at all hours. After hanging up, he would rate them. Several women referred to him as "Mr. Macho." He was also a heavy drinker. Jody once cautioned him as he drank and drove that the combination was illegal. "Fuck the law," he answered. For his crimes, he eventually received multiple death sentences.

Discussion of "Mr. Macho"

Hank Allen's terrible behavior has been punished by the criminal justice system, and many readers may wonder about the appropriateness of trying to assess his behavior from the perspective of psychiatric diagnosis. This case provides vivid examples of extremely antisocial behavior that is symptomatic of several mental disorders.

Perhaps the most frightening aspect of this man's behavior is that the link between sexual arousal and sadistic behavior is so extreme that it involves killing his victims. Such behavior is a symptom of Sexual Sadism (DSM-IV-TR, p. 574), a paraphilia in which the person is sexually excited by the psychological or physical suffering of a victim.

Hank's sadism is not only in the service of sexual excitement. He also demonstrates a lifelong pattern of cruel, demeaning, and aggressive behavior. He has been physically cruel in order to establish dominance in relationships, he humiliates and demeans other people, he gets other people to do what he wants by intimidating them, and he is fascinated by violence and weapons. This personality pattern was described in the DSM-III-R appendix diagnosis of Sadistic Personality Disorder. Unfortunately (at least from our perspective), this category was entirely removed from DSM-IV.

Finally, Hank demonstrates a lifelong pattern of irresponsible and antisocial behavior, beginning with stealing and truancy as a child and, as an adult, engaging in robbery, assault, and murder. This pattern indicates Antisocial Personality Disorder (DSM-IV-TR, p. 706).

It is hard to know how to interpret the abnormal findings on the brain scan and on the neuropsychological and neuropsychiatric tests. We are not sure whether they were merely the result of his frequent head trauma or whether they reflected an underlying brain abnormality that itself was a factor in the development of his pathological behavior.

One could discuss at some length the childhood experiences that undoubtedly were a factor in the evolution of Hank's psychopathology and criminal behavior. As is often the case in people who physically victimize others, he was himself psychologically and physically abused as a child.

Follow-Up

Mr. Macho decided to represent himself in several of the murder trials. He was sentenced to death in more than one state. Five years after his arrest, he now awaits execution.

Junior Executive

A 28-year-old junior executive was referred by a senior psychoanalyst for "supportive" treatment. She had obtained a master's degree in business administration and moved to California 1½ years earlier to begin work in a large firm. She complained of being "depressed" about everything: her job, her husband, and her prospects for the future.

She had had extensive psychotherapy previously. She had seen an "analyst" twice a week for 3 years while in college, and a "behaviorist" for 1½ years while in graduate school. Her complaints were of persistent feelings of depressed mood, inferiority, and pessimism, which she claims to have had since she was 16 or 17. Although she did reasonably well in college, she consistently ruminated about those students who were "genuinely intelligent." She dated during college and graduate school, but claimed that she would never go after a guy she thought was "special," always feeling inferior and intimidated. Whenever she saw or met such a man, she acted stiff and aloof, or actually walked away as quickly as possible, only to berate herself afterward and then fantasize about him for many months. She claimed that her therapy had helped, although she still could not remember a time when she didn't feel somewhat depressed.

Just after graduation, she married the man she was going out with at the time. She thought of him as reasonably desirable, though not "special," and married him primarily because she felt she "needed a husband" for companionship. Shortly after their marriage, the couple started to bicker. She was very critical of his clothes, his job, and his parents; he, in turn, found her rejecting, controlling, and moody. She began to feel that she had made a mistake in marrying him.

Recently she has also been having difficulties at work. She is assigned the most menial tasks at the firm and is never given an assignment of importance or responsibility. She admits that she frequently does a "slipshod" job of what is given her, never does more than is required, and never demonstrates any assertiveness or initiative to her supervisors. She views her boss as self-centered, unconcerned, and unfair, but nevertheless admires his success. She feels that she will never go very far in her profession because she does not have the right "connections," and neither does her husband; yet she dreams of money, status, and power.

Her social life with her husband involves several other couples. The man in these couples is usually a friend of her husband's. She is sure that the women find her uninteresting and unimpressive and that the people who seem to like her are probably no better off than she.

Under the burden of her dissatisfaction with her marriage, her job, and her social life, feeling tired and uninterested in "life," she now enters treatment for the third time.

Discussion of "Junior Executive"

This woman's marriage and occupational functioning are severely affected by her chronically depressed mood, low self-esteem, and pessimism. Although she now complains also of loss of interest and energy, it is unlikely that this represents a significant change from her usual condition. Because her depression is not severe enough to meet the criteria for a Major Depressive Episode and the mood disturbance and associated symptoms have persisted for more than 2 years, the diagnosis of Dysthymic Disorder is considered. Because this woman's depression did not begin with a Major Depressive Episode, and there is no evidence of a Manic or Hypomanic episode, the diagnosis of Dysthymic Disorder (DSM-IV-TR, p. 380) would be made. In this case, the onset of the mood disturbance in adolescence would be noted as Early Onset.

Many clinicians would regard this patient's depressive symptoms as an expression of a Personality Disorder rather than a Mood Disorder. They would argue that it is impossible to separate her depressive symptoms from the characteristic and persistent way in which she relates to the world and to herself and that treatment should be focused on her characterological style as well as on the affective symptoms. However, in classifying Dysthymic Disorder under the broad rubric of Mood Disorders, DSM-IV-TR makes no assumption that the optimal treatment is necessarily biological or should be directed merely at symptom relief.

This woman exhibits several features that suggest the diagnosis of Self-Defeating Personality Disorder, which had only had a semi-official status in an appendix of DSM-III-R. Does she choose people and situations that lead to disappointment, incite rejecting responses from others, fail to accomplish tasks crucial to her objectives, and reject people who are interested in her? Even if the answer to these questions is yes, the diagnosis of Self-Defeating Personality Disorder requires a judgment that the self-defeating behaviors do not occur only when the person is depressed. In this case, it seems that she is always depressed, so it would have been difficult to make this judgment with any degree of certainty. After much controversy, Self-Defeating Personality Disorder was eliminated entirely from DSM-IV.

No Fluids

Ann, a 32-year-old medical secretary in Dublin, Ireland, is referred to a clinic for treatment of depression. She confides that the reason she is depressed is that for the last 5 months, she has been afraid that she will urinate in public. She has never actually done this; and in the safety of her own home, she considers the idea that it will actually happen to her to be nonsensical.

When Ann is away from home, the fear dominates her thinking, and she takes precautions to prevent its happening. She always wears sanitary napkins, never travels far from home, limits her intake of fluids, has stopped drinking alcohol, and has had her desk at work relocated near a toilet. For the 2 weeks before the consultation, she was unable to go to work because the fear had become so intense.

Ann vaguely recalls that her deceased father also had a fear of urinating in public. Before leaving for work each day, he urinated several times and avoided taking any fluids. Her younger sister has been successfully treated for a cleansing ritual.

Ann had psychiatric treatment 10 years ago when she began to fear that she had contracted syphilis, even though there was no clinical or laboratory evidence of infection. Up until 5 months ago, she had never feared that she would urinate in public. In addition to these specific fears, she has always been an anxious, insecure person, considered by her family to be overly cautious and perfectionistic. For the past year she has been upset about her boyfriend's impending return to his home country, after completing his medical studies in Ireland. She was divorced 5 years previously and is now living with her 7-year-old-son and mother. Her mother disapproves of her boyfriend, and Ann has felt increasing pressure to end the relationship. She believes that the onset of her current difficulties coincided with the stress of her relationship with her mother and the threat of her boyfriend's departure from the country.

When interviewed, Ann is visibly anxious. She remarks that she has been feeling despondent about her problems. She has trouble sleeping and has no energy during the day. Although her appetite is poor, she has not lost any weight.

Discussion of "No Fluids"

Ann has markedly restricted her usual activities because of a fear that she will involuntarily urinate in public. The fear of being in situations from which escape might be difficult in the event of developing an embarrassing or incapacitating symptom is called Agoraphobia. Usually Agoraphobia is a complication of Panic Disorder, in which the person avoids certain situations that he or she associates with having had a panic attack. Much more rarely, there is no history of Panic Disorder, and the fear is of developing some specific symptom such as loss of bladder control (as in Ann's case), vomiting, or cardiac distress. In such cases the diagnosis is Agoraphobia Without History of Panic Disorder (DSM-IV-TR, p. 443).

A reader may wonder why Ann's condition is not diagnosed as Social Phobia: a persistent fear of a situation in which she is exposed to possible scrutiny by others and fears that she may do something (e.g., urinate) that will be humiliating or embarrassing. In Social Phobia, the person is attempting to accomplish a voluntary activity (e.g., speaking, eating, writing, urinating) and fears that the normal activity will be impaired by signs of anxiety (e.g., be unable to speak, choke while eating, tremble while writing, be unable to urinate). In contrast, in Agoraphobia Without History of Panic Disorder, the person is afraid of suddenly developing a symptom that is unrelated to the activity that he or she is trying to accomplish (e.g., cardiac distress while shopping, involuntary urination when away from home, dizziness while crossing the street).

Ann is also depressed and has several symptoms of the depressive syndrome, including poor appetite, insomnia, and decreased energy. We suspect a Major Depressive Episode, but because there is inadequate information to determine whether the full criteria are met, we note Depressive Disorder Not Otherwise Specified (DSM-IV-TR, p. 381).

Follow-Up

Ann was treated with an antidepressant. Her fear that she might urinate in public lessened after 10 days of treatment, and a behavioral program was then instituted to correct her repertoire of avoidance behaviors. Before her boyfriend left the country, Ann and her son moved away from her mother, and she was able to lead a more independent life. Her medication was phased out after 2 months, and the fear that she would urinate in public did not return. The psychiatrist attributed her initial improvement to the medication, and her continued improvement to the behavioral program and the changes that she made in her life circumstances, particularly moving away from her mother.

JOE COLLEGE

A 19-year-old college freshman spends an afternoon drinking beer in a bar with fraternity brothers. After 8 or 10 glasses, he becomes argumentative with one of his larger companions and suggests that they step outside and fight. Normally a quiet, unaggressive person, he now speaks in a loud voice and challenges the larger man to fight with him, apparently for no good reason. When the fight does not develop, he becomes morose and spends long periods looking into his beer glass. He seems about to cry. After more beers, he begins telling long, indiscreet stories about former girlfriends. His attention drifts when others talk. He tips over a beer glass, which he finds humorous, laughing loudly until the bartender gives him a warning look. He starts to get up and say something to the bartender, but trips and falls to the floor. His friends help him to the car. Back at the fraternity house, he falls into a deep sleep, waking with a headache and a bad taste in his mouth. He is again the quiet, shy person his friends know him to be.

Discussion of "Joe College"

Although intoxication in the physiologic sense occurs in social drinking, maladaptive behavior is required for the mental disorder diagnosis of a Substance-Induced Intoxication. In this case there is evidence of disinhibition of aggressive impulses (picking a fight), impaired judgment (telling indiscreet stories), mood lability (argumentative, then crying and morose), and physiologic signs of intoxication (incoordination and unsteady gait). This is therefore Alcohol Intoxication (DSM-IV-TR, p. 215), as obviously alcohol is the offending substance.

We are not told if this kind of behavior occurs repeatedly. If it did, the diagnosis of Alcohol Abuse, or even Alcohol Dependence, should be considered.

HIGH-STRUNG

Jane Berenson, a 36-year-old vice-president of a Detroit department store, responded to an advertisement describing a new clinic specializing in the treatment of sleep problems. Ever since college she has had difficulty falling asleep most nights. She feels "mentally hyperactive" at bedtime and is unable to stop thinking about significant experiences of the day, particularly her interactions with dissatisfied customers. When she thinks she has accomplished too little during a particular day, she feels she does not "deserve" to go to bed. Any evening excitement (e.g., an interesting movie, a lively party) leaves her unable to simmer down for hours thereafter. Occasionally, in the middle of the night, she awakens feeling wide awake and again finds herself ruminating about the day's events. When she sleeps poorly, she feels "high-strung" and tense the following day. The insomnia has worsened during the past year, coincident with more stress at work.

Her business involves occasionally "wining and dining" other executives, but she finds that late meals or alcohol intake aggravates the insomnia. She has noticed that on days when she has cocktails with dinner, she invariably awakens in the middle of the night, feeling wide awake and slightly sweaty. Business travel also worsens her sleep. She finds herself in a state of unrelieved overstimulation when her job requires "running from city to city" for extended periods.

Ms. Berenson was divorced 3 years ago after 10 years of marriage. She has a wide circle of friends and enjoys socializing with them. Relaxing alone, however, has long been considered "dead time."

Both of her parents and a sister have had problems with alcohol. She is the only one in her family to be steadily employed.

During the last year she has been in once-a-week psychotherapy to try to understand why she is "so driven." This has not helped her insomnia. She has also tried sleeping pills, which leave her "hung over" the following day.

Discussion of "High-Strung"

This woman has a long-standing problem in falling asleep at night and frequently awakening during the night and being unable to return to sleep. The frequency and severity of the sleep difficulty and resulting daytime fatigue is clearly clinically significant, justifying a diagnosis of insomnia. Although there is a suggestion of obsessive-compulsive personality traits (excessive devotion to work and productivity to the exclusion of leisure activities and friendships), because there is no other sleep disorder or other mental disorder, general medical condition, or use of a substance that can account for the disturbance, the diagnosis is Primary Insomnia (DSM-IV-TR, p. 604).

This case demonstrates a frequently associated feature of Primary Insomnia: that the person is hyperalert in the evening and ruminates about the day's activities.

Follow-Up

The patient was taught by the sleep clinic to use various meditation procedures, to avoid stimulating evening activities, and to take hot baths at bedtime. She was told to discontinue any use of alcohol, which, although it might make it easier for her to fall asleep, would make it harder for her to stay asleep. She was able to decrease her night work obligations. With this regimen her sleep greatly improved, although she occasionally still had trouble sleeping when she traveled.

ASHAMED

A 27-year-old engineer requested consultation because of irresistible urges to exhibit his penis to female strangers.

The patient, an only child, had been reared in an orthodox Jewish environment. Sexuality was strongly condemned by both parents as being "dirty." His father, a schoolteacher, was authoritarian and punitive, but relatively uninvolved in the home. His mother, a housewife, was domineering, controlling, and intrusive. She was preoccupied with cleanliness and bathed the patient until he was 10. The patient remembers that he feared he might have an erection in his mother's presence during one of his baths; however, this did not occur. His mother was opposed to his meeting and dating girls during his adolescence. He was not allowed to bring girls home; according to his mother, the proper time to bring a woman home was when she was "his wife, and not before." Despite his mother's antisexual values, she frequently walked about the house partially disrobed in his presence. To his shame, he found himself sexually aroused by this stimulation, which occurred frequently throughout his development.

As an adolescent the patient was quiet, withdrawn, and studious; teachers described him as a "model child." He was friendly, but not intimate, with a few male classmates. Puberty occurred at age 13, and his first ejaculation occurred at that age during sleep. Because of feelings of guilt, he resisted the temptation to masturbate, and between the ages of 13 and 18 orgasms occurred only with nocturnal emissions.

He did not begin to date women until he moved out of his parents' home, at the age of 25. During the next two years he dated from time to time, but was too inhibited to initiate sexual activity.

At age 18, for reasons unknown to himself, during the week before final exams, he first experienced an overwhelming desire to engage in exhibitionism, for which he now sought consultation. He sought situations in which he was alone with a woman he did not know. As he would approach her, he became sexually excited. He would then walk up to her and display his erect penis. He found that her shock and fear further stimulated him, and usually he would then ejaculate. At other times he fantasized past encounters while masturbating.

He felt guilty and ashamed after exhibiting himself and vowed never to repeat it. Nevertheless, the desire often overwhelmed him, and the behavior recurred frequently, usually at periods of tension. He felt desperate, but was too ashamed to seek professional help. Once, when he was

24, he had almost been apprehended by a policeman, but managed to run away.

For the last 3 years, the patient has managed to resist his exhibitionistic urges. Recently, however, he met a woman, who has fallen in love with him and is willing to have intercourse with him. Never having had intercourse before, he felt panic lest he fail in the attempt. He likes and respects his potential sex partner, but also condemns her for being willing to engage in premarital relations. He has once again started to exhibit himself and fears that, unless he stops, he will eventually be arrested.

Discussion of "Ashamed"

One could discuss at great length the childhood experiences that may have contributed to the development of this disorder in this patient. Regarding the diagnosis, however, there can be little speculation. Recurrent intense sexual urges and sexually arousing fantasies involving the exposure of one's genitals to a stranger, acted upon or causing marked distress or interpersonal difficulty, establishes the diagnosis of Exhibitionism (DSM-IV-TR, p. 569).

Many clinicians would assume that there is also a coexisting personality disorder, but without more information about the patient's personality functioning, such a diagnosis cannot be made.

RADAR MESSAGES

Alice Davis, a 24-year-old copy editor who has recently moved from Colorado to New York, comes to a psychiatrist for help in continuing her treatment with a mood stabilizer, lithium. She describes how, 3 years previously, she was a successful college student in her senior year, doing well academically and enjoying a large circle of friends of both sexes. In the midst of an uneventful period in the first semester, she began to feel depressed; experienced loss of appetite, with a weight loss of about 10 pounds; and had both trouble falling asleep and waking up too early.

After about 2 months, these problems seemed to go away; but she then began to feel increasingly energetic, requiring only 2–5 hours of sleep at night, and to experience her thoughts as "racing." She started to see symbolic meanings in things, especially sexual meanings, and began to suspect that innocent comments on television shows were referring to her. Over the next month, she became increasingly euphoric, irritable, and overtalkative. She started to believe that there was a hole in her head through which radar messages were being sent to her. These messages could control her thoughts or produce emotions of anger, sadness, or the like, that were beyond her control. She also believed that her thoughts could be read by people around her and that alien thoughts from other people were intruding themselves via the radar into her own head. She described hearing voices, which sometimes spoke about her in the third person and at other times ordered her to perform various acts, particularly sexual ones.

Her friends, concerned about Alice's unusual behavior, took her to an emergency room, where she was evaluated and admitted to a psychiatric unit. After a day of observation, Alice was started on an antipsychotic, chlorpromazine, and lithium. Over the course of about 3 weeks, she experienced a fairly rapid reduction in all of the symptoms that had brought her to the hospital. The chlorpromazine was gradually reduced, and then discontinued. She was maintained thereafter on lithium alone. At the time of her discharge, after 6 weeks of hospitalization, she was exhibiting none of the symptoms reported on admission; however, she was noted to be experiencing some mild hypersomnia, sleeping about 10 hours a night, and experiencing a loss of appetite and some feeling of being "slowed down," which was worse in the mornings. She was discharged to live with some friends.

Approximately 8 months after her discharge, Alice was taken off lithium by the psychiatrist in the college mental health clinic. She continued to do fairly well for the next few months, but then began to experience a gradual reappearance of symptoms similar to those that had necessitated her hospitalization. The symptoms worsened, and after 2 weeks she was readmitted to the hospital with almost the identical symptoms that she had had when first admitted.

Alice responded in days to chlorpromazine and lithium; and, once again, the chlorpromazine was gradually discontinued, leaving her on lithium alone. As with the first hospitalization, at the time of her discharge, a little more than a year ago, she again displayed some hypersomnia, loss of appetite, and the feeling of being "slowed down." For the past year, while continuing to take lithium, she has been symptom free and functioning fairly well, getting a job in publishing and recently moving to New York to advance her career.

Alice's father, when in his 40s, had had a severe episode of depression, characterized by hypersomnia, anorexia, profound psychomotor retardation, and suicidal ideation. Her paternal grandmother had committed suicide during what also appeared to be a depressive episode.

Discussion of "Radar Messages"

Alice was functioning at a high level before the development of a depressive episode, followed shortly by an episode with characteristic manic symptoms: euphoric and irritable mood, decreased need for sleep, pressured speech, and the subjective experience that her thoughts were racing. At the height of the illness, she developed bizarre delusions (her emotions and thoughts were being controlled by radar messages sent through a hole in her head) and auditory hallucinations (both command hallucinations and voices speaking about her in the third person). These psychotic symptoms are characteristic of the active phase of Schizophrenia, but in this case are considered part of a psychotic mood disorder because they occur exclusively during the manic mood disturbance.

In the absence of any evidence of abuse of a substance, such as a stimulant, or a general medical condition, such as hyperthyroidism, directly causing the mood disturbance, this syndrome is considered a Manic Episode (DSM-IV-TR, p. 362). The occurrence of a single Manic Episode, even in the absence of any Major Depressive Episodes, is sufficient for a diagnosis of Bipolar Disorder, which would be subtyped as Single Manic Episode as we do not have sufficient evidence of a prior Major Depressive Episode.

The most recent episode of mood disturbance, which necessitated Alice's second hospitalization, was also a Manic Episode, so the current subtype is Most Recent Episode Manic (DSM-IV-TR, p. 389). Finally, the current severity of the disorder, which is coded in the fifth digit, is In Full Remission, in that she has been essentially free of symptoms for the past 6 months (even though taking lithium prophylactically).

There is no evidence of any Personality Disorder (Axis II) or of a physical disorder (Axis III) that is relevant to the Axis I diagnosis.

Follow-Up

In the last 7 years, Alice has had two Manic Episodes, one requiring hospitalization and one managed as an outpatient. Currently she

> continues to take lithium and is pursuing a Ph.D. in creative writing at a New England university.

PEACEABLE MAN

The patient is a 20-year-old man who was brought to the hospital, trussed in ropes, by his four brothers. This is his seventh hospitalization in the last 2 years, each for similar behavior. One of his brothers reports that he "came home crazy," threw a chair through a window, tore a gas heater off the wall, and ran into the street. The family called the police, who apprehended him shortly thereafter as he stood, naked, directing traffic at a busy intersection. He assaulted the arresting officers, escaped from them, and ran home screaming threats at his family. There his brothers were able to subdue him.

On admission, the patient was observed to be agitated, with his mood fluctuating between anger and fear. He had slurred speech and staggered when he walked. He remained extremely violent and disorganized for the first several days of his hospitalization, then began having longer and longer lucid intervals, still interspersed with sudden, unpredictable periods in which he displayed great suspiciousness, a fierce expression, slurred speech, and clenched fists.

After calming down, the patient denied ever having been violent or acting in an unusual way ("I'm a peaceable man") and said he could not remember how he got to the hospital. He admitted using alcohol and marijuana socially, but denied phencyclidine (PCP) use except for once, experimentally, 3 years previously. Nevertheless, blood and urine tests were positive for phencyclidine, and his brother believes "he gets dusted every day."

According to his family, the patient was perfectly normal until about 3 years before. He made above-average grades in school, had a part-time job and a girlfriend, and was of a sunny and outgoing disposition. Then, at age 17 he had his first episode of emotional disturbance. This was of very sudden onset, with symptoms similar to the present episode. He quickly recovered entirely from that first episode, went back to school, and graduated from high school. From subsequent episodes, however, his improvement was less and less encouraging.

After 3 weeks of the current hospitalization, the patient is sullen and watchful, and quick to remark sarcastically on the smallest infringement of the respect due him. He is mostly quiet and isolated from others, but is easily provoked to fury. His family reports that "this is as good as he gets" and that he has returned to his baseline functioning. When he was at home, he kept himself physically clean, but mostly lay around the house, did no housework, and had not held a job for nearly 2 years. The family does not know how he obtains spending money or how he spends his time outside the house.

Discussion of "Peaceable Man"

The hospitalization was occasioned by acute effects of PCP on the central nervous system: violence, bizarre and disorganized behavior, psychomotor agitation, emotional lability, slurred speech, and ataxia. This is a typical picture of Phencyclidine Intoxication (DSM-IV-TR, p. 281).

In addition, there is a history of regular use of PCP, resulting in many similar episodes of disturbed behavior. This patient is frequently intoxicated when he would be expected to be working (lies around the house, does no work), spends a great deal of time recovering from the effects of PCP use, continues to use PCP despite knowledge that it causes him to get into trouble over and over again, and has given up important social and occupational activities because of PCP use. These behaviors indicate the additional diagnosis of Phencyclidine Dependence (DSM-IV-TR, p. 279). Although we count only three of the required symptoms for PCP Dependence, we suspect that additional information would confirm that he has more symptoms. Moreover, the criterion referring to withdrawal symptoms probably does not apply to PCP. Certainly there is extreme impairment in the patient's social and occupational functioning, and we note the severity of the Dependence as Severe. Even though all of the symptom criteria for Phencyclidine Abuse are met, this diagnosis is preempted by the diagnosis of Phencyclidine Dependence.

WEALTHY WIDOW

A wealthy 72-year-old widow is referred by her children against her will, as they think she has become "senile" since the death of her husband

6 months previously. After the initial bereavement, which was not severe, the patient had resumed an active social life and become a volunteer at local hospitals. The family encouraged this, but over the past 3 months have become concerned about her going to bars with some of the hospital staff. The referral was precipitated by her announcing her engagement to a 25-year-old male nurse, to whom she planned to turn over her house and a large amount of money. The patient's three sons, by threat and intimidation, have made her accompany them to this psychiatric evaluation. While one of her sons is talking to the psychiatrist, the patient is heard accusing the other two of trying to commit her so they can get their hands on her money.

Initially in the interview the patient is extremely angry at her sons and the psychiatrist, insisting that they don't understand that for the first time in her life she is doing something for herself, not for her father, her husband, or her children. She then suddenly drapes herself over the couch and asks the psychiatrist if she is attractive enough to capture a 25-year-old man. She proceeds to elaborate on her fiancé's physique and sexual abilities and describes her life as exciting and fulfilling for the first time. She is overtalkative and repeatedly refuses to allow the psychiatrist to interrupt her with questions. She says that she goes out nightly with her fiancé, to clubs and bars and that although she does not drink, she thoroughly enjoys the atmosphere. They often go on to an after-hours place and end up breakfasting, going to bed, and making love. After only 3 or 4 hours of sleep, she gets up, feeling refreshed, and then goes shopping. She spends about $700 a week on herself and gives her fiancé, about $500 a week, all of which she can easily afford.

The patient agrees that her behavior is unusual for someone of her age and social position, but states she has always been conventional and now is the time to change, before it is too late. She refuses to participate in formal testing, saying, "I'm not going to do any stupid tests to see if I am sane." She has no obvious memory impairment and is correctly oriented in all areas. According to the family, she has no previous history of emotional disturbance.

Discussion of "Wealthy Widow"

As the story unfolds, many readers will wonder, as we did, whether this poor lady simply has avaricious children rather than a mental disorder. It does seem, however, that her alternately irritable and expansive mood, pressure of speech, decreased need for sleep, and poor judgment (signing her house over to someone she has met only recently) represent more than a new start in life for someone who has been too "conventional." In fact, all of these symptoms, in the absence of a general medical condition or substance responsible for the disturbance, or a non-mood psychotic disorder, suggest a Manic or Hypomanic Episode. In a Manic Episode there is marked impairment in occupational functioning, or usual activities or relationships with others; in a Hypomanic Episode there is an unequivocal change in functioning observable by others, but marked impairment is not present. We believe that, even though she is wealthy, the widow's plan to sign her house over to her new lover does represent marked impairment in her relationships with others (she would not agree). Thus, the diagnosis is Bipolar I Disorder, Single Manic Episode, Moderate (DSM-IV-TR, p. 388).

Bipolar I Disorder first appearing at age 72 is certainly uncommon. One would want to be careful to rule out the possibility of a physical disorder, such as a brain tumor or degenerative central nervous system disorder, that might be causing a Mood Disorder Due to a General Medical Condition. Because the workup to rule out a physical disorder has not yet been done, the qualifying term *Provisional* is added to this diagnosis.

THE JERK

Leon is a 45-year-old postal employee who was evaluated at a clinic specializing in the treatment of depression. He claims to have felt constantly depressed since the first grade, without a period of "normal" mood for more than a few days at a time. His depression has been accompanied by lethargy, little or no interest or pleasure in anything, trouble concentrating, and feelings of inadequacy, pessimism, and resentfulness. His only periods of normal mood occur when he is home alone, listening to music or watching TV.

On further questioning, Leon reveals that he cannot ever remember feeling comfortable socially. Even before kindergarten, if he was asked to speak in front of a group of his parents' friends, his mind would "go blank." He felt overwhelming anxiety at children's social functions, such as birthday parties, which he either avoided or, if he went, attended in total silence. He could answer questions in class only if he wrote down the answers in advance; even then, he frequently mumbled and couldn't get the answer out. He met new children with his eyes lowered, fearing their scrutiny, expecting to feel humiliated and embarrassed. He was convinced that everyone around him thought he was "dumb" or "a jerk."

As he grew up, Leon had a couple of neighborhood playmates, but he never had a "best friend." His school grades were good, but suffered when oral classroom participation was expected. As a teenager he was terrified of girls, and to this day he has never gone on a date or even asked a girl for a date. This bothers him, although he is so often depressed that he feels he has little energy or interest in dating.

Leon attended college and did well for a while, then dropped out as his grades slipped. He remained very self-conscious and "terrified" of meeting strangers. He had trouble finding a job because he was unable to answer questions in interviews. He worked at a few jobs for which only a written test was required. He passed a civil service exam at age 24 and was offered a job in the post office on the evening shift. He enjoyed this job as it involved little contact with others. He was offered several promotions but refused them because he feared the social pressures. Although by now he supervises a number of employees, he still finds it difficult to give instructions, even to people he has known for years. He has no friends and avoids all invitations to socialize with co-workers. During the past several years, he has tried several therapies to help him get over his "shyness" and depression.

Leon has never experienced sudden anxiety or a panic attack in social situations or at other times. Rather, his anxiety gradually builds to a constant high level in anticipation of social situations. He has never experienced any psychotic symptoms.

Discussion of "The Jerk"

Leon comes to the clinic complaining of lifelong depression. Indeed, he has been depressed and has experienced only limited interest and enjoyment ever since he was a child. Although his depressed mood has been associated with pessimism, low energy, and difficulty concentrating, other symptoms of a Major Depressive Episode, such as appetite and sleep disturbance, have not been present. This chronic mild depression is diagnosed as Dysthymic Disorder (DSM-IV-TR, p. 380), which is further qualified as Early Onset (before age 21).

In addition, Leon has lifelong social anxiety that makes it difficult for him to maintain even the most minimal social contact. His fear is that he will have nothing to say and will be thought of as "a jerk." This fear seems to be independent of his Dysthymic Disorder and therefore justifies the additional diagnosis of Social Phobia, Generalized Type (including most social situations) (DSM-IV-TR, p. 456).

This patient illustrates a frequent problem in diagnosing the Axis I disorder of Social Phobia, Generalized Type, in that the symptoms overlap considerably with those of Avoidant Personality Disorder. Leon has certainly displayed a pervasive pattern of social inhibition, feelings of inadequacy, and hypersensitivity to negative evaluation throughout his life. He believes he is socially inept, avoids occupational activities that involve significant interpersonal contact, and is inhibited in new interpersonal situations because of feelings of inadequacy. He undoubtedly is also preoccupied with being rejected in social situations and is probably unwilling to become involved with people unless he is certain of being liked. Therefore, we make the diagnosis of Avoidant Personality Disorder on Axis II (DSM-IV-TR, p. 721). Future research is needed to clarify whether Avoidant Personality Disorder and Social Phobia, Generalized Type, merely reflect different perspectives on the same disorder.

THE DIRECTOR

A 36-year-old film director had had frequent difficulty falling asleep since early childhood. He went to bed between 11:30 P.M. and 3:30 A.M. and arose at irregular times before 1:00 P.M. His sleep was lighter at the beginning of the night, when he was easily disturbed by random noise or his wife's shifting in bed. Later in the night he slept more soundly, and he felt his deepest sleep came at about 8:00 A.M. He felt groggy for half an hour or longer upon first arising and was not able to function well in the early part of the day.

The patient was currently free of scheduled work obligations except for a morning meeting once a week. This further lessened his motivation to get out of bed in the morning. In the evening, however, he experienced a surge of productive energy. His mind was enjoyably active, and he delayed bedtimes to capitalize on his high work capacity. On fishing trips he would arise at 5:00 A.M. and take a nap at 9:00 A.M. The discrepancy between his and others' sleep schedules on weekends and other social inconveniences caused by his sleep schedule motivated his seeking help.

The patient drank two to five cups of coffee daily, more during occasional work crises. He had a frequently stuffed nose, and occasionally used pseudoephedrine for stimulation, as well as a nasal decongestant (such medications often have long-lasting stimulant effects).

Both of the patient's parents and two brothers were chronic abusers of alcohol. He had survived a childhood full of severe physical and emotional trauma. Further, his mother abused sedatives and had had a 2-year depressive episode during which she remained in bed. His mother, sister, and one brother had made near-lethal suicide attempts, and his father had killed himself. Despite this background, the patient had graduated with high marks from a prestigious university and had done well in graduate school and in his subsequent work. His history revealed, however, that in college he frequently had been unable to get to morning classes.

The patient lived with his wife, who was a writer, and his young daughter. He thought his major problems were indecisiveness and being too ready to please during contract negotiations, to the detriment of his own interests. He thought his childhood misfortunes had diminished his self-confidence.

At the evaluation, the man was casually dressed, ingratiating, and friendly. Despite professions of self-doubt, he was forward, frank, and engaging. The psychiatrist recommended that he keep a sleep chart for 1 month.

The sleep chart revealed bedtimes that were progressively delayed from 9:00 P.M. or 10:00 P.M. until about 3:15 A.M. over 5-day to 7-day cycles. Arising times were even less regular in pattern, generally becoming later at the end of three cycles. Usually some obligation required the patient to get up even after a late bedtime, causing him to take an afternoon nap or to retire at around 10:00 P.M. Thereafter he would fail to fall asleep for some hours. After 1 or 2 such days, the cycle would begin again (see Figure 1–1).

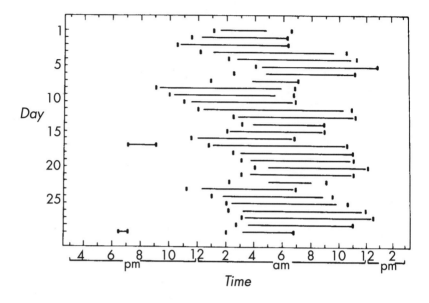

Figure 1–1. The director's sleep–wake pattern. Day (Y axis) and time (X axis) of sleep. First vertical mark on each line indicates when he first tried to sleep, horizontal line when he estimated he slept, and subsequent vertical line when he arose from bed. Note 2½-hour to 3-hour periods between bedtime and sleep onset, days 8 and 22, and evening naps, days 17 and 29.

Discussion of "The Director"

This patient shows the characteristic features of Circadian Rhythm Sleep Disorder, Delayed Sleep Phase Type (DSM-IV-TR, p. 629). There is a mismatch between his normal circadian sleep–wake pattern and the sleep–wake schedule for his environment. The mismatch is that his preferred sleep onset and offset are several hours later than those of people he works and socializes with (i.e., his sleep schedule is delayed relative to the conventional societal sleep–wake schedule). The patient's sleep chart suggests that his normal underlying circadian rhythm, which is somewhat longer than 24 hours, is not reset by external cues that ordinarily induce a 24-hour sleep–wake rhythm.

The lack of regular work hours, the "night person" pattern of greater evening productivity, and the subjectively deeper sleep in the early morning hours are all typical of patients with this problem. The lack of scheduled work obligations removed an important pacemaker for the sleep–wake schedule, unmasking the delaying tendency. The patient's use of stimulants contributed to his evening productivity and to difficulty in falling asleep earlier.

Follow-Up

The patient was treated first by withdrawal of stimulants and establishment of a regular arising hour of 7:00 A.M. daily. This lessened both his morning impairment and his evening sense of arousal. However, within a few weeks he gradually drifted back to late bedtimes and late arising times, and was again using caffeine-containing beverages during work crises. He was then treated with triazolam, 0.25 mg, at 11:30 P.M. (This short-acting benzodiazepine can reportedly resynchronize circadian rhythms that have been displaced [e.g., by jet lag].) He subsequently fell asleep regularly and, unexpectedly, awoke about 6:00 A.M. with a feeling of great alertness. He kept a regular schedule and reported that he accomplished more, despite the lessening of his evening energy surge.

The patient's fear of insomnia and work impairment disappeared. He gradually reduced his drug dosage, but a decrease from 0.25 mg to 0.125 mg of triazolam caused a sense of decreased concentration the following afternoon. On the reduced dosage he slept slightly longer each night and continued to function well.

THE SAILOR

Psychiatric consultation is requested by an emergency room physician for an 18-year-old male who has been brought into the hospital by the police. The youth appears exhausted and shows evidence of prolonged exposure to the sun. He identifies the current date incorrectly, giving it as September 27 instead of October 1. It is difficult to get him to focus on specific questions, but with encouragement he supplies a number of facts. He recalls sailing with friends, apparently about September 25, on a weekend cruise off the Florida coast, when bad weather was encountered. He is unable to recall any subsequent events and does not know what became of his companions. He has to be reminded several times that he is in a hospital, as he expresses uncertainty as to his whereabouts. Each time he is told, he seems surprised.

There is no evidence of head injury or dehydration. Electrolytes and cranial nerve examination are unremarkable. Because of the patient's apparent exhaustion, he is permitted to sleep for 6 hours. Upon awakening, he is much more attentive, but is still unable to recall events after September 25, including how he came to the hospital. There is no longer any doubt in his mind that he is in the hospital, however, and he is able to recall the contents of the previous interview and the fact that he had fallen asleep. He is able to remember that he is a student at a southern college, maintains a B average, has a small group of close friends, and has a good relationship with his family. He denies any previous psychiatric history and says he has never abused drugs or alcohol.

Because of the patient's apparently sound physical condition, a sodium amytal interview is performed. During this interview he relates that neither he nor his companions were particularly experienced sailors capable of coping with the ferocity of the storm they encountered. Although he had taken the precaution of securing himself to the boat with a life jacket and tie line, his companions had failed to do this and had been washed overboard in the heavy seas. He completely lost control of the boat and felt he was saved only by virtue of good luck and his lifeline. He had been able to consume a small supply of food that was stowed away in the cabin over a 3-day period. He never saw either of his sailing companions again. He was picked up on October 1 by a Coast Guard cutter and brought to shore, and subsequently the police had brought him to the hospital.

Discussion of "The Sailor"

The differential diagnosis of acute memory loss begins with a consideration of a Cognitive Disorder, such as Delirium, Dementia, or Amnestic Disorder, which may be caused by head trauma, cerebrovascular accidents, or drug use. The normal physical and neurological examination and the absence of a history of drug use rule out these possibilities in this patient. With the amobarbital interview it becomes clear that the amnestic period developed following a particularly traumatic and life-threatening experience. Amnesia (an episode of sudden inability to recall important personal information that is too extensive to be considered "forgetfulness") that does not occur exclusively during the course of Dissociative Identity Disorder (Multiple Personality Disorder) and is not caused by Delirium, Dementia, or Amnestic Disorder justifies the diagnosis of Dissociative Amnesia (DSM-IV-TR, p. 523). In this case, the circumscribed nature of the amnesia and the perplexity and disorientation during the amnestic period, all following a psychologically stressful event, are quite characteristic.

CRY ME A RIVER

A 38-year-old clerical worker described to a psychiatrist how she had been experiencing a disabling sleep problem for a year and a half. She usually goes to bed at 6:00 P.M. and sleeps straight through until 7:00 A.M. The reason that she comes for help now is that last month her driver's license was suspended after she fell asleep while driving her car out of a parking lot and hit a telephone pole. As a result, she now has to arise at 6:00 A.M. to use public transportation to arrive in time for work at 8:15 A.M. Upon arising she typically feels groggy and "out of it." During the day she remains sleepy. She frequently falls asleep on buses, missing her stop. She recently took a sales job after work, from 6:00 P.M. until 10:00 P.M. two nights a week, in an attempt to remain on her feet at least some of the time that she is away from her office job. On weekends she remains in bed asleep all day, arising only to go to the toilet or for meals, except on an occasional Saturday when she does her routine chores.

The patient does not believe that she snores during sleep (as would be likely in a Breathing-Related Sleep Disorder), and she denies nightmares (as in Nightmare Disorder), sleepwalking (as in Sleepwalking Disorder), or sudden loss of muscle tone (cataplexy) or feelings of paralysis upon awakening, both symptoms of Narcolepsy.

Before the onset of her sleep problem, the patient generally required only 6–7 hours of sleep a night. During the first year of her "sleepiness" she began to treat herself with caffeine, drinking up to 10 cups of coffee and 1–2 liters of cola daily.

In addition to the sleepiness, the patient has had severe, recurrent periods of depression since approximately age 13. For several months before the evaluation, she was having crying spells in her office. These sometimes would come on so suddenly that she had no time to run to the rest room to hide them. She acknowledged trouble concentrating on her job and noted that she was getting little pleasure from her work, which she used to enjoy. She had been harboring angry and pessimistic feelings for the past several years, and noted that these were more severe recently as she had allowed her diabetes and weight to get out of control. She felt guilty that she was physically damaging herself and slowly dying in this way. She sometimes thought that she deserved to be dead.

She had been treated from age 18 to age 33 with psychotherapy, during which time her depression gradually worsened. More recently she had been given trials of antidepressants, including imipramine, desipramine, and fluoxetine, which had each made improvements in mood and wakefulness that lasted several months. She tended to fall asleep during evening group psychotherapy sessions.

The patient's diabetes was diagnosed at age 11. She first lost control of her weight and her blood sugar during her teenage years, regained it, but has frequently lost control since then. At this evaluation she weighed about 30% above her ideal weight, was on 52 units of insulin daily, but neither kept regular mealtimes nor tested her blood or urine. Results of recent random blood-sugar determinations were abnormally high. Significant diabetic retinopathy had developed, compelling her to use a magnifying glass for reading. She had mild hypertension without apparent diabetic kidney disease and took one diuretic tablet daily.

The patient had done poorly in high school and had gone to business school for 4 years but had failed to graduate. She had had some hope of a romantic relationship, but never had a steady boyfriend. She lives at home with her mother and has no close friends outside her family. On close questioning, it became apparent that the onset of the sleep problems and the beginning of the most recent period of depression had coincided.

The patient's family history revealed that one of her five siblings took a nap each afternoon and slept 7 hours nightly. Otherwise, there was no history of Sleep Disorder, diabetes, or treatment for depression in the patient's family.

As the patient described her problem to the psychiatrist, she gazed continually downward and conversed in a low monotone. She answered questions dutifully, but without elaboration. She shed copious tears.

The patient was admitted to the hospital for studies. Nursing observations documented that the patient slept 12–15 hours daily. She was much impaired in tests of vigilance, which involved her pushing a button whenever the letter "X" appeared in a series of letters visually presented at one per second; she averaged 4% correct responses during two trials, compared with a normal score of 66%–78%. She had an average multiple sleep latency (i.e., onset of sleep after lights out) of 8.5 minutes during four polygraphically recorded daytime naps, a result consistent with only mild sleepiness. Nocturnal sleep monitoring revealed an abnormally short REM latency of 2 minutes and an abnormal increase (42%) in the amount of REM sleep. The nocturnal sleep monitoring revealed no other abnormality. The patient had only 2% wakefulness, much less than expected in a prolonged recording; this was consistent with her daytime sleepiness. She continued to sleep for 9½ hours, until she had to be awakened so the laboratory could be used for daytime purposes.

Discussion of "Cry Me a River"

Although this patient experiences recurrent periods of depression, her predominant complaints are of excessive daytime sleepiness (falls asleep on buses, remains in bed all day on weekends) and prolonged transition to the fully awake state (feels groggy and "out of it" on awakening). The sleep laboratory findings (prolonged sleep, impaired vigilance, short rapid eye movement [REM] latency, increased REM activity) confirm her complaints of hypersomnia.

In this case there is no evidence that the hypersomnia is better accounted for by insomnia or that it occurs exclusively during the course of another sleep disorder (e.g., Narcolepsy, Breathing-Related Sleep Disorder) or that it is the result of the direct physiological effects of a general medical condition or substance use. The magnitude of her excessive sleepiness is compatible with that seen in Primary Hypersomnia. However, because the onset of her sleep disturbance seems to have coincided with the most recent recurrence of her depression, it seems reasonable to conclude that the hypersomnia is related to the Mood Disorder. Therefore, the principal diagnosis is Hypersomnia Related to Major Depressive Disorder (DSM-IV-TR, p. 650). The recurrent episodes of depression warrant the additional Axis I diagnosis of Major Depressive Disorder, Recurrent (DSM-IV-TR, p. 376).

The reason a separate diagnosis is given for the sleep disturbance caused by the Mood Disorder is that the hypersomnia is the predominant complaint and is sufficiently severe to warrant independent clinical attention. Otherwise, it would be considered merely a symptom of the Major Depressive Disorder and would not require a separate diagnosis.

PERPETUAL PATIENT

In 1945, at the age of 18, the patient became apprehensive about leaving home to go to an out-of-state college for her freshman year. One day in September, while with her mother shopping for college clothes, she began to have episodes in which she would stop walking and become stiff for a few moments without explanation, then proceed to talk and act appropriately. The next day she became more silent. Sometimes she made inappropriate remarks, but at other times she acted and talked quite normally. Silences, refusal to eat, and inappropriate comments such as "Daddy, kill me" precipitated a consultation, and then hospitalization, almost on the day that the patient was to have been admitted to college.

In the early days of hospitalization, the patient vaguely suggested that she might be having auditory hallucinations and at times gave "confused" or silly answers that were out of keeping with her 121 IQ score on psychological testing. When by herself, she would write coherent letters and short stories that were regarded as publishable. Partly because of the "lack of progress" and the bizarreness of her behavior at times, she was diagnosed as having Catatonic Dementia Praecox.

Early in her hospitalization the patient received individual psychotherapy four times a week. She continued to receive psychotherapy in and out of the institution, with a series of nine therapists, for the next 20 years. From the beginning of her hospitalization, she was frequently negativistic, precipitated physical fights, mutilated herself in many minor ways, and self-induced vomiting. These behaviors contributed to her receiving a great deal of attention in a public institution with limited staff. She stated that she wanted to try every form of therapy there was, "even lobotomy," and her wishes were carried out, except for the lobotomy. She received a dozen electroconvulsive treatments, four dozen insulin subcoma treatments, dance therapy, occupational therapy, recreational therapy, psychodrama (loved it), group psychotherapy, and art therapy, in addition to individual psychotherapy and lots of attention from ministers and priests.

After the first 3 stormy years of her hospitalization, the patient was transferred to the care of a woman psychiatrist, became much calmer, registered at a local university, and did well at her studies. Nevertheless, "hysterical" vomiting, violence, and other bizarre acts would take place whenever discharge from the institution was mentioned. In 2 more years, working primarily with women therapists, she held a job and acted ap-

propriately and eventually accepted discharge to a female psychotherapist as "recovered" at age 24.

One evening, after 6 uneventful years and satisfactory occupational
functioning, the patient appeared at the hospital, distraught at being unable to reach her therapist by phone, and asked to be readmitted. She
was admitted despite the difficulties in determining the genuineness of
her behavior and of her statements about suicide and "confusion." A series of many forms of psychotherapies, including individual psychotherapy, commenced immediately and lasted nearly a decade.

When the patient was 40, a change in the approach to her evaluation
and treatment was initiated when it was decided that she had a "hysterical personality." For the next 5 years, a series of efforts to place her in the
community was blocked by negativism, threats, minor self-mutilations, self-
induced vomiting, occasional inappropriate comments, and other attention-
getting behavior, none of which was "rewarded," however, with individual therapy, psychodrama, and so on. Eventually, when she was in her
mid-40s, she was discharged, despite complaints that she was not ready.
When told that the discharge was being carried out over her objections,
the patient vomited; but the therapist stated that she would be discharged nevertheless. She pulled down her pants and defecated in the
office, but was still discharged. In the decade since she was discharged,
she has continued to function outside the institution, usually with the
support of a boarding home.

Discussion of "Perpetual Patient"

This woman was able to engage the attention of countless dedi-
cated mental health professionals over many years. Her remarkable
illness persisted despite a trial of nearly every known treatment.
The pattern of her symptoms, from the start, did not correspond to
any recognizable illness, and she seemed able to produce them at
will (e.g., defecation in public when her discharge was imminent).
Over the years her behavior seems to have been designed to achieve
one goal: continuing to be treated as a psychiatric patient.

In the past such a case might have been called Hysteria because
of the exaggerated, self-dramatizing nature of the symptoms. These
histrionic features were also noted by the hospital personnel who took

care of this patient. In DSM-IV (and DSM-IV-TR) the intentional production of psychological symptoms for the purpose of assuming the
patient role (and the absence of external incentives for the behavior,
as in Malingering) is called Factitious Disorder With Predominantly
Psychological Signs and Symptoms (DSM-IV-TR, p. 517).

In addition to the factitious production of symptoms, this woman's long-term functioning is characterized by excessive emotional-
ity and attention-seeking; in her relationships with people she is
vain, demanding, and dependent. These features suggest the additional diagnosis of Histrionic Personality Disorder. However, there is
insufficient information about other symptoms of the disorder, such
as inappropriate seductiveness and consistent use of physical appearance to attract attention. We therefore would add the diagnosis
of Personality Disorder Not Otherwise Specified (with histrionic
features) (DSM-IV-TR, p. 729).

I AM VISHNU

Mr. Nehru is a single, unemployed 32-year-old man who migrated from
India to the United States when he was age 13. His brother brought him to
the emergency room of an Atlanta, Georgia, hospital after neighbors complained that he was standing in the street harassing people about his religious beliefs. To the psychiatrist he keeps repeating, "I am Vishnu. I am
Krishna."

Mr. Nehru has been living with his brother and sister-in-law for the
past 7 months, attending an outpatient clinic. During the last 4 weeks, his
behavior has become increasingly disruptive. He awakens his brother at
all hours of the night to discuss religious matters. He often seems to be
responding to voices that only he hears. He neither bathes nor changes
his clothes.

Mr. Nehru's first episode of emotional disturbance was 5 years ago.
Medical records are not available, but from the brother's account, it
seems to have been similar to the present episode. There have been two
other similar episodes, each requiring hospitalization for a few months.
Mr. Nehru admits that, starting about 5 years ago and virtually continuously since then, he has been troubled by "voices" that he hears throughout the day. There are several voices, which comment on his behavior
and discuss him in the third person. They usually are either benign ("Look

at him now. He is about to eat.") or insulting in content ("What a fool he is. He doesn't understand anything!").

Between episodes, according to both his outpatient psychiatrist and his brother, Mr. Nehru is a quiet, somewhat withdrawn person, but popular in his neighborhood because he helps some of his elderly neighbors with shopping and yard work. At these times his mood is unremarkable. However, he claims that, because of the "voices," he cannot concentrate sufficiently to hold a job. He sometimes reads books, but watches little TV, because he hears the voices coming out of the TV and is upset that the TV shows often refer to him.

For the past 6 weeks, with increasing insistence, the voices have been telling Mr. Nehru that he is the new Messiah, Jesus, Moses, Vishnu, and Krishna, and should begin a new religious epoch in human history. He has begun to experience surges of increased energy, "so I could spread my gospel," and needs very little sleep. According to his brother, he has become more preoccupied with the voices and disorganized in his daily activities.

When interviewed, Mr. Nehru is euphoric and his speech is rapid and hard to follow. He paces up and down the ward and, upon seeing a doctor, grabs his arm, puts his face within 2 inches of the doctor's, and talks with great rapidity and enthusiasm about his religious "insights." In the middle of a speech on his new religion, he abruptly compliments the doctor on how well his shirt and tie match. When limits are placed on his behavior, he becomes loud and angry. In addition to his belief that he is the Messiah, he feels that the hospital is part of a conspiracy to suppress his religious message. Although he seems to enjoy his "voices," he sometimes complains about them and makes references to "those damned voices." He states that he feels that his religious insights, euphoria, and energy have been put into him by God.

Discussion of "I Am Vishnu"

Mr. Nehru has a chronic illness characterized by prominent hallucinations that are so intrusive that he cannot concentrate enough to be able to work. These hallucinations seem to have been persistently present since his illness began 5 years ago. In addition, there have been four episodes (including the current one) with symptoms that fulfill the criteria for a Manic Episode: he is euphoric, grandiose, and irritable and has pressured speech and increased energy.

If we did not know that between these Manic Episodes Mr. Nehru is continuously hearing voices, we would have no trouble in making the diagnosis of Bipolar I Disorder. However, the diagnosis of Bipolar I Disorder excludes cases in which there are delusions or hallucinations for as long as 2 weeks in the absence of prominent mood symptoms. Thus, the continuous voices during the times when Mr. Nehru is not manic rule out the diagnosis of Bipolar I Disorder.

If we were diagnosing Mr. Nehru's condition between these episodes, we would note that the prominent hallucinations, with no apparent relation to depression or elation, fulfill the symptomatic criteria for Schizophrenia. We would then have to consider the differential diagnosis between Schizophrenia with a superimposed Bipolar Disorder Not Otherwise Specified and Schizoaffective Disorder. The key question for the diagnosis of Schizophrenia is whether the total duration of all of the episodes of a mood syndrome (in his case, Manic Episodes) has been brief relative to the total duration of the whole illness. We do not know exactly how long each of Mr. Nehru's Manic Episodes lasted, but it is unlikely that the total time is more than 6 months, compared with the 5 years' total duration of the psychotic illness. Is this brief? Because DSM-IV-TR does not provide more precise guidelines, we are inclined to give more weight to the prominent manic symptoms that seem to have been present with each exacerbation of his psychotic illness. We therefore provisionally diagnose Schizoaffective Disorder, Bipolar Type (DSM-IV-TR, p. 323) and note the need to rule out Schizophrenia.

AGITATED BUSINESSMAN

This agitated 42-year-old businessman was admitted to the psychiatric service after a 2½-month period in which he found himself becoming increasingly distrustful of others and suspicious of his business associates. He was taking their statements out of context, "twisting" their words, and making inappropriately hostile and accusatory comments; he had, in fact, lost several business deals that had been "virtually sealed." Finally, the patient fired a shotgun into his backyard late one night when he heard noises that convinced him that intruders were about to break into his house and kill him.

One and one-half years previously, the patient had been diagnosed as having Narcolepsy because of daily irresistible sleep attacks and episodes of sudden loss of muscle tone when he became emotionally excited, and had been placed on an amphetaminelike stimulant, methylphenidate. He became asymptomatic and was able to work quite effectively as the sales manager of a small office-machine company and to participate in an active social life with his family and a small circle of friends.

In the 4 months before admission, the patient had been using increasingly large doses of methylphenidate to maintain alertness late at night because of an increasing amount of work that could not be handled during the day. He reported that during this time he often could feel his heart race and had trouble sitting still.

Discussion of "Agitated Businessman"

The primary symptoms are palpitations, psychomotor agitation, hypervigilance, paranoid ideation about his co-workers, and delusions of reference (the patient acted on his belief that noises indicated the presence of intruders who were about to kill him). The presence of psychotic symptoms during these periods of drug-induced intoxication and the absence of any evidence of a preexisting psychotic disorder indicate Methylphenidate-Induced Psychotic Disorder (DSM-IV-TR, p. 342). Because the clinical picture is dominated by delusions rather than hallucinations, With Delusions is noted. Had there not been any psychotic symptoms, and had the patient sought help for the other symptoms, such as hypervigilance and psychomotor agitation, the diagnosis would have been the residual category Methylphenidate Intoxication (DSM-IV-TR, p. 227).

Narcolepsy (DSM-IV-TR, p. 615), although traditionally considered a neurologic disorder, is a sleep disorder in DSM-IV (and DSM-IV-TR) and is noted on Axis I.

I Could Be Dying

Bill Ainsworth awoke in the middle of the night gasping for breath, sweating, shaking, and experiencing palpitations. He felt his pulse; it was 120. He thought, "I could be dying." It was his third attack of the week and at least his tenth that month that had awakened him from sleep. The problem, which had begun 2 years previously when he turned 50, was getting much worse: not only was he having trouble staying asleep because of similar attacks, but after such nights he felt tired all day. He decided to take a friend's advice and seek help from a psychiatrist who specialized in sleep problems.

The psychiatrist elicited this additional history. Attacks of panic occurring during the day had begun at age 12 and had recurred every few months since that time. They did not begin to occur during sleep until the patient turned age 50, 2 years earlier. A few months ago the attacks had become much rarer, after the patient had discontinued drinking the 8 to 10 beers he had drunk every weekend for most of his adult life. His weight had fallen from 227 pounds to a mildly overweight 181 pounds, and the mild hypertension he had had for several years disappeared.

In addition to the recurrent attacks, for most of his life the patient had also felt anxious in anticipation of particular situations, including being shut inside airplanes or elevators or traveling in the middle lane of a road. On a turnpike he counted the exits until he could leave, fearing that he would have a panic attack.

He described a fear of falling apart if he ever got too far from his "support system," his term for a beer cooler, which he carried with him always, although he rarely drank the beer. In anticipation of an airplane flight, however, he would drink six to eight beers. He almost always had a company employee, his son, or a friend accompany him, and particularly disliked plane flights when he was not with a familiar person. The night after he drank, the anxiety attacks almost always occurred, awakening him from sleep.

Mr. Ainsworth ran a successful auto parts business and consulted for several others. Recently, however, anxiety had prevented his accepting a huge government contract to set up an international distribution system for retail stores on military bases. He felt he would be too exposed to scrutiny and would therefore fail. He also worried that some long plane rides would be unavoidable.

During the interview Mr. Ainsworth was highly verbal, informative, cheerful, friendly, and engaging. He talked about uncomfortable subjects frankly and productively. He had two sisters and two daughters who had "agoraphobia"; one of the daughters was housebound.

Initially, the patient was thought to have sleep apnea (recurrent periods of not breathing during sleep), on the basis of the loud snoring that he reported and the awakening provoked by drinking alcohol, relieved by weight loss, and the presence of mild hypertension. (These symptoms are commonly seen in sleep apnea and are presumably related to the pulmonary hypertension that develops from insufficient breathing and oxygen desaturation. No evidence for this emerged from results of sleep laboratory recording, upper airway examination, or daytime vigilance testing.)

Discussion of "I Could Be Dying"

Although this patient's chief complaint is difficulty staying asleep, it is clear that what keeps waking him up are recurrent panic attacks. He wakes up with typical symptoms of panic attacks: the abrupt onset of difficulty breathing, sweating, shaking, rapid heartbeat, and palpitations. The diagnosis of Panic Disorder is made in this case because there are recurrent, unexpected panic attacks with at least four of the characteristic symptoms and concern about the consequences of the attacks (i.e., fear of dying from the attacks).

People with Panic Disorder frequently avoid places or situations from which escape might be difficult or embarrassing or in which help might not be available in the event of having a panic attack (Agoraphobia). This man's history is unusual in that he apparently avoided situations in which he anticipated feeling anxious even before he identified the adult onset of panic attacks. In any case, he currently avoids many of those situations because of fears of having a panic attack. Therefore, the diagnosis of Panic Disorder With Agoraphobia is made (DSM-IV-TR, p. 441).

This case is unusual from two perspectives. First, it is unusual for patients with Panic Disorder to have panic attacks at night. Second, insomnia is rarely caused by panic attacks that awaken the patient. When, as in this case, persistent insomnia is the predominant symptom requiring independent clinical attention and causes day-time fatigue and distress or impairment in functioning, the additional diagnosis of a Sleep Disorder is made. We would therefore also note Insomnia Related to Panic Disorder With Agoraphobia (DSM-IV-TR, p. 650).

Follow-Up

The Panic Disorder With Agoraphobia was treated with a short-acting benzodiazepine. His panic attacks disappeared, and his sleep returned to normal.

SOMETHING HAPPENED

A 25-year-old woman was admitted to a psychiatric unit after being brought to the emergency ward by police officers. She reported that she had been shopping in an exclusive boutique when "something happened." She said that she had no recollection of events between that time and an hour later, when she was arrested for shoplifting in a nearby department store. She protested her innocence and became so agitated, belligerent, and profane that the arresting officers took her to the hospital. At the hospital she reported that 2 years previously she had been arrested for shoplifting and had had amnesia for the act. The charges against her were then dropped because she explained that both the shoplifting and the amnesia resulted from her forgetting to eat after taking her insulin. However, her blood-sugar level on testing in the emergency ward was actually elevated.

The patient rapidly calmed down after admission and appeared asymptomatic for 2 days. When she learned that her discharge was planned for the next day and that the charges against her would not be dropped, she became extremely agitated, angry, and abusive to the staff. Shortly thereafter, she complained of a headache and said she had no recollection of her abusive behavior. Later that evening she accosted a nurse angrily. When the nurse responded and addressed the patient by name, "Elaine," the patient said that her name was "Leslie" and that she would not allow herself to be called "Elaine," whom she described as a "wimp and a loser."

"Leslie's" voice and movement were somewhat different from those of "Elaine." She claimed that she had done the shoplifting and stepped back so that "Elaine" could be caught and humiliated, and that if she had wanted to, she could have evaded detection easily. For the next 2 days, the patient had many apparent switches of personality, accompanied by conspicuous changes in dress, makeup, and deportment. On several occasions "Leslie" was disruptive, and twice "Elaine" reported to nurses that she had found things belonging to other patients in her possession.

There were no consistent differences in blood-sugar levels in the different personalities or changes at the time of the shifts. A neurological workup with extensive electroencephalographic studies proved unremarkable. The patient began to complain that her behavior was out of her control and that she could not be held accountable for it. Each day's progress notes revealed further details of the differences between "Elaine" and "Leslie."

A consultant with considerable experience with Dissociative Identity Disorder (Multiple Personality Disorder) was asked to see the patient. He observed the presence of both "Elaine" and "Leslie" and documented their polarized and clear-cut differences. The personalities were detailed and elaborate as they discussed issues relating to the patient's current legal difficulties. He learned that the patient had an extensive history of discrepant behaviors that she had "forgotten," to which many witnesses would attest, and that her family often remarked that she was "like two different people." He found that these episodes had usually occurred when the patient had engaged in behavior that brought adverse personal consequences upon her. He noted that the patient was on a unit that, by coincidence, had three other patients with that diagnosis and that, beginning the day the patient learned that the charges against her would not be dropped, she had begun to associate with those patients. He learned that she was aware of a case in which the consultant had appeared as a defense witness for a man with Dissociative Identity Disorder arrested under similar circumstances.

An extensive history, taken over several days, and ancillary sources failed to reveal the typical childhood history of a patient with Dissociative Identity Disorder; that is, there was no indication that the patient had experienced child abuse or any other overwhelming traumatic events. Furthermore, the history indicated that the patient, despite the apparently classic nature of her two personalities, had never shown or complained of the wide variety of symptoms suggestive of other mental disorders that is characteristic of Dissociative Identity Disorder and often delays recognition of the diagnosis.

The interviewer also noted that the "Elaine" he was interviewing was somewhat different from the "Elaine" with whom her family and friends were familiar. The usual "Elaine" was pleasant and mild-mannered unless "crossed," at which times she became angry and bellicose: she was not unfailingly mild and good. He also found that the patient was not very hypnotizable, which is quite unusual in patients with Dissociative Identity Disorder. He undertook a prolonged interview in which he covered a wide range of topics over several hours. As the interview proceeded, "Leslie," who was completely consistent in her presentation during her discussion of matters related to the shoplifting and disruptive events on the ward, began to become inconsistent in her voice and manner. She complained that the consultant disbelieved her and was trying to "trick" her. As "Leslie" seemed unable to maintain her presentation, "Elaine" vehemently reproached the consultant for doubting the account offered by "Leslie," for whose past behaviors and current interactions with the consultant she had consistently maintained she had amnesia. At these angry moments her behavior was indistinguishable from "Leslie's." After another hour's interviewing, during which the patient made several efforts to convince the consultant that she had Dissociative Identity Disorder, she ceased to display behaviors typical of the disorder.

Discussion of "Something Happened"

The psychiatrist who consulted on this case provided the following discussion:

> This case illustrates that distinguishing Dissociative Identity Disorder from Malingering can be difficult. Patients with true Dissociative Identity Disorder often do not have the stereotypical features of the disorder, such as polarization of the personalities and clear boundaries and amnestic barriers between and among them. Elaine demonstrates that it is easy to mimic classic Dissociative Identity Disorder behaviors around a unified theme for circumscribed bits of time, but exceedingly difficult to simulate the full spectrum of symptoms in a wide range of contexts over a long period of time.
>
> People motivated to represent themselves as having Dissociative Identity Disorder in order to achieve an understandable

goal (in Elaine's case, to have the authorities drop charges against her) generally draw upon lay sources of information and stress those aspects of the disorder that are obvious and can be made public and be used as "evidence" for the reality of the condition. Usually this is the dramatization of a small number of polarized "personalities" related to the issue that has prompted the evaluation.

Anticipating (correctly) that Elaine could mobilize herself to offer a convincing portrayal of "personalities" with regard to the shoplifting offense, the consultant focused on exploring the presence or absence of the plethora of associated features of the disorder, such as high hypnotizability, relative consistency of the different "personalities," history of the "personalities" before the current difficulties, and a history of being abused in childhood. Elaine had none of these characteristics, and her pathological behavior invariably occurred in situations in which she sought to escape the consequences of illegal or inappropriate actions. She dramatized the manifestations of the "personalities" to create a public record of their behaviors. The consultant became increasingly convinced that she was Malingering (DSM-IV-TR, p. 739).

The consultant considered the likelihood of Antisocial Personality Disorder or Borderline Personality Disorder. He documented strong evidence suggesting both of these conditions, but noted that Elaine, in her efforts to represent herself as a good person intruded upon by "Leslie," minimized her personality difficulties. Therefore, although he suspected that either or both personality disorders might be present, there was insufficient information to document either of them.

Follow-Up

Elaine was placed on probation and never again showed signs of having more than one personality. On one occasion she deliberately manipulated her blood sugar to create the alibi of hypoglycemia for a shoplifting episode that she realized had been observed, but she was unable to escape the consequences of her actions and has not shoplifted again.

Subsequent psychotherapists have made the diagnosis of Borderline Personality Disorder and have been divided as to whether Elaine merited the additional diagnosis of Antisocial Personality Disorder. There has, however, been increasing stability in her life, and she has been steadily employed for the past 3 years.

THE WORKAHOLIC

The patient is a 45-year-old lawyer who seeks treatment at his wife's insistence. She is fed up with their marriage; she can no longer tolerate his emotional coldness, rigid demands, bullying behavior, sexual disinterest, long work hours, and frequent business trips. The patient feels no particular distress in his marriage and has agreed to the consultation only to humor his wife.

It soon develops, however, that the patient is troubled by problems at work. He is known as the hardest-driving member of a hard-driving law firm. He was the youngest full partner in the firm's history and is famous for being able to handle many cases at the same time. Lately, he finds himself increasingly unable to keep up. He is too proud to turn down a new case and too much of a perfectionist to be satisfied with the quality of work performed by his assistants. Displeased by their writing style and sentence structure, he finds himself constantly correcting their briefs and therefore unable to stay abreast of his schedule. People at work complain that his attention to details and inability to delegate responsibility are reducing his efficiency. He has had two or three secretaries a year for 15 years. No one can tolerate working for him for very long because he is so critical of any mistakes made by others. When assignments get backed up, he cannot decide which to address first, starts making schedules for himself and his staff, but then is unable to meet them and works 15 hours a day. He finds it difficult to be decisive now that his work has expanded beyond his own direct control.

The patient discusses his children as if they were mechanical dolls, but also with a clear underlying affection. He describes his wife as a "suitable mate" and has trouble understanding why she is dissatisfied. He is punctilious in his manners and dress and slow and ponderous in his speech, dry and humorless, with a stubborn determination to get his point across.

The patient is the son of two upwardly mobile, extremely hard-working parents. He grew up feeling that he was never working hard enough, that he had much to achieve and very little time. He was a superior student, a "bookworm," awkward and unpopular in adolescent social pursuits. He has always been competitive and a high achiever. He has trouble relaxing on vacations, develops elaborate activity schedules for every family member, and becomes impatient and furious if they refuse to follow his plans. He likes sports but has little time for them and refuses to play if he can't be at the top of his form. He is a ferocious competitor on the tennis courts and a poor loser.

Discussion of "The Workaholic"

Although the marital problem is the entry ticket, it is clear that this fellow has many personality traits that are quite maladaptive. He is cold, rigid, excessively perfectionistic, and preoccupied with details. He is indecisive but insists that others do things his way; his interpersonal relationships suffer because of his excessive devotion to work. These are the characteristic features of Obsessive-Compulsive Personality Disorder (DSM-IV-TR, p. 729).

Follow-Up

The patient has been seen by a psychotherapist off and on for several years. He usually has come back into treatment when there was a crisis at work or at home and dropped out after the crisis was resolved. He has made considerable progress in learning how to play (e.g., he now plays squash) and has bought a vacation home, where he spends frequent weekends. His relationships with his wife and children have improved, and he is generally happier and more relaxed. Moreover, he has been extremely successful at work and has made a great deal of money.

THE OUTDOORSMAN

A 78-year-old, retired lumber-company president sought help for the onset of a series of attacks in which he experienced marked apprehension, restlessness, and the need to be outdoors to relieve his sense of discomfort. He described the most recent event as having occurred at 3:00 A.M. a week earlier: he awoke from sleep and felt "the walls were caving in" on him. He denied that this was related to dreaming and said that he was fully awake at the time. He arose, dressed, and went outside in subzero weather; once outside, he noted gradual improvement (but not full resolution) of his symptoms. Complete resolution took a full day.

In response to pointed questioning, the patient denied dyspnea, palpitations, choking sensations, paresthesias, or nausea. He reported trembling and some sweating, together with intermittent dizziness. He imagined that he would die (or lose consciousness) if he could not "escape" from his house. He spoke of a need "to be active."

On questioning, the patient recalled a similar series of attacks almost 30 years earlier following eye surgery for an injury. He described bilateral patching of his eyes and being confined to bed for days, with his head sandbagged to preclude movement. Once ambulatory, he had experienced these attacks for more than a year.

The patient denied recent sleep dysfunction, change in appetite or weight, crying spells, or decreased energy. He had been taking diazepam for approximately 2 months for feelings of increased nervousness and tension. He had noted mild memory problems of late.

Further inquiry established a problem with balance and intermittent pain in the right arm, and a complaint of indigestion and intermittent diarrhea. The patient had stopped gardening the past summer because of his balance problem. On examination he was found to have a "beefy" red tongue (which he said was painful), difficulty with tandem gait and rapid alternating motion, and a mild intention tremor. He denied urinary incontinence.

Laboratory studies revealed a macrocytic anemia and vitamin B_{12} deficiency. The patient was given B_{12} replacement, and his attacks did not recur.

Discussion of "The Outdoorsman"

This patient describes fairly typical, unexpected panic attacks, suggesting a diagnosis of Panic Disorder. However, careful physical examination and laboratory findings indicate the characteristic features of vitamin B_{12} deficiency caused by pernicious anemia, an acquired vitamin B_{12} malabsorption syndrome. Because the panic attacks disappeared with treatment of the vitamin deficiency, it is reasonable to assume that the correct diagnosis is Anxiety Disorder Due to Pernicious Anemia, With Panic Attacks (DSM-IV-TR, p. 479).

What is puzzling is the history of similar episodes of panic many years ago. In the absence of any known general medical condition or substance causing the panic attacks, at that time we assume that he had Panic Disorder. The current Anxiety Disorder Due to Pernicious Anemia may be a manifestation of an underlying vulnerability to panic attacks.

SUPPLY SERGEANT[*]

The patient, an African American man, was a supply sergeant in the military during the late 1950s. He was caught by the military police stealing a deodorant stick from the post exchange. The army, which had reason to suspect the sergeant of other thefts and was undeterred by constitutional restraints on search and seizure, went to his home and reclaimed every piece of army property the sergeant could not account for. The pile of supplies—uniforms, blankets, picks and shovels, cartons of canned goods, mess kits, and so on—could have filled a trailer truck. It was all photographed on the sergeant's front lawn, and that photo became part of his army medical file.

The army was determined to court-martial the sergeant; but he had been examined by a civilian psychiatrist, who decided that much of what was stolen was of no use to the sergeant and, on the basis of an understanding of the sergeant's psychodynamics, had diagnosed him as having Kleptomania. This civilian psychiatrist was prepared to testify at a court-martial that the stealing resulted from unconscious and irresistible impulses. Unhappy with the civilian psychiatrist's report, the army sent this man to be evaluated at an army hospital. There he was told repeatedly that anything he said could be used against him at the court-martial. The sergeant took the warning rather impassively, and the army psychiatrist set to work gathering a detailed history.

---

[*]From Stone A: "Conceptual Ambiguity and Morality in Modern Psychiatry." *Am J Psychiatry* 137:887–894, 1980.

The sergeant, a very intelligent man, got caught up in telling the story of his life. He had grown up in a southern city during the days of racial segregation. A good and serious student from a deeply religious family, he had done well in school and had gone on to a small college, where he had studied literature. After graduation, despite his hopes and dreams, he had found no appropriate work and eventually was drafted during the Korean War. After the war, seeing no alternatives, he became increasingly bitter. He was convinced that life had cheated him because he was black and that the army, in the work and position it gave him, continued to discriminate against him. Out of this sense of being cheated grew a sense of entitlement, and he came to feel that he was justified in taking whatever he could, whenever he could. He had no sense of being impulsively driven to steal army property; instead, he stole with a sense of entitlement and reparation in protest against the racist world that had deprived him of his hopes.

It is not clear why, despite being warned, the sergeant told all this to the army psychiatrist. At any rate, he did; and the army psychiatrist, after puzzling over the diagnostic possibilities, which included Paranoid Personality and Depression, concluded that the sergeant did not have Kleptomania or any other mental disorder that might excuse him from responsibility. Subsequently, the army psychiatrist, trying to avoid the sergeant's eyes, testified to this at the court-martial. The sergeant sat there in his dress uniform with his medals, his wife, and their small children. He was sentenced to 5 years at hard labor.

Discussion of "Supply Sergeant"

This poignant case illustrates that not all maladaptive behavior is adequately accounted for by the disorders that are included in standard classifications of mental illness. Although stealing by an adult may occur in many disorders (e.g., Schizophrenia, Dementia, Bipolar Disorder), there are only two in which it is likely to be the predominant symptom: Antisocial Personality Disorder and Kleptomania.

The civilian psychiatrist attempted to make a case for the diagnosis of Kleptomania. The army psychiatrist had no difficulty in demonstrating the absence of the characteristic signs of the disorder: Kleptomania is an Impulse-Control Disorder in which the stealing represents a failure to resist an impulse; generally it is preceded by an increasing sense of tension and is followed by the experience of pleasure or release. In this case the sergeant "had no sense of being impulsively driven to steal army property; instead, he stole with a sense of entitlement and reparation in protest against the racist world that had deprived him of his hopes." A diagnosis of Antisocial Personality Disorder would make no sense in view of the absence of any childhood history of antisocial behavior, the sergeant's good work and family functioning in adulthood, and the lack of a pervasive pattern of adult antisocial behavior.

There is a suggestion that this man stole some things that he did not need and that the extent of his stealing probably invited his being caught. In addition, once caught, he made no attempt to protect himself either by distorting his story to lend credence to the diagnosis of Kleptomania or by refusing to cooperate with the army psychiatrist. All this indicates a self-destructive, and therefore maladaptive, aspect of his behavior.

Does the maladaptive nature of his behavior indicate a mental disorder—albeit unspecified—as it does not correspond to any of the specific mental disorders included in the DSM-IV-TR classification? To classify it as such would so broaden the concept of mental disorder that virtually all criminal acts (murder, rape, grand larceny) could be interpreted as symptoms of mental disorder. There is no doubt that careful psychological study of any person who has engaged in a criminal act would reveal the psychological origins of the maladaptive behavior—in this case, the sergeant's sense of entitlement as a reaction to his life in a racist society.

DSM-IV-TR does provide a code for indicating that antisocial behavior in an adult is the focus of attention, but does not result from a mental disorder—the V code Adult Antisocial Behavior (DSM-IV-TR, p. 740).

THREATENING VOICES

A 44-year-old unemployed man who lived alone in a single-room-occupancy hotel was brought to the emergency room by police, to whom he had gone for help, complaining that he was frightened by hearing voices of men in the street below his window talking about him and threatening him with harm. When he looked out the window, the men had always "disappeared."

The patient had a 20-year history of almost daily alcohol use, was commonly "drunk" each day, and often had experienced the "shakes" on awakening. On the previous day he had reduced his intake to 1 pint of vodka because of gastrointestinal distress. He was fully alert and oriented on mental status examination.

Discussion of "Threatening Voices"

This patient is disturbed by auditory hallucinations and he experiences the voices as real. Vivid auditory hallucinations with impaired reality testing that develop shortly after the reduction in heavy ingestion of alcohol in a person who apparently has Alcohol Dependence indicate Alcohol-Induced Psychotic Disorder With Hallucinations (DSM-IV-TR, p. 342). Because the onset is during withdrawal, we would note With Onset During Withdrawal. Alcohol-Induced Psychotic Disorder With Onset During Withdrawal is distinguished from Alcohol Withdrawal Delirium by the absence of a disturbance in attention.

The additional diagnosis of Alcohol Dependence (DSM-IV-TR, p. 213) is made because of a long pattern of daily heavy alcohol use, inability to work because of alcohol use, and frequent withdrawal symptoms (experiencing morning "shakes"). Alcohol Psychotic Disorder With Hallucinations apparently develops only in people with a long history of Alcohol Dependence.

BRUISED

A 25-year-old female graduate student asked for a consultation because of depression and marital discord. The patient had been married for 5 years, during which time both she and her husband were in school. For the past 3 years, her academic performance had been consistently better than his, and she attributed their frequent, intense arguments to this. She noted that she experienced a feeling of sexual excitement when her husband screamed at her or hit her in a rage. Sometimes she would taunt him until he had sexual intercourse with her in a brutal fashion, as if she were being raped. She experienced the brutality and sense of being punished as sexually exciting.

One year before the consultation, the patient had found herself often ending arguments by storming out of the house. On one such occasion she went to a "singles' bar," picked up a man, and got him to slap her as part of their sexual activity. She found the "punishment" sexually exciting and subsequently fantasized about being beaten during masturbation to orgasm. The patient then discovered that she enjoyed receiving physical punishment at the hands of strange men more than any other type of sexual stimulus. In a setting in which she could be whipped or beaten, all aspects of sexual activity, including the quality of orgasms, were far in excess of anything she had previously experienced.

This sexual preference was not the reason for the consultation, however. She complained that she could not live without her husband, yet could not live with him. She had suicidal fantasies stemming from the fear that he would leave her.

She recognized that her sexual behavior was dangerous to herself and felt mildly ashamed of it. She was unaware of any possible reasons for its emergence and was not sure she wished treatment for "it," because it gave her so much pleasure.

Discussion of "Bruised"

Fantasies of being humiliated, beaten, bound, or otherwise made to suffer may increase sexual excitement for some people whose sexual life is in all other respects unremarkable. However, when sexually arousing fantasies of this kind are acted out in a way that is dangerous (as in this case), or if the fantasies are markedly distressing, the diagnosis of Sexual Masochism (DSM-IV-TR, p. 573) is made.

With the limited information available, it is not possible to determine if this patient's marital problem is primarily 1) a symptom of the Sexual Masochism (e.g., does she provoke arguments in order to be sexually aroused?); 2) a symptom of a Personality Disorder; or 3) a problem unrelated to a mental disorder for which the V code Partner Relational Problem would be appropriate.

COFFEE BREAK

A 35-year-old secretary sought consultation for "anxiety attacks." A thorough history revealed that the attacks occurred in mid- to late afternoon, when she became restless, nervous, and easily excited and sometimes was noted to be flushed, sweating, and, according to co-workers, "talking a mile a minute." In response to careful questioning, she acknowledged drinking five or six cups of coffee each day before the time the attacks usually occurred.

Discussion of "Coffee Break"

The temporal association of heavy coffee drinking and the anxiety symptoms indicates the etiological significance of caffeine. In the literature this has been referred to as Caffeinism. In DSM-IV-TR, Caffeine Intoxication (DSM-IV-TR, p. 232) is diagnosed when symptoms such as restlessness, nervousness, flushed face, rambling speech, and excitability are present because of the effect of recent ingestion of caffeine, usually in excess of 250 mg (a single cup of coffee has 100–150 mg; tea is about half as strong; a glass of cola is about a third as strong).

Although the symptoms suggest an Anxiety Disorder, such a diagnosis is not made when the disturbance is caused by a known specific organic factor.

CAR SALESMAN

A 29-year-old car salesman was referred by his girlfriend, a psychiatric nurse, who suspected he had a Mood Disorder, even though the patient was reluctant to admit that he might be a "moody" person. According to him, since age 14 he has experienced repeated alternating cycles that he terms "good times and bad times." During a "bad" period, usually lasting 4–7 days, he oversleeps 10–14 hours daily and lacks energy, confidence, and motivation—"just vegetating," as he puts it. Often he abruptly shifts, characteristically upon waking up in the morning, to a 3-day to 4-day stretch of overconfidence, heightened social awareness, promiscuity, and sharpened thinking ("Things would flash in my mind"). At such times he indulges in alcohol to enhance the experience, but also to help him sleep. Occasionally the "good" periods last 7–10 days but culminate in irritable and hostile outbursts, which often herald the transition back to another period of "bad" days. He admits to frequent use of marijuana, which he claims helps him "adjust" to daily routines.

In school, A's and B's alternated with C's and D's, with the result that the patient was considered a bright student whose performance was mediocre overall because of "unstable motivation." As a car salesman his performance has also been uneven, with "good days" canceling out the "bad days"; yet even during his "good days," he is sometimes argumentative with customers and loses sales that appeared sure. Although considered a charming man in many social circles, he alienates friends when he is hostile and irritable. He typically accumulates social obligations during the "bad" days and takes care of them all at once on the first day of a "good" period.

Discussion of "Car Salesman"

This patient has had numerous periods during the last 2 years in which he has had some symptoms characteristic of both the depressive and the manic syndromes. Characteristics of the "good days" are overconfidence, increased activity, and poor judgment (promiscuity). These periods come perilously close to meeting the criteria for Manic Episodes, but they are not sufficiently severe to cause marked impairment in social or occupational functioning, which is required for the diagnosis of a Manic Episode. Similarly, the "bad days," characterized by oversleeping and lack of energy, confidence, and motivation, are not of sufficient severity and duration to meet the criteria for a Major Depressive Episode. Moreover, the brief cycles follow each other irregularly though chronically. Therefore, in the absence of any substance use or general medical condition that could cause the disturbance, the appropriate diagnosis is Cyclothymic Disorder (DSM-IV-TR, p. 400).

If a clear-cut Manic Episode had occurred after at least 2 years of Cyclothymic Disorder, the additional diagnosis of superimposed Bipolar I Disorder would be made. If there were a clear history of a Major Depressive Episode, then the diagnosis of Bipolar II Disorder would be made instead of Cyclothymic Disorder. The presence of

Hypomanic Episodes precludes a diagnosis of Major Depressive Disorder; the presence of a Major Depressive Episode rules out the diagnosis of Cyclothymic Disorder.

Additional diagnoses of Alcohol Abuse and Cannabis Abuse are suspected, but insufficient information is available to make them.

Follow-Up

This patient was stabilized on lithium, married the nurse, and did well for a year. He then ceased taking the lithium on his own and had several extramarital affairs that led to his separation and divorce. He was forced to seek psychiatric help upon his ex-wife's insistence that resumption of treatment with lithium be a precondition for reconciliation. When next seen, the patient was in the midst of a moderately severe Major Depressive Episode. Lithium was reinstituted. The couple remarried 3 months later, and the patient was doing reasonably well when last seen.

UNFAITHFUL WIFE

A woman in her late 40s took an overdose of drugs. When she recovered, she confided to her family doctor that during the previous 18 months, her husband had become increasingly jealous and accusatory. Recently his accusations had been totally irrational, and he was saying that she had multiple lovers, that she got out of bed at night to go to them, and that she was communicating with them by lights and mirrors. Wrong-number telephone calls were "evidence" that men were contacting her, and he believed that cars passing the house at night flashed their headlights as a signal to her. He put tape on the windows and doors, nailed doors shut, and closely measured the location of every piece of furniture. Any change resulted in a tirade about her unfaithfulness. He refused to accept any food or cigarettes from her. During this time her husband did not physically assault her, and their sexual activity remained at its usual level; but he appeared increasingly distressed and haggard and lost 15 pounds.

The wife was so wretched about her husband's behavior that she considered leaving him, but she was afraid he might become violent. She admitted her overdose was a "cry for help."

The husband was referred for psychiatric assessment and complied willingly. He gave an account similar to his wife's, but with total conviction about her infidelity. Despite his vehemence and his belief in all the various pieces of "evidence," he seemed to have some awareness that something was wrong with him. An interview with a daughter who lived at home corroborated her mother's innocence and her father's irrationality.

The marriage had been stable until the onset of this problem, although the husband had drunk heavily as a young man and sometimes assaulted his wife. His heavy drinking and violent behavior had ceased in his mid-30s, and he had generally been a good husband and provider. He had never used street drugs at any time. His wife described him as always being "pig-headed," but he was not normally unduly argumentative and had never previously evinced jealousy. He had attended school up to the seventh grade; he was probably of low-to-average intelligence. His family history included many relatives with alcoholism, but no other mental disorders.

Discussion of "Unfaithful Wife"

All of this man's difficulties stem from his unfounded belief that his wife has been unfaithful. It hardly needs to be stated that this is not a bizarre delusion. The persistence of a nonbizarre delusion of jealousy with behavior that is otherwise unremarkable, in the absence of other psychotic symptoms (e.g., prominent hallucinations, disorganized speech), a Mood Disorder, or a general medical condition that could account for the disturbance, indicates the diagnosis Delusional Disorder, Jealous Type (DSM-IV-TR, p. 329).

Follow-Up

The patient was unexpectedly agreeable to treatment and was started on an antipsychotic drug, which he continues to take 3 years later. On two occasions this drug has been withdrawn, but after 1–2 weeks he reports, "I'm beginning to get funny ideas about the wife again," and he voluntarily resumes the medication. Not long after commencing treatment with the neuroleptic, he had an episode of depression, which responded to a tricyclic antidepressant in addition to the antipsychotic. The antidepressant was subsequently withdrawn, and the depression has not recurred.

MARTIAL ARTS

John Marshall, a single, 32-year-old white man, was referred for psychiatric evaluation by juvenile court prior to termination of his parental rights for his 7-year-old son, Richard. Mr. Marshall had been involved with child protective services and in dependency and neglect proceedings for 7 years. During that time he had one charge of physical abuse of children other than his son and two charges of spouse abuse brought against him. He has had no other legal involvement.

Child protective services initially worked with Mr. and Mrs. Marshall when their son was living with them. However, by the time he was age 3, Richard was afraid of water, not toilet-trained, extremely withdrawn, unable to play, and had bilateral optic nerve damage, which was thought to be related to repeated, severe shaking as an infant. He is now legally blind. At 3, Richard was placed in foster care. It was discovered that his father had locked him in closets for long periods of time and had prevented his mother from caring for him.

Since Richard has been in foster care, his father was expected to provide child support. Mr. Marshall is regularly employed but has paid none of the child support and has not bought any gifts for his son at any time. He is known to have some discretionary income, which he tends to use to buy magazines, such as *Soldier of Fortune,* or to otherwise indulge his continuing interest in the martial arts. He is fascinated by guns, knives, and other weapons, which he describes as "tools of status." He enjoys these "toys" and finds that they "make my adrenaline flow." He fantasizes about becoming a mercenary and joining the Foreign Legion.

Mr. Marshall freely admits beating up two children, ages 6 and 7, for whom he was baby-sitting and giving them bruises and a black eye. He believes this was justified because one of the two children lied to him. He addresses his son as "brat" or "rug rat" during visits. In front of Richard he describes in great detail his own abusive upbringing and plays with sharp knives during these discussions. When he was sent to parenting classes to improve his relationship with Richard, he distracted the class by telling long, dramatic stories about various devious deeds, such as breaking the necks of geese in the city park. He was eventually asked to leave parenting classes.

Mr. Marshall met his common-law wife when she was working in a massage parlor. She attempted to leave him at various times, but he followed her whenever she moved out and caused such a disruption at her new place of residence that she was evicted. He also harassed her at work and threatened repeatedly that if she left him, he would get her fired. He did, in fact, precipitate her being fired on several occasions. He would call her workplace, telling her boss that he was a detective investigating her for embezzlement, fraud, or child abuse (all of these allegations were untrue). Shortly after she left him for the last time, Mr. Marshall called her workplace, leaving a message that he was a representative of the foster home where their son was staying and that Richard had been mortally injured in an auto accident (untrue). Mrs. Marshall eventually filed spouse abuse charges against him.

Mr. Marshall met a new girlfriend at parenting class. He became abusive of this woman soon after moving in with her, and she filed charges against him. He continued to harass her, following her to work, calling her there, and being very disruptive. On one occasion he followed her into her workplace, cornered her in a room without windows, and "karate-chopped" at various supplies, saying that he would do the same to her. He did not actually touch her.

Mr. Marshall is the eldest of six step-siblings. He had no contact with his natural father. His stepfather was a career military man, and the family therefore moved frequently during Mr. Marshall's childhood. He denies observing any spouse abuse in his own home when he was growing up, but says that his stepfather had a violent temper and sometimes beat him for no reason. These beatings frequently resulted in bruises and cuts. Mr. Marshall became interested in karate at age 14 as a means of defending himself against his father.

He denies any conduct problems at home or at school during childhood or adolescence. He obtained a B average in high school and was involved in various sports. Nevertheless, he never felt he won acknowledgment or praise from his father. Following high school, Mr. Marshall attended college for 2 years, studying police science.

Mr. Marshall does not have a drug or alcohol problem, and there is no family history of drug or alcohol abuse. He is not aware of having been depressed at any time in his life and has made no suicidal gestures. He feels unjustly treated by the child protective services and juvenile court. Although Social Services reports that he frightens the foster mother, the social worker, and his own grandmother, he perceives himself as being picked on by child protective services.

He believes that the allegations against him are insignificant or false and that he will eventually get custody of his son. He laughs when he describes being told that his son has significant visual problems and will never see well enough to drive.

During the interview, Mr. Marshall was somewhat demanding, attempting to manipulate meeting times for evenings or weekends. He was demeaning of the Social Services worker in this case and of his ex-wife, but not of the interviewer. Formal mental status testing indicated normal cognition, abstractions, concentration, and fund of general information, with poor judgment.

Discussion of "Martial Arts"

Mr. Marshall's long-standing pattern of cruel and aggressive behavior suggests the diagnosis of Antisocial Personality Disorder. However, he denies the childhood antecedents of that disorder (e.g., truancy, fighting, stealing, and conduct problems at school) that are required for the diagnosis.

As an adult, Mr. Marshall is physically cruel, humiliates and demeans people, uses harsh discipline, lies for the purpose of harming others, and is fascinated by weapons and violence. When this kind of behavior is the predominant personality pathology and is not for the purpose of sexual arousal (as in Sexual Sadism), the diagnosis of Sadistic Personality Disorder has been applied. Mental health professionals rarely encounter people with this condition except when they are referred, as in this case, because of court proceedings in which they are accused of abusing a wife (in almost all cases they are men) or child. In forensic settings the condition is not rare, particularly among perpetrators of violent crimes against people.

Sadistic Personality Disorder was included in an appendix of DSM-III-R but eliminated (mistakenly, we believe) from DSM-IV because of the small number of published validity studies. Such a case in DSM-IV-TR would be diagnosed as Personality Disorder Not Otherwise Specified (DSM-IV-TR, p. 729).

BRIDGE BOY

An 18-year-old high-school senior was brought to the emergency room by police after being picked up wandering in traffic on the Triborough Bridge. He was angry, agitated, and aggressive and talked of various people who were deliberately trying to "confuse" him by giving him misleading directions. His story was rambling and disjointed, but he admitted to the police officer that he had been using "speed." In the emergency room he had difficulty focusing his attention and had to ask that questions be repeated. He was disoriented as to time and place and was unable to repeat the names of three objects after 5 minutes. The family gave a history of the patient's regular use of "pep pills" over the past 2 years, during which time he was frequently "high" and did very poorly in school.

Discussion of "Bridge Boy"

The history of regular use of "pep pills" immediately raises the question of the presence of an Amphetamine-Related Disorder. Although persecutory delusions are present, the disorientation, attention disturbance, and increased psychomotor activity indicate Amphetamine Intoxication Delirium (DSM-IV-TR, p. 145), which, because it involves a global cognitive disturbance, takes precedence over the diagnosis of an Amphetamine-Induced Psychotic Disorder.

Although we do not have much information about his pattern of amphetamine use, his regular use during the school day undoubtedly contributed to his poor school performance. Thus, we make an additional diagnosis of Amphetamine Abuse (DSM-IV-TR, p. 225).

ON STAGE

Harry is a 33-year-old man who lives in Seattle with his wife. He has been employed as a salesperson for an insurance company since graduating from college. He came to a private psychiatrist, recommended by a friend, complaining of "anxiety at work."

Harry describes himself as having been outgoing and popular throughout his adolescence and young adulthood, with no serious problems until his third year of college. He then began to become extremely tense and nervous when studying for tests and writing papers. His heart would pound; his hands would sweat and tremble. Consequently, he often did not write the required papers or, when he did, would submit them after the date due. He could not understand why he was so nervous about doing papers and taking exams when he had always done well in these tasks in the past. As a result of his failure to submit certain papers and his late submission of others, his college grades were seriously affected.

Soon after graduation, Harry was employed as a salesperson for an insurance firm. His initial training (attending lectures, completing reading assignments) proceeded smoothly. However, as soon as he began to take on clients, his anxiety returned. He became extremely nervous when anticipating phone calls from clients. When his business phone rang, he would begin to tremble and sometimes would not even answer it. Eventually, he avoided becoming anxious by not scheduling appointments and by not contacting clients whom he was expected to see.

When asked what it was about these situations that made him nervous, he said that he was concerned about what the client would think of him: "The client might sense that I am nervous and might ask me questions that I don't know the answers to, and I will feel foolish." As a result, he would repeatedly rewrite and reword sales scripts for telephone conversations because he was "so concerned about saying the right thing. I guess I'm just very concerned about being judged."

Although never unemployed, Harry estimates that he has been functioning at only 20% of his work capacity, which his employer tolerates because a salesman is paid only on a commission basis. For the last several years, Harry has had to borrow large sums of money to make ends meet.

Although financial constraints have been a burden, Harry and his wife entertain guests at their home regularly and enjoy socializing with friends at picnics, parties, and formal affairs. Harry lamented, "It's just when I'm expected to do something. Then it's like I'm on stage, all alone, with everyone watching me."

Discussion of "On Stage"

Harry's problem is crippling anxiety whenever he feels that he is performing. In college this happened when he had to write papers or take exams. At work it happens whenever he has to talk to clients, either on the phone or face to face. What he fears is that people will observe his anxiety and make him "feel foolish." Significantly, he has no anxiety in social situations that he does not define as "being on stage," and he has never experienced sudden attacks of panic in situations that he did not expect to cause him anxiety (as in Panic Disorder).

A marked and persistent fear of one or more social or performance situations in which the person is exposed to unfamiliar people or to possible scrutiny by others and fears that he or she will act in a way that will be humiliating or embarrassing is the essential feature of Social Phobia (DSM-IV-TR, p. 456). Social Phobia may be limited to a specific phobic stimulus (as in this case) or may be generalized to almost all social situations. The most common specific Social Phobia is fear of public speaking. Usually fear of public speaking is limited to formal presentations and does not include, as in this case, fear of talking on the telephone. Less common specific Social Phobias are fear of eating in public, fear of writing in public, and fear of using public lavatories. In the Generalized type of Social Phobia, the phobic situation includes most social situations (see "Mail Sorter," p. 181). Because Harry is able to enjoy social activities in which he does not feel he is being judged, he does not have the Generalized Type of Social Phobia.

UNDERGROUND SEX

Charles was 45 when he was referred for psychiatric consultation by his parole officer following his second arrest for rubbing up against a woman in the subway. According to Charles, he had a "good" sexual relationship with his wife of 15 years when he began, 10 years ago, to touch women in the subway. A typical episode would begin with his decision to go into the subway to rub against a woman, usually in her 20s. He would select the woman as he walked into the subway station, move in behind her, and wait for the train to arrive at the station. He would be wearing plastic wrap around his penis so as not to stain his pants after ejaculating while rubbing up against his victim. As riders moved on to the train, he would follow the woman he had selected. When the doors closed, he would begin to push his penis up against her buttocks, fantasizing that they were having inter-course in a normal, noncoercive manner. In about half of the episodes, he would ejaculate and then go on to work. If he failed to ejaculate, he would either give up for that day or change trains and select another victim. Ac-cording to Charles, he felt guilty immediately after each episode but would soon find himself ruminating about and anticipating the next encounter. He estimated that he had done this about twice a week for the last 10 years and thus had probably rubbed up against approximately a thousand women.

During the interview, Charles expressed extreme guilt about his be-havior and often cried when talking about fears that his wife or employer would find out about his second arrest. However, he had apparently never thought about how his victims felt about what he did to them.

His personal history did not indicate any obvious mental problems other than being rather inept and unassertive socially, especially with women.

Discussion of "Underground Sex"

The recurrent touching and rubbing up against a nonconsenting person for the purpose of sexual arousal and gratification is called Frotteurism (DSM-IV-TR, p. 570) and is classified as one of the Paraphilias. In some classic textbooks Frotteurism (rubbing) is dis-tinguished from Toucherism (fondling), but both are included in the DSM-IV-TR category of Frotteurism. No cases of the disorder have ever been reported in females.

Charles's behavior is typical of that seen in this disorder. A crowded place where there is a wide selection of victims is selected (e.g., subway, sports event, mall). In such a setting the initial rub-bing of the woman may not be immediately noticed; the victim usually does not protest because she is not absolutely sure what has happened. This probably explains why Charles has been ar-rested only twice.

What we do not know is the kind of sexual fantasies that Charles had for years before he actually engaged in the acts of Frotteurism. However, as is common in the disorder, while he en-gaged in the act he fantasized about a loving sexual relationship with the victim.

STUBBORN PSYCHIATRIST

Dr. Wilson, a 34-year-old psychiatrist, is 15 minutes late for his first appointment. He has recently been asked to resign from his job in a mental health center because, according to his boss, he is frequently late for work and meetings, has missed appointments, has forgotten about assignments, is late with his statistics, refuses to follow instructions, and seems unmotivated. Dr. Wilson was surprised and resentful—he thought he had been doing a particularly good job under trying circumstances and experienced his boss as excessively obsessive and demanding. Nonetheless, he reports a long-standing pattern of difficulties with authority.

The patient had a childhood history of severe and prolonged temper tantrums that were a legend in his family. He had been a bossy child who demanded that other kids "play his way" or else he wouldn't play at all. With adults, particularly his mother and female teachers, he was sullen, insubordinate, oppositional, and often unmanageable. He had been sent to an all-boys preparatory school that had primarily male teachers, and he gradually became more subdued and disciplined. He continued, however, to stubbornly want things his own way and to resent instruction or direction from teachers. He was a brilliant but erratic student, working only as hard as he himself wanted to; he "punished" teachers he didn't like by not doing their assignments. He was argumentative and self-righteous when criticized, and claimed that he was not being treated fairly.

Dr. Wilson is unhappily married. He complains that his wife does not understand him and is a "nitpicker." She complains that he is unreliable and stubborn. He refuses to do anything around the house and often forgets to complete the few tasks he has accepted as within his responsibility. Tax forms are submitted several months late; bills are not paid. The patient is sociable and has considerable charm, but friends generally become annoyed at his unwillingness to go along with the wishes of the group (e.g., if a restaurant is not his choice, he may sulk all night or "forget" to bring his wallet).

Discussion of "Stubborn Psychiatrist"

Whenever Dr. Wilson feels that demands are being made on him, either socially or occupationally, he passively resists through characteristic maneuvers such as procrastination (e.g., tax returns are late, bills are not paid), forgetfulness (e.g., forgets errands for wife and assignments at work), and sulking when asked to do something he doesn't want to do. His behavior has resulted in impaired work performance and marital difficulties. Such a long-standing pattern of resistance to demands for adequate performance in role functioning, not limited to situations in which assertive behavior is not encouraged or is actually punished (e.g., in the military service), would have qualified for the DSM-III-R diagnosis of Passive-Aggressive Personality Disorder. However, concern that passive-aggressive behavior can be an important clinical feature of some people with personality problems, but is not multifaceted as is generally the case with the other personality disorders, led to its demotion in DSM-IV to the appendix of "Criteria Sets and Axes Provided for Further Study" (DSM-IV-TR, p. 791). This case, then, would have to be diagnosed as Personality Disorder Not Otherwise Specified (DSM-IV-TR, p. 729).

Follow-Up

The patient was treated once a week, for 5 years, with psychotherapy that was in part behavioral and in part psychodynamic. The behavior therapy aspect of his treatment consisted of assertiveness training and specific assignments (e.g., an instruction to do his monthly report the minute it appeared on his desk, and then use the therapy session to discuss the feelings engendered by having done it). When he stopped treatment, the patient was doing very well professionally and reported being much happier.

HOUSE PAINTER

A 46-year-old house painter is admitted to the hospital with a history of 30 years of heavy drinking. He has had two previous admissions for detoxification, but his family states that he has not had a drink in several weeks and he shows no signs of alcohol withdrawal. He looks malnourished, however, and on examination is found to be ataxic and to have a bilateral sixth cranial nerve palsy. He appears confused and mistakes one of his physicians for a dead uncle.

Within a week the patient walks normally, and there is no longer any sign of a palsy. He seems less confused and can now find his way to the bathroom without direction. He remembers the names and birthdays of his siblings, but has difficulty naming the past five United States presidents. More striking, he has great difficulty in retaining information for longer than a few minutes. He can repeat a list of numbers immediately after he has heard them, but a few minutes later does not recall being asked to perform the task. Shown three objects (keys, comb, ring), he cannot recall them 3 minutes later. He does not seem worried about this. Asked if he can recall the name of his doctor, he replies, "Certainly," and proceeds to call the doctor "Dr. Masters" (not his name), whom, he claims, he first met in the Korean War. He tells a long untrue story about how he and "Dr. Masters" served as fellow soldiers.

The patient is calm, alert, and friendly. Because of his intact immediate memory and spotty but sometimes adequate remote memory, one can be with him for a short period and not realize he has a severe memory impairment. Although treated with high doses of thiamine, the short-term memory deficit persists and appears to be irreversible.

Discussion of "House Painter"

Confusion, ataxia, and sixth cranial nerve palsy, with a history of heavy alcohol use, are diagnostic of the neurological disorder Wernicke's encephalopathy, noted on Axis III. As is often the case, when this responds to treatment with thiamine, the patient is left with memory impairment, as manifested by the inability to learn new information or recall previously learned information. In an effort to mask the memory impairment, the person may confabulate (i.e., fabricate facts or events in response to questions about situations that are not recalled). The memory impairment warrants a diagnosis of Alcohol-Induced Persisting Amnestic Disorder (DSM-IV-TR, p. 179). If multiple cognitive deficits were present, rather than just memory loss, then a diagnosis of Alcohol-Induced Persisting Dementia (DSM-IV-TR, p. 170) would be appropriate.

The history of years of heavy drinking and two admissions for detoxification make the additional diagnosis of Alcohol Dependence in Early Partial Remission (DSM-IV-TR, p. 213) extremely likely.

LATIN AMERICAN BUSINESSMAN

Mr. Zeigler is a married, 55-year-old Latin American businessman who is hospitalized with an 8-month history of diarrhea, fatigue, and weight loss. He has sought help from several institutions in both the United States and Europe, but his illness remains undiagnosed. A psychiatric consultation is requested because both the patient and his physician think he is depressed and wonder what role this might play in his weight loss and overall condition.

Mr. Zeigler gives a detailed history of his family's emigration from Europe when he was a child, his personal success in business, and the progressive difficulty he has been experiencing because of his weight loss and fatigue. He has lost 85 pounds over the 8 months and now has to force himself to eat. In the past, eating had been a great pleasure for him, and he considered himself a gourmet. Although he complains of some difficulty with his memory and concentration, he continues to manage a multinational business and to conduct complex financial deals. He says he feels sad but is hopeful the diagnosis can be made quickly. He conducts himself in the same autocratic manner in the hospital that he is accustomed to displaying in business and with his family. He has many interests, including an active sex life, which he wishes to resume once he regains his strength.

Mrs. Zeigler confirms her husband's history and speaks of his complete control of his business and of all of the family's financial affairs. She describes how this has created conflicts with her sons, who resent their father's unyielding control, even though they work in the family company. It is her opinion that her husband is depressed and that this is the cause of most of his symptoms. In response to questions about his activities, she agrees that his fatigue seems the only obstacle to pursuing his interests. She cannot answer any questions about his sex drive because she stopped having sex with him 10 years before this illness. He accepted this, and she presumed he frequented prostitutes.

Over the next few days Mr. Zeigler's condition deteriorates markedly, and he is thought to have had a stroke because of some slurred speech and a slight weakness of the right side of his body. He then becomes short of breath and is admitted to the intensive care unit. A chest

X-ray suggests *Pneumocystis carinii* pneumonia, which is confirmed by bronchoscopy. He does not respond to trimethoprim/sulfamethoxazole and is started on pentamidine. While in the intensive care unit Mr. Zeigler is delirious, frequently hallucinating, and often incoherent in both Spanish and English. His children fly to the United States, as he is not expected to survive. This prediction proves to be incorrect, and his pneumonia resolves after several weeks of treatment. A CT scan of the brain suggests a central nervous system infection with toxoplasmosis, and examination of the stomach by endoscopy leads to the diagnosis of gastrointestinal *Isospora*. Surprisingly, all of these infections respond to treatment.

It is now clear that Mr. Zeigler has acquired immunodeficiency syndrome (AIDS), and his physician presents this diagnosis to him along with an inquiry about his sexual experiences. Mr. Zeigler is enraged by his doctor's "implication" of homosexuality and adamantly denies any homosexual activity. He discusses his adaptation to his wife's decision to cease sexual activity with him. He has frequented prostitutes in the Far East, where he traveled regularly on business. It seems impossible to him that he might have AIDS, although he admits to having contracted syphilis 4 years before his current illness. On discharge, Mr. Zeigler is given the diagnosis of AIDS, with the only clear risk factor his sexual contact with prostitutes.

Six months later Mr. Zeigler and his wife return to the United States for further evaluation of his mental status. His wife is concerned that he has become depressed because he is no longer able to handle his financial affairs. She feels his personality has undergone a radical change, as he no longer seems to care about anything, in spite of the fact that his appetite has returned to normal and he has regained much of his lost weight. Much of his time is now spent sitting idly in their garden.

When examined, Mr. Zeigler appears to be in good physical health. However, his mental condition has obviously deteriorated; and it is not possible to conduct an interview in English, whereas previously he had spoken several languages fluently. He smiles pleasantly, but is both disoriented and confused, even in Spanish. This surprises even his wife, since she had not been aware of this change in his cognitive functioning. He has poor short-term memory and cannot perform simple calculations. His remote memory is intact, although his wife feels that he has confused some historical events. Mr. Zeigler seems unaware that there are any deficits in his intellectual functioning. Medical evaluation does not reveal any active infections.

Discussion of "Latin American Businessman"

This sad case illustrates one aspect of the current epidemic of human immunodeficiency virus (HIV) disease. In retrospect, when Mr. Zeigler first presented with diarrhea, fatigue, and weight loss, he already had AIDS-Related Complex. His loss of memory and difficulty concentrating were most likely the early manifestations of neuropsychological impairment resulting from HIV disease. On his last visit, his impairment in memory and abstract thinking, severe enough to interfere with his work, were evidence of Dementia Due to HIV Disease, Without Behavioral Disturbance (DSM-IV-TR, p. 168). A diagnosis of HIV Infection would be noted on Axis III.

Because many of the symptoms of a Major Depressive Episode can be seen in patients with general medical conditions (fatigue, impaired appetite and weight loss, insomnia), this differential diagnosis is often difficult. The possible presence of a Major Depressive Episode on Mr. Zeigler's first visit was suggested by his admitted sadness, fatigue, weight loss, and disturbed concentration. However, the magnitude of the weight loss (85 pounds) in the absence of profound depressed mood and anhedonia is not what one would expect in a Major Depressive Episode.

Follow-Up

Mr. Zeigler returned to his country, where he died of an unknown infection several months later.

PERFECT RELATIONSHIP

Jim Healy, a 35-year-old social science researcher, has just received multiple sentences of life imprisonment after his third conviction for a series of rapes.

Jim was reared in a chaotic family. His father was physically abusive toward his mother and toward women in general. Both parents were sexually promiscuous, sometimes in his presence. On at least one occasion as a child, he was sodomized by his father. Growing up, often feeling alone and unloved, he began fantasizing about a "perfect relationship" with an ideal woman whom he could "sweep off her feet." As time passed, such fantasies and urges began to assume an eroticized, obsessional quality. Initially, he would imagine himself coercing an unwilling woman into sexual activities that she would then come to enjoy. He would then fantasize a continuing, caring relationship. Often he would masturbate while having these fantasies.

Though Jim understood that the scenario in his fantasies was unlikely, he nevertheless began to be preoccupied with sexually exciting urges to act upon these fantasies. When he was 16, he committed his first rape. After each rape, he would promise himself "never again," but in time, as his preoccupations and urges were rekindled, he would repeat the cycle.

Although he would often threaten women with a knife to obtain their compliance, he never physically hurt them and used the minimal amount of force necessary. Any obvious signs of suffering or anguish would diminish rather than enhance his erotic arousal. During the course of each rape, he would invariably throw away his weapon and assure the woman that he did not intend to injure her or cause her harm.

When reading magazines or watching movies depicting scenes of females in positions of subjugation or bondage, he would become erotically aroused, fantasizing that they were enjoying the experience, but he would not become thus aroused if the women seemed to be suffering or to be in genuine distress.

When tested in prison with a penile plethysmograph, Jim developed an erection when presented with stimuli depicting females in positions of subjugation or bondage, but his arousal was diminished if they seemed to be suffering. Laboratory testing of his blood revealed an elevated level of serum testosterone.

Apart from his convictions for rape, Jim has never been convicted or even accused of any other type of criminal activity. He has no history of outpatient or inpatient psychiatric treatment. He has a stable work history. He has never abused alcohol or any other drugs.

Discussion of "Perfect Relationship"

Jim has committed repeated rapes. Rape is by definition a coercive act and a traumatic experience for the person who is raped. Recognizing that rape is an antisocial and criminal act should not preclude an investigation of the motivation or mental state of the rapist. Most rapes are probably committed by men with quite ordinary (nonparaphilic) sexual preferences, many of whom would meet the criteria for Antisocial Personality Disorder. More rarely, rape is committed by men with Mental Retardation, a psychotic disorder, drug intoxication, or Dissociative Identity Disorder. However, some rapists, particularly serial rapists, have an aberrant sexual drive, a Paraphilia, a disorder in which there are intense sexual urges and sexually arousing fantasies involving either nonhuman objects or the suffering or humiliation of oneself, one's partner, children, or other nonconsenting persons.

Jim showed no evidence of other antisocial behavior. Although he had raped often, he had never engaged in any other criminal acts. He had a reasonably stable work and social history, and the other criteria necessary to make a diagnosis of Antisocial Personality Disorder were absent. His acts of rape could not be explained as a function of Mental Retardation, drug intoxication, a psychotic disorder, or Dissociative Identity Disorder.

Jim experienced recurrent eroticized urges and fantasies about coercing women sexually. Such fantasies and urges had been present for many years, and he had repeatedly acted upon them. Unlike a person with Sexual Sadism, he was not erotically aroused by inflicting pain, humiliation, or suffering; in fact, his erotic arousal was inhibited by any signs of anguish or distress in the victim. However, his rape behavior can best be understood as a manifestation of a specific Paraphilia because his erotic arousal depended on having a nonconsenting partner. During the development of DSM-III-R, the term *Paraphilic Coercive Disorder* was suggested for this particular kind of Paraphilia, but the category has never been officially recognized. Therefore, Jim's disorder would be coded as a Paraphilia Not Otherwise Specified (DSM-IV-TR, p. 576).

Follow-Up

While in prison, Jim was treated with behavioral therapy utilizing masturbatory satiation, in which he was required to masturbate repeatedly to the fantasies of coercive situations that he had previously found sexually arousing. He was also given pharmacological treatment with a testosterone-lowering medication. This combined therapy diminished his aberrant erotic arousal pattern, as evidenced both by less time spent fantasizing rape situations and diminished physiologic arousal as measured by the penile plethysmograph.

When last seen in prison, 2 years after his incarceration, Jim was still receiving the medication and reported that, at least for now (in prison), he was free of both fantasies and urges to rape.

MYSTERY MASTERY

Donna Marks, a 28-year-old lawyer, described her problems to a psychiatrist. She frequently felt anxious and upset around bedtime. On these nights it would take her an hour or more to fall asleep. She dreaded going to bed and would engross herself in reading murder mysteries until late hours. Her bedtime varied from 7:00 P.M. to 2:00 A.M. On awakening in the morning, she felt groggy and incapacitated, hardly able to crawl out of bed. Some mornings she missed work completely. She slept until noon on weekends. Worry about her tardiness getting to work motivated her to seek a consultation.

Donna had had bronchial asthma since age 18 months. Her mother had constantly worried that Donna would die during the night. As a teenager Donna used epinephrine inhalers to remain awake until 1:00 A.M. to 3:00 A.M., reading. She remembers her father screaming at her to turn out the lights. She always considered the late night hours, when everyone else was asleep, a "safe time," free from interference by others.

Donna was particularly prone to nocturnal asthma attacks, which typically occurred around 4:00 A.M. Wheezing at night led to feelings of terror and fear of dying ("I feel out of control"). The current treatment for her asthma was aminophylline 400 mg/day plus 2 puffs on a beclomethasone inhaler twice daily. She also used an albuterol inhaler irregularly, sometimes at bedtime. About once a year, an exacerbation of asthma would require a short course of systemic steroids.

Donna drank five to eight cups of coffee daily. Alcoholic beverages precipitated wheezing and aggravated the delay in onset of sleep. Short-acting sedatives at bedtime caused a noticeable decrease in her ability to concentrate on work the following day. Evening relaxation exercises precipitated fears of being alone with a breathing problem and made her feel like "a skeleton with a pair of lungs."

During the consultation, Donna was articulate, smiling and cheerful and had a full range of affect. She seemed to enjoy her own idiosyncrasies. She was quite talkative, organized, and informative and easily able to discuss her feelings. She noted that it was ironic that she feared death so much yet loved to read about murders in fiction. "I guess it's been my way of feeling some sense of control."

Discussion of "Mystery Mastery"

The effects of the coffee and the drugs that Donna takes for asthma (xanthines, beta-agonists, and steroids) all exert long-lasting stimulation effects likely to interfere with good sleep quality. In addition, the alcohol that she takes, after an initial sedative effect, often lightens sleep 5 or 6 hours following ingestion.

When many substances contribute to the insomnia, the clinician should diagnose, for each drug judged to have a significant role in the insomnia, [Substance]-Induced Sleep Disorder, Insomnia Type (DSM-IV-TR, p. 660). In this case we would probably note the contribution of xanthines, beta-agonists, and caffeine.

BINOCULARS

A 25-year-old male business executive requests psychiatric consultation because of his repeated need to peep at women undressing or engaging in sexual activity. The patient was apprehended for this activity in the past, and the personnel office at his place of work found out about it. He was advised that treatment of his problem was mandatory and that he would lose his job if the behavior were repeated. He did not seek professional assistance and continued to engage in voyeuristic activity. Recently, he was almost caught again, and because of this now seeks a consultation.

The patient is an articulate, handsome man who has no difficulty attracting sexual partners. He dates frequently and has sexual intercourse once or twice a week with a variety of partners. In addition, however, he is frequently drawn to certain types of situations he finds uniquely arousing. He owns a pair of high-powered binoculars and uses these to peep into neighboring apartments. Sometimes he is rewarded for his efforts, but more frequently is not. He then leaves his apartment and goes to rooftops of large apartment buildings, where he searches with his binoculars until he finds a woman undressing or engaging in sexual activity. He has no desire to enter the apartments he peeps into, and he denies experiencing impulses to rape. If he finds a scene in which he can watch a woman undressing or engaging in sexual activity, he masturbates to orgasm while watching, or immediately afterward, and then returns home. He experiences the voyeuristic situation, in its entirety, as uniquely pleasurable, despite the fact that he sometimes encounters potentially hazardous situations. On more than one occasion he has been nearly apprehended by building staff or police, who took him to be a potential burglar or assailant; once he was chased from a "lovers' lane" by an irate man wielding a tire iron; another time he was discovered peeping into a bedroom window in a rural area and barely escaped being shot.

The patient was reared in a family that included three older sisters. His father was puritanical, religious, and generally punitive in his attitudes toward the patient. The patient's mother was allegedly warm, expressive, and flirtatious toward men, but not toward the patient. He felt he was his mother's favorite child and wondered whether he would ever fall in love with a woman who measured up to her. He has never been in love or experienced a durable, deep attachment to a woman.

The patient's family was sexually straight-laced. Family members did not disrobe in front of each other, for example; and the parents avoided open displays of activity that could be interpreted as erotic. Still, the patient recalls that, between age 7 and age 10, he watched his mother and sisters undress "as much as possible."

The patient began "peeping," along with many other boys, at age 10, while at summer camp. He is unable to explain why this particular stimulus subsequently had a unique appeal for him whereas other boys seemed to become less interested in peeping as they became more interested in sexual intercourse. He has used binoculars to search for erotically stimulating scenes since age 11, but did not leave his home to do so until age 17.

The patient notices some relationship between presumed psychological stress and his voyeuristic activity; for example, at times of major life change, such as moving out of his parents' home or finishing a college semester, the activity increased. He is not, however, aware of any relationship between anxiety about having sexual intercourse and the desire to engage in voyeuristic activity. He feels that anxiety is often present in the voyeuristic situation, but it is only a fear of being apprehended. He feels no guilt or shame about his voyeurism and considers it harmless.

He is concerned, however, that he might someday go to jail unless he alters his sexual behavior, and for that reason seeks help.

Discussion of "Binoculars"

There is no question that this patient repeatedly engages in voyeuristic activities for the purpose of achieving sexual excitement. When a person acts on recurrent and intense voyeuristic urges or is markedly distressed by them, or if they cause interpersonal difficulty, the diagnosis of Voyeurism is made (DSM-IV-TR, p. 575).

Many people have voyeuristic impulses, but no clinician would consider making a diagnosis of Voyeurism in someone who occasionally was sexually aroused by observing an unsuspecting neighbor disrobe or by watching pornography, in which the actors pretend to be unaware that they are being observed. In this case, however, the impulses are recurrent and intense, and even the patient is able to recognize the potentially disastrous consequences of his continued voyeuristic behavior.

This case illustrates that people with Paraphilias may also get pleasure from nonparaphilic heterosexual intercourse.

CONTRACT ON MY LIFE

Mr. Polsen, a 42-year-old married African American postal worker and father of two, is brought to the emergency room by his wife because he has been insisting that "there is a contract out on my life."

According to Mr. Polsen, his problems began 4 months ago when his supervisor at work accused him of tampering with a package. Mr. Polsen denied that this was true and, because his job was in jeopardy, filed a protest. At a formal hearing, he was exonerated and, according to him, "This made my boss furious. He felt he had been publicly humiliated."

About 2 weeks later, Mr. Polsen noticed that his co-workers were avoiding him. "When I'd walk toward them, they'd just turn away like they didn't want to see me." Shortly thereafter, he began to feel that they were talking about him at work. He never could make out clearly what they were saying, but he gradually became convinced that they were avoiding him because his boss had taken out a contract on his life.

This state of affairs was stable for about 2 months, until Mr. Polsen began noticing several "large white cars," new to his neighborhood, driving up and down the street on which he lived. He became increasingly frightened and was convinced that the "hit men" were in these cars. He refused to go out of his apartment without an escort. Several times when he saw the white cars he would panic and run home. After one such incident, his wife finally insisted that he accompany her to the emergency room.

Mr. Polsen was described by his wife and brother as a basically well-adjusted, outgoing man who enjoyed being with his family. He had served with distinction in Vietnam. He saw little combat there, but was pulled from a burning truck by a buddy seconds before the truck blew up.

When interviewed, Mr. Polsen was obviously frightened. Aside from his belief that he was in danger of being killed, his speech, behavior, and demeanor were in no way odd or strange. His predominant mood was anxious. He denied having hallucinations and all other psychotic symptoms except those noted above. He claimed not to be depressed and, although he noted that he had recently had some difficulty falling asleep, he said there had been no change in his appetite, sex drive, energy level, or concentration.

Discussion of "Contract on My Life"

Mr. Polsen's anxiety stems from his belief that his boss has taken a contract out on his life. There is no reason to believe this; thus, we must conclude that he has a delusion. Because contract killers are sometimes hired in real life, the delusion is nonbizarre. Mr. Polsen has no auditory or visual hallucinations, no manic or depressive syndrome, and no evidence of a general medical condition or the use of a substance that might have caused the disturbance. His behavior, apart from the delusion and its ramifications, is not odd or bizarre. These are the characteristics of Delusional Disorder (DSM-IV-TR, p. 329). Because the content of his delusion involves the theme of being malevolently treated in some way, the disorder is specified as Persecutory Type.

People with the Persecutory Type of Delusional Disorder are often reluctant to seek help. Mr. Polsen, however, was frightened enough to allow his wife to take him to the emergency room.

Follow-Up

Mr. Polsen was hospitalized. During the first week of hospitalization, he received an antipsychotic drug. He remained delusional, however, and in fact became convinced that several of the other patients on the ward with Italian names were part of the "hit team" sent to kill him. Over the ensuing 3 weeks, with continued treatment, these beliefs faded. At discharge, 1 month after admission, he stated: "I guess my boss has called off the contract. He couldn't get away with it now without publicity."

Mr. Polsen was followed up over a period of 18 months, during which time he had two relapses into more active delusions, all with the same content, and each relapse occurring after he stopped taking his medication. Both episodes resolved relatively rapidly with outpatient treatment with an antipsychotic drug.

BLOOD IS THICKER THAN WATER

Matthew is a 34-year-old single man who lives with his mother and works as an accountant. He is seeking treatment because he is very unhappy after having just broken up with his girlfriend. His mother had disapproved of his marriage plans, ostensibly because the woman was of a different religion. Matthew felt trapped and forced to choose between his mother and his girlfriend, and because "blood is thicker than water," he had decided not to go against his mother's wishes. Nonetheless, he is angry at himself and at her and believes that she will never let him marry and is possessively hanging on to him. His mother "wears the pants" in the family and is a very domineering woman who is used to getting her way. Matthew is afraid of disagreeing with his mother for fear that she will not be supportive of him and he will then have to fend for himself. He criticizes himself for being weak, but also admires his mother and respects her judgment—"Maybe Carol wasn't right for me after all." He alternates between resentment and a "Mother knows best" attitude. He feels that his own judgment is poor.

Matthew works at a job several grades below what his education and talent would permit. On several occasions he has turned down promotions because he didn't want the responsibility of having to supervise other people or make independent decisions. He has worked for the same boss for 10 years, gets on well with him, and is, in turn, highly regarded as a dependable and unobtrusive worker. He has two very close friends whom he has had since early childhood. He has lunch with one of them every single workday and feels lost if his friend is sick and misses a day.

Matthew is the youngest of four children and the only boy. He was "babied and spoiled" by his mother and elder sisters. He had considerable separation anxiety as a child—he had difficulty falling asleep unless his mother stayed in the room, mild school refusal, and unbearable homesickness when he occasionally tried "sleepovers." As a child he was teased by other boys because of his lack of assertiveness and was often called a baby. He has lived at home his whole life except for 1 year of college, from which he returned because of homesickness. His heterosexual adjustment has been normal except for his inability to leave his mother in favor of another woman.

Discussion of "Blood Is Thicker Than Water"

This patient has allowed his mother to make the important decision as to whether he should marry his girlfriend, and this seems to be merely one instance of a pattern of subordinating his own needs and wishes to those of his domineering mother. At work he demonstrates lack of initiative and reluctance to rely on his own judgment and abilities by avoiding promotions and working below his potential. He apparently feels uncomfortable when he is alone, and he has always worried about being left to take care of himself. He is afraid of disagreeing with his mother. This dependent and submissive behavior is severe enough to interfere significantly with his social and occupational functioning and therefore to justify the diagnosis Dependent Personality Disorder (DSM-IV-TR, p. 725).

Follow-Up

Matthew's therapist treated him with a combination of behavior therapy and psychodynamic psychotherapy for several years. He was also seen in group therapy. After a year of therapy, he moved out of his mother's house and married his girlfriend. When last heard from, he said he was fairly happy in his marriage.

MAIL SORTER

Andy, a 25-year-old single man, lives with his mother and brother. He works as a mail sorter at the post office, a job he has had since he dropped out of college after 2 years. He came to an anxiety disorders clinic after reading a newspaper advertisement of the availability of free treatment if he participated in a research study of anxiety disorders. His chief complaint is of "nervousness." He says that right now he is "just going through the motions" and wants "to lead a normal life and go back to college."

During his adolescence and young adulthood, Andy had no close friends and usually preferred to be by himself. When he entered college, he formed several close friendships but became "super self-conscious" when speaking to strangers, classmates, and sometimes even friends. He would feel nervous, and his face would become so "stiff" that he had difficulty speaking. He had a "buzzing" in his head, felt as if he were "outside [his] body," had hot flashes, and perspired. These "panic attacks" (his term) came on suddenly, within seconds, and only when he was with people. When a classmate spoke to him, he sometimes "couldn't hear" what the classmate was saying because of his nervousness.

Outside class, Andy began to feel increasingly uncomfortable in social situations. "I think that I was afraid of saying or doing something stupid." He began to turn down invitations to parties and to withdraw from other social activities (e.g., a bowling league). Eventually, he dropped out of college entirely.

Andy explains that the reason he chose to work at the post office is that the job does not require him to deal with people. When asked about other things that make him nervous, he says he tries to avoid using public lavatories and feels more comfortable in a public bathroom when the lights are dim, when there are few people present, and when he can use a stall rather than a urinal.

Andy has two long-standing "best" friends with whom he socializes regularly and feels completely comfortable. However, he hasn't dated since college, and he totally avoids group settings, such as weddings and dances. He has no problem with authority figures, and even welcomes constructive criticism from his supervisor at the post office. "My problem is nervousness, not obstinacy."

Discussion of "Mail Sorter"

Andy says that he has "panic attacks," and it is true that he gets sudden attacks of intense anxiety. However, these always occur in situations that he knows are frightening to him. Thus, the attacks are quite different from the unexpected attacks of panic that occur in Panic Disorder. Andy's anxiety occurs in a variety of different social situations in which he fears that he will do something or act in a way that will be humiliating or embarrassing. This is the hallmark of a Social Phobia, Generalized Type (DSM-IV-TR, p. 456). This diagnosis is given only, as in Andy's case, when the distress significantly interferes with the person's normal routine, occupational functioning, or social activities or relationships, or there is marked distress about having the phobia.

The diagnosis of Social Phobia is given only when the fear is unrelated to another disorder. For example, the diagnosis would not be given to a patient with Panic Disorder who was afraid of having a panic attack in public, or to a patient with Parkinson's disease who was afraid of trembling in public.

Andy's chief complaint is "nervousness," and therefore his evaluation focuses on a differential diagnosis of his anxiety symptoms. Were he to seek treatment for the interpersonal problems that have constricted his life, the focus would be on his personality functioning and would have suggested the diagnosis of Avoidant Personality Disorder (DSM-IV-TR, p. 721). In fact, his symptoms probably meet the criteria for that disorder in view of his avoidance of activities that involve interpersonal contact, preoccupation with being criticized or rejected, and feelings of inadequacy. Most people with the Generalized Type of Social Phobia report that the difficulties have persisted in a more or less stable form since childhood or adolescence. For this reason, it may well be that Generalized Social Phobia and Avoidant Personality Disorder are the same condition, viewed from different perspectives.

PROFESSOR

A 33-year-old college professor presented with the complaint that he had never been able to ejaculate while making love. He had no trouble in attaining and maintaining an erection and no difficulties in stimulating his partner to her orgasm, but he could never be stimulated himself to ejaculation and would finally give up in boredom. He has always been able to reach ejaculation by masturbation, which he does about twice a week; but he has never been willing to allow a partner to masturbate him to orgasm. Previously he resisted all of his girlfriend's attempts to persuade him to seek medical or psychological help, as he felt that intravaginal ejaculation was unimportant unless one wanted children.

The patient's current relationship is in jeopardy because his girlfriend is eager to marry and have children. He has never wanted to have children and is reluctant to become a father, but the pressures from his girlfriend have forced him to seek therapy. Throughout the interview his attitude toward the problem is one of distance and disdain. He describes the problem as though he were a neutral observer, with little apparent feeling.

Discussion of "Professor"

This professor has an unusual sexual problem. He is able to have an erection without any difficulty, has no problem in sustaining the erection during intercourse (as would be the case in Male Erectile Disorder), but is unable to have an orgasm during intercourse. Significantly, he has no trouble having an orgasm when he masturbates, which excludes the possibility that a general medical condition accounts for the problem. Persistent inhibition of the male orgasm phase not caused exclusively by an general medical condition or medication (such as a side effect of certain antidepressants) is called Male Orgasmic Disorder (Inhibited Male Orgasm) (DSM-IV-TR, p. 552). We note the condition is Due to Psychological Factors, Lifelong (not acquired after a period of normal functioning) and Generalized (not limited to a specific situation).

There is a suggestion of coldness and hyperintellectualization, traits often present in men with this disorder. Perhaps on the basis of more information, a diagnosis of Obsessive-Compulsive Personality Disorder might also be warranted.

COCAINE

Al Santini, a 39-year-old restaurant owner, is referred by a marriage counselor to a private outpatient substance abuse treatment program for evaluation and treatment of a possible "cocaine problem." According to the counselor, attempts to deal with the couple's marital problems have failed to produce any signs of progress over the past 6 or 7 months. The couple continues to have frequent, explosive arguments, some of which have led to physical violence. Fortunately, neither spouse has been seriously injured, but the continuing chaos in their relationship has led to a great deal of tension at home and appears to be contributing to the acting-out behavior and school problems of their two children, ages 9 and 13.

Several days ago the patient admitted to the counselor and to his wife that he had been using cocaine "occasionally" for at least the past year. The wife became angry and tearful, stating that if her husband failed to obtain treatment for his drug problem, she would separate from him and inform his parents of the problem. He reluctantly agreed to seek professional help, insisting that his cocaine use was "not a problem" and that he felt capable of stopping his drug use without entering a treatment program.

During the initial evaluation interview, Al reports that he is currently using cocaine, intranasally, 3–5 days a week, and that this pattern has been continuing for at least the past 2 years. On average, he consumes a total of 1–2 grams of cocaine weekly, for which he pays $80 per gram. Most of his cocaine use occurs at work, in his private office or in the bathroom. He usually begins thinking about "coke" while driving to work in the morning. When he arrives at work, he finds it nearly impossible to avoid thinking of the cocaine vial in his desk drawer. Although he tries to distract himself and postpone using it as long as possible, he usually snorts his first "line" within an hour of arriving at work. On some days he may snort another two or three lines over the course of the day. On other days, especially if he feels stressed or frustrated at work, he may snort a line or two every hour from morning through late afternoon. His cocaine use is sometimes fueled by offers of the drug from his business partner, whom the patient describes as a more controlled, infrequent user of the drug.

Al rarely uses cocaine at home, and never in the presence of his wife or children. Occasionally he snorts a line or two on weekday evenings or weekends at home when everyone else is out of the house. Al denies current use of any other illicit drug, but reports taking 10–20 mg of an antianxiety drug, diazepam (prescribed by a physician friend), at bedtime on days when cocaine leaves him feeling restless, irritable, and unable to fall asleep. When diazepam is unavailable, he drinks two or three beers instead.

He first tried cocaine 5 years ago at a friend's party. He enjoyed the energetic, euphoric feeling and the absence of any unpleasant side effects, except for a slightly uncomfortable "racing" feeling in his chest. For nearly 3 years thereafter he used cocaine only when it was offered by others and never purchased his own supplies or found himself thinking about the drug between episodes of use. He rarely snorted more than four or five lines on any single occasion of use. During the past 2 years his cocaine use escalated to its current level, coincident with a number of significant changes in his life. His restaurant business became financially successful; he bought a large home in the suburbs; he had access to large sums of cash; and the pressures of a growing business made him feel entitled to the relief and pleasures offered by cocaine.

He denies any history of alcohol or drug abuse problems. The only other drug he has ever used is marijuana, which he smoked infrequently in college but never really liked. He also denies any history of other emotional problems and, except for marriage counseling, reports that he has never needed help from a mental health professional.

During the interview, Al remarks several times that although he thinks that his cocaine use "might be a problem," he does not consider himself to be "addicted" to it and is still not sure that he really requires treatment. In support of this view, he lists the following evidence: 1) His current level of cocaine use is not causing him any financial problems or affecting his standard of living. 2) He is experiencing no significant drug-related health problems that he is aware of, with the possible exception of feeling lethargic the next day following a day of heavy use. 3) On many occasions he has been able to stop using cocaine on his own, for several days at a time. 4) When he stops using the drug, he experiences no withdrawal syndrome and no continuous drug cravings. On the other hand, he does admit the following: 1) He often uses much more cocaine than intended on certain days. 2) The drug use is impairing his functioning at work because of negative effects on his memory, attention span, and attitude toward employees and customers. 3) Even when he is not actively intoxicated with cocaine, the aftereffects of the drug cause him to be short-tempered, irritable, and argumentative with his wife and children, leading to numerous family problems, including a possible break-up of his marriage. 4) Although he seems able to stop using cocaine for a few days at a time, somehow he always goes back to it. 5) As soon as he starts to use cocaine again, the craving and the preoccupation with the drug are immediately as intense as before he stopped using it.

At the end of the interview, Al agrees that although he came for the evaluation largely under pressure from his wife, he can see the potential benefits of trying to stop using cocaine on a more permanent basis. With a saddened expression, he explains how troubled and frightened he feels about the problems with his wife and children. He says that although marital problems existed before he started snorting cocaine, his continuing drug use has made them worse, and he now fears that his wife might leave him. He also feels extremely guilty about not being a "good father." He spends very little time with his children and often is distracted and irritable with them because of his cocaine use.

Discussion of "Cocaine"

Al, like many people with a serious drug problem, does not like to think of himself as "addicted." However, Al's use of cocaine illustrates the core concept of psychoactive substance dependence: a cluster of cognitive, behavioral, and physiologic symptoms indicating that the person has impaired control of psychoactive substance use and continues use of the substance despite adverse consequences. Al cannot stop himself from taking the first hit of cocaine in the morning; he uses it more often than he plans to; he keeps returning to it after stopping for a few days; he experiences withdrawal symptoms (lethargy); and he has reduced important social activities with his family because of mood changes caused by his taking cocaine. Therefore the diagnosis is Cocaine Dependence, With Physiological Dependence (DSM-IV-TR, p. 242).

Follow-Up

Al entered the outpatient treatment program. His treatment included individual, group, and marital counseling combined with supervised urine screening and participation in a self-help group (Cocaine

Anonymous). He initially had difficulty in fully acknowledging and accepting the seriousness of his drug dependency problem. He harbored fantasies about returning to "controlled" cocaine use and disputed the program's requirement of total abstinence from all mood-altering substances, arguing that because he had never experienced problems with alcohol, he saw no reason to deny himself an occasional drink with dinner or at social gatherings. During the first 3 months of treatment, he had two short "slips" back to taking cocaine, one of which was precipitated by drinking a glass of wine, which led to an intense craving for cocaine.

Subsequently, Al remained completely abstinent for the duration of the program (12 months) and became increasingly committed to maintaining a drug-free lifestyle. His relationships with his wife and children improved considerably. The violent arguments had stopped immediately with the cessation of cocaine use, and spending more time with his children became much easier without the negative influence of cocaine on his mood and mental state.

Three years later Al was still abstinent. He was no longer in treatment, but continued to attend Cocaine Anonymous meetings at least two or three times every week. If he were diagnosed at this time, the Cocaine Dependence would be specified as Sustained Full Remission because of the absence of any of the signs or symptoms of Cocaine Dependence for over 12 months.

CHILD PSYCHIATRIST

Dr. Crone, a single, 35-year-old child psychiatrist, has been arrested and convicted of fondling several neighborhood boys, ages 6 to 12. Friends and colleagues were shocked and dismayed, as he had been considered by all to be particularly caring and supportive of children. Not only had he chosen a profession involving their care, but he had been a Cub Scout leader for many years and also a member of the local Big Brothers.

Dr. Crone is from a stable family. His father, who had also been a physician, was described as a workaholic, spending little time with his three children. Dr. Crone never married and, when interviewed by a psychiatrist as part of his presentence investigation, admitted that he experienced little, if any, sexual attraction toward females, either adults or children. He also denied sexual attraction toward adult men. In presenting the history of his psychosexual development, he reported that he had become somewhat dismayed as a child when his boyfriends began expressing rudimentary awareness of an attraction toward girls. His "secret" at the time was that he was attracted more to other boys and, in fact, during childhood often played "doctor" with other boys, eventually progressing to mutual masturbation with some of his boyfriends.

His first sexual experience was at age 6, when a 15-year-old male camp counselor performed fellatio on him several times over the course of the summer—an experience that he had always kept to himself. As he reached his teenage years, he began to suspect that he was homosexual. As he grew older, he was surprised to notice that the age range of males who attracted him sexually did not change, and he continued to have recurrent erotic urges and fantasies about boys between the ages of 6 and 12. Whenever he masturbated, he would fantasize about a boy in that age range, and on a couple of occasions over the years had felt himself to be in love with such a youngster.

Intellectually, Dr. Crone knew that others would disapprove of his many sexual involvements with young boys. He never believed, however, that he had caused any of these youngsters harm, feeling instead that they were simply sharing pleasurable feelings together. He yearned to be able to experience the same sort of feelings toward women, but he never was able to do so. He frequently prayed for help and that his actions would go undetected. He kept promising himself that he would stop, but the temptations were such that he could not. He was so fearful of destroying his reputation, his friendships, and his career that he had never been able to bring himself to tell anyone about his problem.

Discussion of "Child Psychiatrist"

Dr. Crone experiences recurrent intense sexual urges and sexually arousing fantasies involving sexual activity with prepubescent boys. He has acted on these fantasies and urges on many occasions. This alone is sufficient to make the diagnosis of Pedophilia (DSM-IV-TR, p. 572). The diagnosis would also be made if Dr. Crone had never acted on these fantasies and urges but was markedly distressed by them or if they caused interpersonal difficulties.

In DSM-III the diagnosis of Pedophilia required that the deviant sexual behavior be the preferred source of sexual arousal. Beginning with DSM-III-R and continuing in DSM-IV (and DSM-IV-TR), this is not required because, in many cases of people who act on pedophilic (and other paraphilic) impulses, the deviant behavior may alternate with other paraphilic or with more ordinary sexual behavior. In Dr. Crone's case, we note that his deviant behavior is directed toward the same sex. This has prognostic significance in that the recidivism rate for people with Pedophilia involving a preference for the same sex may be roughly twice that of those who prefer the opposite sex. We also note that he is exclusively aroused by young boys and, as is usually the case, boys within a relatively narrow age range. Thus, the diagnosis is further specified as Sexually Attracted to Males, Exclusive Type.

Dr. Crone, like many other men with Pedophilia who do not also have Sexual Sadism, has a genuine interest in children and justified his behavior with the rationalization that he was not harming them in any way.

EMILIO

Emilio is a 40-year-old man who looks 10 years younger. He is brought to the hospital, his twelfth hospitalization, by his mother because she is afraid of him. He is dressed in a ragged overcoat, bedroom slippers, and a baseball cap and wears several medals around his neck. His affect ranges from anger at his mother ("She feeds me shit . . . what comes out of other people's rectums") to a giggling, obsequious seductiveness toward the interviewer. His speech and manner have a childlike quality, and he walks with a mincing step and exaggerated hip movements. His mother reports that he stopped taking his medication about a month ago and has since begun to hear voices and to look and act more bizarrely. When asked what he has been doing, he says, "Eating wires and lighting fires." His spontaneous speech is often incoherent and marked by frequent rhyming and clang associations (speech in which sounds, rather than meaningful relationships, govern word choice).

Emilio's first hospitalization occurred after he dropped out of school at age 16, and since that time he has never been able to attend school or hold a job. He has been treated with neuroleptics during his hospitalizations but doesn't continue to take medication when he leaves, so he quickly becomes disorganized again. He lives with his elderly mother, but sometimes disappears for several months at a time and is eventually picked up by the police as he wanders in the streets. There is no known history of drug or alcohol abuse.

Discussion of "Emilio"

The combination of a chronic illness with marked incoherence, inappropriate affect, auditory hallucinations, and grossly disorganized behavior leaves little doubt that the diagnosis is chronic Schizophrenia (DSM-IV-TR, p. 312). The course would be noted as Continuous because Emilio apparently never has prolonged remissions of his psychosis. The prominence of his disorganized speech and behavior, his grossly inappropriate affect, and the absence of prominent catatonic symptoms indicate the Disorganized Type (DSM-IV-TR, p. 315).

Follow-Up

Emilio has been hospitalized five more times in the 10 years following this admission to the hospital. During each of his hospitalizations, he was treated with high doses of antipsychotic drugs and within a few weeks began to behave appropriately and to be able to ignore the voices of his auditory hallucinations. During the first hospitalization, he was able to establish a relationship with a therapist and talk thoughtfully and with a full range of appropriate affect about his unhappy life, his inability to do any work because "nobody wants me," and his desire to be taken care of. However, soon after leaving the hospital, Emilio stopped taking his medication, failed to keep clinic appointments, and within a few months was again grossly disorganized and psychotic.

Emilio's last psychiatric hospitalization was 2 years ago, when he was age 48. His mother was now too feeble to care for him, and arrangements were made for him to live in an adult home after he left the hospital—supported by welfare, and with medication managed by the staff of the institution. In that setting he does fairly well.

WORMS

Ms. Green, a 62-year-old retired librarian, complains to her doctor that "the worms are still at it."

Four years ago, when taking a bath, Ms. Green noted what she thought were lots of "little worms" floating in the bath water. Soon thereafter she began to experience the feeling of these worms "digging under my skin." Multiple visits to doctors, to whom she brought samples of the "worms," could uncover no evidence of parasites. She received symptomatic treatment for itching. To her exasperation, the doctors persisted in telling her that her samples were only flakes of dry skin. She refused a psychiatric consultation. She soon began to feel that her co-workers and friends avoided her because of her worms. She reduced her previously rather numerous social activities. She became so upset by the worms that she eventually decided to take early retirement from her job, which she had held for over 30 years. She denied symptoms of depression during this time.

Ms. Green's condition was apparently unchanged until 9 months ago when, in church, she noticed that all the rosaries within a few yards of her were rotating in a clockwise direction. She began to see other evidence that she was giving off a "magnetic field." She explains that this is a result of the worms entering her spinal cord and traveling up and down, which "creates a magnetic current."

Ms. Green is a pleasant, articulate woman with full range of affect and coherent, goal-directed speech. She denies other unusual experiences, such as hearing voices, or any symptoms of depression. She has become more socially isolated recently as she feels the "magnetic field" makes other people uncomfortable. Otherwise, she maintains active correspondence with several people, likes to knit and read, and volunteers time at her old library, where they say her work continues to be of high quality.

Discussion of "Worms"

Had we seen Ms. Green early in her illness, when she was complaining only of being infested with "worms," we would have concluded that she had a nonbizarre delusion, and made a diagnosis of Delusional Disorder. Seeing her now, however, we have to take into account that her delusion involves phenomena that her culture would regard as totally implausible: the worms create a magnetic current that causes rosaries to rotate. She now has a prominent bizarre delusion, so the diagnosis of Delusional Disorder is no longer appropriate.

The chronic bizarre delusion of greater than 6 months' duration in the absence of a mood disturbance suggests Schizophrenia. However, Schizophrenia is an illness that invariably involves marked disturbance in social and occupational functioning. Ms. Green did reduce her social activities, but is still described as functioning well in her work and maintaining social contact, at least by mail. We are therefore more comfortable with the diagnosis of Psychotic Disorder Not Otherwise Specified (DSM-IV-TR, p. 343).

EVENING SHIFT

A 30-year-old warehouse worker had experienced episodes of poor sleep for the preceding 5 years whenever he had to work on the evening shift. Every 2 weeks he alternated between working the evening shift (3:00 P.M. to 11:00 P.M.) and the day shift (7:00 A.M. to 3:00 P.M.). When he worked the evening shift, he would go to bed about 2 hours after work, around 1:00 A.M. About half the time it would take him 1–2 hours to fall asleep. When this happened, he typically would awaken at 5:00 A.M., his normal time for getting up to go to work the day shift. He would have a snack and then return to bed and drift in and out of sleep until arising between 8:30 A.M. and 11:00 A.M. On weekends and holidays, however, he would revert to his normal bedtime, approximately 10:00 P.M., when he would fall into bed exhausted.

When the patient slept poorly at night, he felt sleepy the next day; if he slept well, he felt alert. When he worked the day shift and was on vacation, he slept well and felt alert the next day.

Discussion of "Evening Shift"

Sleep, like most biological functions, follows a rhythm over a period that lasts about 24 hours (circadian rhythm). The sleep rhythm induced by daytime work in this patient persists when he works the evening shift. At these times the mismatch between his circadian rhythm and the demands of his work schedule results in insomnia (trouble falling asleep and staying asleep). His biological clock causes sleepiness at 10:00 P.M. and awakening at about 5:00 A.M. When he works the evening shift, he is forced to stay awake hours beyond his usual bedtime, and he initially awakens at his usual arising time.

If the patient were able to stay on the evening shift for several months and maintain the same sleep times, his biological clock would gradually be reset, so that his sleep schedule would harmonize with the hours of his work day. It is because the hours of his shift keep changing and he is apparently particularly intolerant of the mismatch between his circadian rhythm and his daily work schedule that he cannot sleep during desirable hours.

Sleep problems resulting from a mismatch between the normal sleep–wake schedule for the person's environment and his or her circadian sleep–wake pattern are diagnosed as Circadian Rhythm Sleep Disorder (DSM-IV-TR, p. 629). When the disorder is apparently caused by frequently changing sleep and waking times resulting from changes in work shifts, the Shift Work Type is specified. The diagnosis is confirmed, as in this case, by normal sleep and daytime alertness when the internal sleep schedule conforms again to environmental demands.

Follow-Up

The patient was advised to gradually discontinue eating at night in order to stop reinforcing nocturnal appetite and wakefulness. In addition, he was advised to arise at 8:30 A.M. when he worked the evening shift, no matter how tired he felt. In this way it was hoped that he would feel tired enough at 1:00 A.M. to fall asleep immediately and then have a full night's sleep.

After trying the program, the patient reported that he could not stick to it. He said he became "like a madman" during the night, searching everywhere for his favorite snacks after his wife, with his consent, had hidden them. Nor could he remain awake until 1:00 A.M. on the weekend between the 2 weeks of the evening shift.

The patient did not return for another appointment, but called several months later to report that he had been able to convince his employer to take him off the evening work shift permanently, which completely relieved his sleep problem.

LOVELY RITA

A 36-year-old London meter maid was referred for psychiatric examination by her solicitor. Six months previously, moments after she had written a ticket and placed it on the windshield of an illegally parked car, a man came dashing out of a barbershop, ran up to her, swearing and shaking his fist, swung, and hit her in the jaw with enough force to knock her down. A fellow worker came to her aid and summoned the police, who caught the man a few blocks away and placed him under arrest.

The patient was taken to the hospital, where a hairline fracture of the jaw was diagnosed by X-ray. The fracture did not require that her jaw be wired, but the patient was placed on a soft diet for 4 weeks. Several different physicians, including her own, found her physically fit to return to work after 1 month. The patient, however, complained of severe pain and muscle tension in her neck and back that virtually immobilized her. She spent most of her days sitting in a chair or lying on a bedboard on her bed. She enlisted the services of a solicitor as the Workmen's Compensation Board was cutting off her payments and her employer was threatening her with suspension if she did not return to work.

The patient shuffled slowly and laboriously into the psychiatrist's office and lowered herself with great care into a chair. She was attractively dressed and well made up and wore a neck brace. She related her story with vivid detail and considerable anger directed at her assailant (whom she repeatedly referred to as "that bloody foreigner"), her employer, and the compensation board. It was as if the incident had occurred yesterday. Regarding her ability to work, she said that she wanted to return to the job and would soon be severely strapped financially, but was physically not up to even the lightest office work.

She denied any previous psychological problems and initially described her childhood and family life as storybook perfect. In subsequent interviews, however, she admitted that as a child, she had frequently been beaten by her alcoholic father, and had once had a broken arm as a result, and that she had often been locked in a closet for hours at a time as punishment for misbehavior.

Discussion of "Lovely Rita"

In this case the first question is: Can this woman's pain be entirely accounted for by the nature of her very real physical injury? Evidently, the answer is no, given the extensive assessment by several physicians. The next question is: Is this woman simply attempting to get continued financial support from Workmen's Compensation so that she will no longer have to earn a living? If the answer is yes, this would be an instance of Malingering—that is, the intentional production and presentation of false or grossly exaggerated symptoms in pursuit of external incentives. The apparent genuineness of her suffering and her desire to return to work makes this unlikely.

Although the pain was initially caused by her injury, most physicians who examined the patient thought that she was sufficiently recovered physically and that her persistent complaints of pain were excessive. In addition, there is evidence of specific psychological factors contributing to the severity and maintenance of the pain. The history of the patient's having been physically abused by her father as a child probably produced psychological conflict that was revived by the assault. This might account for the continuation of the pain beyond what would be accounted for by her injury. This leaves us with the diagnosis of Pain Disorder Associated With Both Psychological Factors and a General Medical Condition (DSM-IV-TR, p. 503), as both are judged to play an important role in this case.

NIGHTMARES

Martha, a 35-year-old woman, has had nightmares every night, beginning in her early teenage years. She comes to a sleep specialist at the insistence of her husband, who is fed up with her behavior both while sleeping and while awake. One to four times a night, she awakens out of a dream, the content of which is always disturbing. Often she dreams of yelling at other people or of menacing confrontations. In the dreams she feels angry and frustrated. Typically, she awakes from the dreams feeling extremely tense.

During the day Martha often has uncontrollable outbursts of temper. These can be precipitated by minor frustrations, such as a delay in finding her eyeglasses. In the midst of an outburst she may feel that it is wrong to behave thus, that her outburst is unwarranted, but she is powerless to stop it. After the outburst she apologizes for it.

Martha sleeps excessively, sometimes 12–13 hours consecutively on weekends, and often takes 3-hour to 4-hour naps. She is sleepy while driving on the turnpike, but manages to stay awake by having the temperature cold and the radio "blasting."

She denies having sudden, irresistible attacks of sleepiness, cataplexy (sudden loss of motor power), hypnogogic hallucinations (hallucinations while awakening), or sleep paralysis (motor weakness and brief inability to move upon sudden awakening), all of which are characteristic of narcolepsy. She denies feeling confused or disoriented when she awakens from her dreams (as might be found in impaired arousal states, such as in episodes associated with temporal lobe dysfunction). Her husband notes that she has greatly increased eyelid flutter and eye movements shortly after she has fallen asleep (which might mean abnormally early onset of rapid eye movement [REM] sleep, as is seen in Major Depressive Disorder and drug withdrawal states). She always sleeps restlessly and occasionally hits him suddenly in the middle of the night (a common symptom of Parasomnias).

At the initial evaluation, Martha appeared downcast but did not cry. She was organized and informative. She made three mistakes on serial sevens, but her sensorium was otherwise intact. She described her work as a registrar in a small college, which she considered enjoyable and her "salvation." Her 4-year-old daughter was bright and well.

Martha had smoked a pack of cigarettes a day for 25 years and drank a cup of chocolate and 48 oz of cola beverages daily. She took alcohol only a few times per year.

All-night sleep recording revealed 9 hours of sleep continually interrupted by 10-second to 30-second arousals that frequently began with a K-complex (an arousal pattern) and were mostly unassociated with prior body movements. These happened about 35 times per hour in sleep stages I and II and during REM sleep, but only 4 times per hour during deep sleep. Otherwise, REM latency (the time spent before the initial appearance of REM sleep), density, and amount were normal, and other stages, although interrupted, were of normal pattern and percentage. However, there were no reports of nightmares during the night. (The constant arousals were unusual and possibly related to the abnormalities noted on the electroencephalogram.)

Discussion of "Nightmares"

Martha's recurrent nightmares are a form of Parasomnia, a group of Sleep Disorders in which the predominant symptom is an abnormal event that occurs during sleep or at the threshold between wakefulness and sleep. Martha has Nightmare Disorder (DSM-IV-TR, p. 634), in which there are repeated awakenings from sleep with detailed recall of frightening dreams. These dreams are typically vivid and quite extended and usually include threats to survival, security, or self-esteem. The dreams occur during periods of REM sleep and thus are more likely to appear toward the end of the night.

Martha also has unusually prolonged sleep and daytime sleepiness (hypersomnia). Because the cause of the hypersomnia is not another sleep disorder (e.g., Narcolepsy, Breathing-Related Sleep Disorder) or another mental disorder (such as Major Depressive Disorder) and does not result from the direct physiological effects of a general medical condition or substance, the diagnosis of Primary Hypersomnia (DSM-IV-TR, p. 609) is also made.

It is hard to know how to explain Martha's irritability and temper outbursts. The psychiatrist who treated her suspected that these symptoms might have been manifestations of hypomania.

Follow-Up

Treatment has included psychotherapy, attempts to control dream content through a lucid dreaming routine (in which the dreamer directs the events of the dream or attempts to converse with the characters in it), and trials of an antidepressant and of an anticonvulsant, neither of which helped. A trial of lithium significantly lessened the temper outbursts for a period of 2 weeks, but they then returned, despite dosage increases.

After being seen for 8 months, the patient became discouraged and angry with the therapist and refused further treatment.

PAUL AND PETULA

Paul and Petula have been living together for the last 6 months and are contemplating marriage. Petula describes the problem that has brought them to the sex therapy clinic.

"For the last 2 months he hasn't been able to keep his erection after he enters me."

The psychiatrist turns to Paul and asks him how he sees the problem. Paul, embarrassed, agrees with Petula and adds, "I just don't know why."

The psychiatrist learns that Paul, age 26, is a recently graduated lawyer, and that Petula, age 24, is a successful buyer for a large department store. They both grew up in educated middle-class suburban families. They met through mutual friends and started to have sexual intercourse a few months after they met and had no problems at that time.

Two months later, Paul moved from his family home into Petula's apartment. This was her idea, and Paul was unsure that he was ready for such an important step. Within a few weeks, Paul noticed that although he continued to be sexually aroused and wanted intercourse, as soon as he entered his partner, he began to lose his erection and could not stay inside. They would try again, but by then his desire had waned, and he was unable to achieve another erection.

After the first few times this happened, Petula became so angry that she began punching him in the chest and screaming at him. Paul, who weighs 200 pounds, would simply walk away from his 98-pound lover, which would infuriate her even more.

The psychiatrist learned that sex was not the only area of contention in the relationship. Petula complained that Paul did not spend enough time with her and preferred to go to baseball games with his male friends. Even when he was home, he would watch all the sports events that were available on TV and was not interested in going to foreign movies, museums, or the theater with her. Despite these differences, Petula was eager to marry Paul and was pressuring him to set a date.

Physical examination of the couple revealed no abnormalities, and there was no evidence that either partner was persistently depressed.

Discussion of "Paul and Petula"

Paul and Petula have many problems that a family-oriented clinician would want to focus on, such as Paul's ambivalence about committing himself to a relationship with Petula and her frantic efforts to obtain that commitment. The effect of these problems on Paul's sexual functioning is clear: he is unable to maintain his erection until the completion of sexual activity.

When there is no evidence that the disturbance is caused exclusively by a general medical condition (such as by diabetic neuropathy or certain medications), the diagnosis of Male Erectile Disorder, Due to Psychological Factors, is made (DSM-IV-TR, p. 547). We note that the disorder is Acquired (recent onset), not Lifelong. (Note: When an erectile dysfunction is caused by a general medical condition, the medical condition would be coded as a physical disorder on Axis III.)

Follow-Up

Neither partner was willing to discuss nonsexual problems. They were treated with Masters and Johnson's sensate focus exercises over the next several months. In these exercises, the couple explored nongenital ways of giving physical pleasure to each other without the psychological demands of demonstrating sexual competence. Petula continually pressured Paul to translate the therapy into action. She saw herself as a therapist and teacher and Paul as patient and pupil. Paul passively avoided doing the exercises on many occasions; but over a period of 8 months, Paul's problem with maintaining an erection was gradually resolved. They were married within 3 months after treatment ended.

The Petersens sought treatment twice more over the next 8 years.

On both occasions the underlying issue was again Paul's ambivalence about further committing himself to the relationship (buying a house, having children). Paul had a recurrence of erectile problems and, in addition, a complaint of premature ejaculation on the rare occasions when he could maintain an erection intravaginally. During the treatment, greater attention was given to their relationship, rather than simply focusing on the sexual problem. At last report they had two children and had bought a house in the suburbs, and the sexual problem had again been resolved.

THE BULLY

J.P. is a muscular 24-year-old man who presented himself to the admitting office of a state hospital. He told the admitting physician that he had taken thirty 200-mg tablets of chlorpromazine in the bus on the way over to the hospital. After receiving medical treatment for the "suicide attempt," he was transferred to the inpatient ward.

On mental status examination, the patient told a fantastic story about his father's being a famous surgeon who had a patient die in surgery. The patient's husband then killed J.P.'s father. J.P. stalked his father's murderer several thousand miles across the United States and, when he found him, was prevented from killing him at the last moment by the timely arrival of his 94-year-old grandmother. He also related several other intriguing stories involving his $64,000 sports car, which had a 12-cylinder diesel engine, and about his children, two sets of identical triplets. All these stories had a grandiose tinge, and none of them could be confirmed. The patient claimed that he was hearing voices, as on the TV or in a dream. He answered affirmatively to questions about thought control, thought broadcasting, and other unusual psychotic symptoms; he also claimed depression. He was oriented and alert and had a good range of information except that he kept insisting that it was the Iranians (not the Iraqis) who had invaded Kuwait (referring to the Gulf War that took place in 1990–1991). There was no evidence of any associated features of mania or depression, and the patient did not seem either elated, depressed, or irritable when he related these stories.

It was observed on the ward that J.P. bullied the other patients and took food and cigarettes from them. He was very reluctant to be discharged, and whenever the subject of his discharge was brought up, he renewed his complaints about "suicidal thoughts" and "hearing voices." It was the opinion of the ward staff that the patient was not truly psychotic, but merely feigned his symptoms whenever the subject of further disposition of his case came up. They thought that he wanted to remain in the hospital primarily so that he could bully the other patients and be a "big man" on the ward.

Discussion of "The Bully"

Although this patient would have us believe that he is psychotic, his story, almost from the start, seems to conform to no recognizable psychotic syndrome. That his symptoms are not genuine is confirmed by the observation of the ward staff that he seemed to feign them whenever the subject of discharge was brought up.

Why does this fellow try so hard to act crazy? His motivation is not to achieve some external incentive, such as, for example, avoiding the draft, as would be the case in Malingering; his goal of remaining a patient is understandable only with knowledge of his individual psychology (the suggestion that he is motivated to assume the sick role because he derives satisfaction from being the "big man" on the ward). The diagnosis is, therefore, Factitious Disorder With Predominantly Psychological Signs and Symptoms (DSM-IV-TR, p. 517).

TOUGHING IT OUT

Mindy Markowitz is an attractive, stylishly dressed 25-year-old art director for a trade magazine who comes to an anxiety clinic after reading about the clinic program in the newspaper. She is seeking treatment for "panic attacks" that have occurred with increasing frequency over the past year, often 2 or 3 times a day. These attacks begin with a sudden intense wave of "horrible fear" that seems to come out of nowhere, sometimes during the day, sometimes waking her from sleep. She begins to tremble, is nauseated, sweats profusely, feels as though she is choking, and fears that she will lose control and do something crazy, like run screaming into the street.

Mindy remembers first having attacks like this when she was in high school. She was dating a boy her parents disapproved of and had to do a lot of "sneaking around" to avoid confrontations with them. At the same time, she was under a lot of pressure as the principal designer of her high-school yearbook and was applying to Ivy League colleges. She remembers that her first panic attack occurred just after the yearbook went to press and she was accepted by Harvard, Yale, and Brown. The attacks lasted only a few minutes, and she would just "sit through them." She was worried enough to mention them to her mother; but because she was otherwise perfectly healthy, she did not seek treatment.

Mindy has had panic attacks intermittently over the 8 years since her first attack, sometimes not for many months, but sometimes, as now, several times a day. There have been extreme variations in the intensity of the attacks, some being so severe and debilitating that she has had to take a day off from work.

Mindy has always functioned extremely well in school, at work, and in her social life, apart from her panic attacks and a brief period of depression at age 19 when she broke up with a boyfriend. She is a lively, friendly person who is respected by her friends and colleagues both for her intelligence and creativity and for her ability to mediate disputes.

Mindy has never limited her activities, even during the times that she was having frequent, severe attacks, although she might stay home from work for a day because she was exhausted from multiple attacks. She has never associated the attacks with particular places. She says, for example, that she is as likely to have an attack at home in her own bed as on the subway, so there is no point in avoiding the subway. Whether she has an attack on the subway, in a supermarket, or at home by herself, she says, "I just tough it out."

Discussion of "Toughing It Out"

Mindy describes classic, unexpected panic attacks. They hit her unpredictably with a sudden burst of fear and the characteristic symptoms of autonomic arousal: sweating, trembling, nausea, and choking, all severe enough to make her fear she will lose control. Unlike most patients who have such severe panic attacks (see "I Could Be Dying," p. 141), she has never associated particular situations, such as crowded places or public transportation, with having the attacks. Therefore, she does not show any symptoms of agoraphobic avoidance. Thus, the diagnosis is Panic Disorder Without Agoraphobia (DSM-IV-TR, p. 440).

TOY DESIGNER

A 45-year-old toy designer was admitted to the hospital following a series of suicidal gestures culminating in an attempt to strangle himself with a piece of wire. Four months before admission, his family had observed that he was becoming depressed: when at home he spent long periods sitting in a chair, he slept more than usual, and he had given up his habits of reading the evening paper and puttering around the house. Within a month he was unable to get out of bed in the morning to go to work. He expressed considerable guilt, but could not make up his mind to seek help until forced to do so by his family. He had not responded to 2 months of outpatient antidepressant drug therapy and had made several half-hearted attempts to cut his wrists before the serious attempt that precipitated the admission.

Physical examination revealed signs of increased intracranial pressure, and a computed tomographic scan showed a large frontal-lobe tumor.

Discussion of "Toy Designer"

Depressed mood, suicidal gestures, increased sleep, loss of interest, and guilt all suggest a Major Depressive Episode. Although the patient's symptoms are identical to those seen in a Major Depressive Episode, it is reasonable to infer that the disturbance is caused by the frontal-lobe tumor; thus, the diagnosis is Mood Disorder Due to Brain Tumor, With Major Depressive–Like Episode (DSM-IV-TR, p. 404).

Some clinicians might prefer to consider this diagnosis provisional, pending the results of surgery. If the depression lifts after removal of the brain tumor, the diagnosis of a Mood Disorder caused by the brain tumor would be supported. If the depression persists following surgery, the diagnosis would remain equivocal, as there would be no way to definitely rule out a Major Depressive Disorder that developed coincidentally.

The frontal-lobe tumor is, of course, noted on Axis III.

Follow-Up

The patient underwent surgery, and the tumor was removed. Two years following surgery, his wife described to the surgeon how hopeful she initially was following the surgery because her husband's depression seemed to lift. However, he never regained interest in returning to work and has spent all of his time at home. Although the patient makes few complaints, his wife describes him as lacking his former enthusiasm and "spark." In addition, he seems to have trouble concentrating while reading the paper.

The diagnosis at follow-up is changed from the original diagnosis of Mood Disorder Due to Brain Tumor. The predominant disturbance now is a marked change in personality, as manifested by the patient's apathy and indifference. Personality changes are common in Dementia; but in this patient, despite some difficulty in concentrating, there is no evidence of a global deterioration in intellectual functioning. Thus, the follow-up Axis I diagnosis is Personality Change Due to Brain Tumor, Apathetic Type (DSM-IV-TR, p. 190). The general medical condition, postsurgical removal of the frontal-lobe tumor, is noted on Axis III.

FREAKING OUT

In the middle of a rainy October night in 1970, a family doctor in a Chicago suburb was awakened by an old friend who begged him to get out of bed and come quickly to a neighbor's house, where he and his wife had been visiting. The caller, Lou Wolff, was very upset because his wife, Sybil, had smoked some marijuana and was "freaking out."

The doctor, extremely annoyed, arrived at the neighbor's house to find Sybil lying on the couch looking quite frantic, unable to get up. She said she was too weak to stand and that she was dizzy, having palpitations, and could feel her blood "rushing through [her] veins." She kept asking for water because her mouth was so dry she could not swallow.

She was sure there was some poison in the marijuana. Sybil was relieved to see the doctor, because she had believed the neighbors would not let her husband call him for fear of being arrested for possession of marijuana, and she was sure that without medical help, she would die.

Sybil, age 42, was the mother of three teenage boys. She worked as a librarian at a university. She was a very controlled, well-organized woman who prided herself on her rationality. She had smoked marijuana, a small amount, only once before, and the only reaction she had detected was that it made her feel "slightly mellow." It was she who had asked the neighbors to share some of their high-quality homegrown marijuana with her, because marijuana was a big thing with the students and she "wanted to see what all the fuss was about."

Her husband said that she took four or five puffs of a joint and then wailed, "There's something wrong with me. I can't stand up." Lou and the neighbors tried to calm her, telling her she should just lie down and she would soon feel better; but the more they reassured her, the more convinced she became that something was really wrong with her and that her husband and neighbors were just trying to cover it up.

The doctor examined her. The only positive findings were that her heart rate was increased and her pupils dilated. Adopting his best bedside manner, he said to her, "For Christ's sake, Sybil, you're just a little stoned. Go home to bed and stop making such a fuss." Sybil seemed reassured. He then walked into another room and told Lou, "If that doesn't work, we'll have to take her to the emergency room."

Discussion of "Freaking Out"

Sybil's bad experience with marijuana (cannabis) included characteristic physical symptoms such as dry mouth and increased heart rate. It was the mental symptoms, however, that caused her husband to seek help. Sybil became extremely anxious and had paranoid ideation (thinking that the marijuana was poisoned and that her neighbors would not let her husband call the doctor). This maladaptive reaction to the recent use of cannabis indicates Cannabis Intoxication (DSM-IV-TR, p. 238).

In diagnosing this case, we considered whether Sybil's paranoid ideation could justify a diagnosis of Cannabis-Induced Psychotic Disorder; we decided the answer was no. First of all, the neighbors might well have been reluctant to call the doctor as they would have had to admit that they were smoking an illegal substance. Second, Sybil was reassured by the doctor that the marijuana did not contain poison, whereas, by definition, a delusion is a false belief that is firmly held, even despite evidence to the contrary.

Follow-Up

Sybil was helped into her car by Lou (she still couldn't stand up) and went home to bed. She stayed in bed for 2 days, feeling "spacey" and weak, but no longer terribly anxious. She realized that, because the marijuana was homegrown, there was no reason to think that it contained any poison. However, she still believed her neighbors did not want to call the doctor because they were afraid of the police. She vowed never to smoke marijuana again.

CHARLES

A 25-year-old patient, who called himself Charles, requested a "sex change operation." He had for 3 years lived socially and been employed as a man. For the last 2 of these years, he had been the housemate, economic provider, and husband-equivalent of a bisexual woman who had fled from a bad marriage. Her two young children regarded Charles as their stepfather, and there was a strong affectionate bond between them.

In social appearance the patient passed as a not-very-virile man whose sexual development in puberty might be conjectured to have been extremely delayed or hormonally deficient. His voice was pitched low, but not baritone. His shirt and jacket were bulky and successfully camouflaged tightly bound, flattened breasts. A strap-on penis produced a masculine-looking bulge in the pants; it was so constructed that, in case of social necessity, it could be used as a urinary conduit in the standing position. Without success the patient had tried to obtain a mastectomy so that in summer he could wear only a T-shirt while working outdoors as a heavy construction machine operator. He had also been unsuccessful in trying to get a prescription for testosterone to produce male secondary sex characteristics and suppress menses. The patient wanted a hysterectomy and oophorectomy and as a long-term goal looked forward to obtaining a successful phalloplasty.

The history was straightforward in its account of progressive recognition in adolescence of being able to fall in love only with a woman, following a tomboyish childhood that had finally consolidated into the transsexual role and identity.

Physical examination revealed normal female anatomy, which the patient found personally repulsive, incongruous, and a source of continual distress. The endocrine laboratory results were within normal limits for a female.

Discussion of "Charles"

The diagnosis of Gender Identity Disorder (DSM-IV-TR, p. 581) is certainly suggested by the first sentence, which indicates that the person desperately wants to get rid of his primary sex characteristics and acquire the sex characteristics of the other sex because of persistent discomfort and sense of inappropriateness about his assigned sex. This case also demonstrates the other characteristic features of the disorder when present in an adult: a strong and persistent cross-gender identification manifested by dressing, living socially, and being employed as a man. As is almost always the case, there is no evidence of physical intersex or genetic abnormality.

The diagnosis is further specified as Adult Type to indicate current age and, with regard to the predominant history of sexual orientation, Sexually Attracted to Females.

Adults who have developed the desire to physically change their sex (previously referred to as Transsexualism) almost invariably report having had a gender identity problem beginning in childhood, although the onset of the full syndrome is (as with Charles) most often in late adolescence or early adult life.

CAT NAPS

Nora, a 24-year-old graduate student, complained of episodes of severe sleepiness that forced her to take naps. Sometimes when she attempted to stay awake, she was unable to do so; she had fallen asleep at the dinner table and even when walking. She had trouble staying alert enough to get off at the right bus stop. In fact, she was unable to remain seated without becoming sleepy, slept through classes, and failed her courses in graduate school.

Nora is bothered by frequent cataplexy, in which she becomes limp and briefly unable to move after sudden emotional arousal. This occurred, for example, when she discovered that her cat had urinated on her rug and when she had become enraged with her roommate. On another occasion she almost had a car accident when another driver did something that annoyed her and she almost lost control of the car.

As she falls asleep at night, Nora sees vivid scenes that seem real and feels that someone else is in the room. She still feels awake, however, and knows that there is really no one there. Her sleep is frequently punctuated by nightmares. She then wakes up feeling very hungry and has a snack.

Extremely bothersome to Nora is her continual automatic behavior, in which she suddenly discovers that she has accomplished very little after a lengthy period of work on a task. For example, she spent 2 hours unsuccessfully trying to fix her glasses and was unaware of this until her roommate interrupted her and pointed it out. The automatic behavior makes it difficult for her to change from one task to another, so it sometimes takes her 2 hours to get out of the house in the morning or to get ready for bed at night. Delays in getting to bed prevent her from getting a good night's sleep, which further aggravates her daytime sleepiness. Her roommates grew weary of her undependability, and she had to move back to her parents' home.

Previous treatment with a drug regimen consisting of an antidepressant, a stimulant, and a bedtime sedative was unsuccessful.

Discussion of "Cat Naps"

Nora's problem of sleep attacks and excessive daytime sleepiness is an example of hypersomnia. Her daytime sleep attacks, cataplexy, hypnogogic (when falling asleep) hallucinations, automatic behavior, nightmares, and disturbed sleep are the characteristic features of Narcolepsy (DSM-IV-TR, p. 615). Although traditionally this disorder has been regarded as a neurological disorder, to facilitate the differential diagnosis of hypersomnia, in DSM-IV-TR it is included in the Sleep Disorders section as an Axis I disorder.

> ## Follow-Up
>
> Nora was instructed to keep records of her in-bed times, nap times, cataplexy attacks, episodes of night eating, and automatic behavior. Psychotherapy was focused on examining the details of her failure to adhere to prescribed bedtimes, forgetting to take medication, and other behaviors that worsened her situation. She was withdrawn from the sedative, and her treatment with an antidepressant and a stimulant was empirically adjusted on the basis of the record she kept of her behavior.
>
> Nora's symptoms gradually disappeared, and she was able to move out of her parents' house, get a job, reestablish a social life, and return to graduate school.

A PRAYING ATHLETE

Richard Gramm, a 24-year-old African American man, was, when brought to the emergency room, mute and rigid. The friends who had brought him stated that he was playing basketball with them at the student athletic building when he suddenly put his head down on the floor, made sounds as if he were praying, and became "frozen." When interviewed an hour later, Richard would only say, "I am communicating directly with God."

According to his friends, Richard had been getting "hyper" recently, but they emphatically denied that he either used drugs or drank to excess. A call to his girlfriend, whose name and number were provided by his friends, revealed the following.

Richard had been doing well, with no evidence of unusual behavior, up until 1 week prior to admission. He had been living with his girlfriend, going to school, and working at a part-time job. One week before admission, he began to say "odd" things, usually of a religious nature. He also stopped sleeping at night and became sexually demanding of his girlfriend. He had begun working out even more than usual at the gym in order to "burn off excess energy." His girlfriend said that he had had similar symptoms when he was hospitalized 1 year previously. At that time he left the hospital against medical advice and had become increasingly depressed for about 3 months. He did not seek professional help. He withdrew from social activities at school and would spend up to 14 hours a day sleeping. Just when his girlfriend had decided to break up with him, he spontaneously returned to his normal self. She described him as a friendly, outgoing, energetic young man who was interested in school and athletics and performed well both academically and at work.

Toxicology screening in the emergency room proved negative, as did other medical tests. Physical examination revealed an extremely healthy, athletic young man who was largely mute and held his body in a rigid posture. The hospital chart noted one previous psychiatric admission a year before. The diagnosis was "Atypical Psychosis, rule out some kind of organic or drug psychosis." Richard had been in the hospital only 4 days, during which time he was observed to have auditory hallucinations and a delusion that he was communicating directly with God.

During the first few days of the current hospitalization, Richard was observed to alternate between "rigid posturing" and "mild hyperactivity." He would spontaneously become "unstuck" and begin pacing actively around the unit, talking about his newfound faith in religion to "anyone he could corral."

Discussion of "A Praying Athlete"

The bizarre behavior (becoming mute and rigid) that is the reason for Richard's admission to the hospital is a catatonic symptom. Traditionally, catatonic symptoms have been understood to be evidence of either Schizophrenia or unusual forms of a central nervous disorder. Now it is recognized that catatonic symptoms are also seen in Manic Episodes of Bipolar Disorder (DSM-IV-TR, p. 418).

Richard continues to have catatonic symptoms (rigid posturing) when he is in the hospital, but at other times he has the classic symptoms of a Manic Episode: his mood is expansive (we suspect that is what was meant by his friends' describing him as "hyper," "talking to anyone he could corral" about his religious ideas, and his girlfriend's description of him as sexually demanding); he is grandiose (communicates with God); he is hyperactive (paces); and he does not sleep. In addition, there is a history of what seems to be a Major Depressive Episode: he was extremely depressed and socially withdrawn and slept 14 hours a day.

Also characteristic of Bipolar Disorder is the rapid develop-ment of the Manic Episode and the full return to usual functioning between episodes of mood disturbance. Richard's delusion of com-municating with God is a typical mood-congruent, grandiose de-lusion. Therefore, we diagnose Bipolar I Disorder, Most Recent Episode Manic, Severe With Mood-Congruent Psychotic Features, With Catatonic Features (DSM-IV-TR, p. 389).

Follow-Up

An antipsychotic, thiothixene, and a mood stabilizer, lithium carbon-ate, were prescribed, and Richard's lithium level rapidly increased to therapeutic levels over the next 5 days. During this time his catatonic episodes became less frequent and his hyperactivity between epi-sodes decreased in amplitude. Twelve days after admission, Rich-ard's mental status was essentially normal, without hallucinations or active delusions. He was discharged, with follow-up through the university clinic. Richard had a mild depression about 1 month after discharge from the hospital. This was managed by increasing his lith-ium dosage. During the year of follow-up, no further psychotic symp-toms or depressive or Manic Episodes occurred.

USEFUL WORK

An 85-year-old man is seen by a social worker at a senior citizens' center for evaluation of health-care needs for himself and his bedridden wife. He is apparently healthy, with no evidence of impairment in thinking or mem-ory. He has been caring for his wife, but has been reluctantly persuaded to seek help because her condition has deteriorated, and his strength and en-ergy have decreased with age.

A history is obtained from the subject and his daughter. He has never been treated for mental illness and in fact has always claimed to be "im-mune to psychological problems" and to act only on the basis of "ratio-nal" thought. He had a moderately successful career as a lawyer and businessman. He has been married for 60 years, and his wife is the only person for whom he has ever expressed tender feelings and is probably the only person he has ever trusted. He has always been extremely careful about revealing anything of himself to others, assuming that they are out to take something away from him. He refuses obviously sincere offers of help from acquaintances because he suspects their motives. He never reveals his identity to a caller without first questioning him as to the nature of his business. Throughout his life there have been numerous occasions on which he has displayed exaggerated suspiciousness, sometimes of almost delusional proportions (e.g., storing letters from a client in a secret safe deposit box so that he could use them as evidence in the event that the client attempted to sue him for mismanagement of an estate).

He has always involved himself in "useful work" during his waking hours and claims never to have time for play, even during the 20 years he has been retired. He spends many hours monitoring his stock market investments and has changed brokers several times when he suspected that minor errors on monthly statements were evidence of the brokers' attempt to cover up fraudulent deals.

Discussion of "Useful Work"

This gentleman demonstrates pervasive and unwarranted distrust and suspiciousness of others. He expects to be exploited or deceived by others (e.g., assuming others are out to take something from him; first questioning callers before revealing his identity). He reads hidden threatening meanings into benign events (has changed brokers several times when he misinterpreted minor errors on his statements). He questions the loyalty or trustworthiness of others (his wife is the only person he has ever trusted). He is reluctant to confide in others (has always been extremely careful about revealing anything about himself). These lifelong features, in the absence of any evidence of persistent persecutory delusions or any other psychotic symptoms, characterize Paranoid Personality Disorder (DSM-IV-TR, p. 694).

This case illustrates the ego-syntonic nature of the disturbance. For this reason, treatment is rarely sought. It also demonstrates the frequently associated features of inability to relax (never has time for recreation) and restricted affectivity (has pride in being "rational").

> This patient has several schizoid features, but not enough to warrant the additional diagnosis of Schizoid Personality Disorder.

Music Lessons

Gary and Norma came to a sexual disorders clinic a few weeks after Norma had attended the funeral of her uncle. At the funeral she suddenly recalled childhood experiences with her uncle that made her think there might be a psychological basis for her sexual problems.

Gary and Norma were having sex approximately once every 1–2 months, and only at Gary's insistence. Their sexual activity consisted primarily of Gary stimulating Norma to orgasm by manually caressing her genitals while he masturbated himself to orgasm. Norma had a strong aversion to the male genitals and refused to touch his penis. The couple had recently discontinued attempts at penile-vaginal intercourse because Norma often had spasms of her vagina that made entry of the penis painful and difficult, if not impossible.

There were other problems in the marriage. Gary worked long hours and spent much of his free time visiting his widowed mother and doing errands or household chores for her. He also had a compulsive gambling problem and went to the race track three or four times a week. As their income was not large, Gary's gambling losses caused severe financial problems.

Norma had always had a strong aversion to looking at or touching her husband's penis. During the interview she explained that she had had no idea of the origin of this aversion until her uncle's recent funeral. At the funeral she was surprised to find herself becoming angry as the eulogy was read. Her uncle had been a world-famous concert musician and was widely respected and admired. As Norma became angrier, she suddenly recalled having been sexually molested by him when she was a child. From the ages of 9 to 12, her uncle had been her music teacher. The lessons included "teaching [her] rhythm" by having her caress his penis in time with the beating of the metronome. This repelled her, but she was too frightened to tell her parents about it. She finally refused to continue lessons at age 12, without ever telling her parents why. At some point during her adolescence, she said, she "forgot what he did to me."

Discussion of "Music Lessons"

Norma's traumatic sexual experiences with her uncle when she was a child apparently made it impossible for her as an adult to experience sexual activity as pleasurable. Norma is repelled by male genitalia and avoids sexual activity with her husband. Because, in Norma's case, this is not a symptom of another Axis I disorder, such as Major Depressive Disorder, the diagnosis of Sexual Aversion Disorder, Due to Psychological Factors, Lifelong Type, Generalized Type, is made (DSM-IV-TR, p. 542). In addition, she has persistent, involuntary spasms of the vaginal muscles that are so severe that coitus is impossible. This indicates a diagnosis of Vaginismus, Due to Psychological Factors, Lifelong Type, Generalized Type (DSM-IV-TR, p. 558).

LOAN SHARKS

A 48-year-old male attorney was interviewed while he was being detained awaiting trial. He had been arrested for taking funds from his firm, which he stated he had fully intended to return after he had a "big win" at gambling. He appeared deeply humiliated and remorseful about his behavior, although he had a previous history of near-arrests for defrauding his company of funds. His father had provided funds to extricate him from these past financial difficulties, but refused to assist him this time. The patient had to resign from his job under pressure from his firm. This seemed to distress him greatly as he had worked diligently and effectively at his job, although he had been spending more and more time away from work in order to pursue gambling.

The patient had gambled on horse racing for many years. He spent several hours each day studying the results of the previous day's races in the newspaper. He had been losing heavily recently and had resorted to illegal borrowing in order to increase his bets and win back his losses (called "chasing" in gambling circles). He was now being pressured by "loan sharks" for payment. He stated that he embezzled the money to pay off these illegal debts because the threats of the "loan sharks" were so frightening to him that he could not concentrate or sleep. He admitted to problems with his friends and wife after he had borrowed from them.

They were now alienated and giving him little emotional support because they no longer had any faith in his repeated promises to limit his gambling. His wife had decided to leave him and live with her parents.

During the interview the patient was tense and restless, at times having to stand up and pace. He said he was having a flare-up of a duodenal ulcer. He was somewhat tearful throughout the interview and said that although he realized his problems stemmed from his gambling, he still had a strong urge to gamble.

Discussion of "Loan Sharks"

This man is preoccupied with gambling, which has led to his being arrested for embezzlement and defaulting on debts and the disruption of his marriage. After losing money gambling, he borrows more to gamble again ("chasing"). He has destroyed relationships and lost his job because of his gambling. He relies on others to support his gambling habit. All of these features are clearly beyond the bounds of "recreational gambling" and indicate a disturbance in impulse control, Pathological Gambling (DSM-IV-TR, p. 674).

The essential features of this disorder are in many ways parallel to the features of dependence on a psychoactive substance. In both cases the person has impaired control over the behavior and continues it despite severe adverse consequences.

Although this patient has engaged in antisocial behavior, a diagnosis of Antisocial Personality Disorder is not appropriate because the antisocial behavior is limited to attempts to obtain money to pay off gambling debts and there is neither a childhood history of antisocial behavior nor evidence of impaired occupational and interpersonal functioning other than that associated with his gambling.

A complete diagnostic assessment would also make note of the duodenal ulcer (recorded on Axis III), which is apparently being exacerbated by the stress associated with his out-of-control gambling, recorded on Axis I as a Mental Disorder Affecting Duodenal Ulcer (DSM-IV-TR, p. 734).

A MAN WHO SAW THE AIR

A 20-year-old undergraduate presented with a chief complaint of seeing the air. The visual disturbance consisted of perception of white pinpoint specks in both the central and peripheral visual fields too numerous to count. They were constantly present and were accompanied by the perception of trails of moving objects left behind as they passed through the patient's visual field. Attending a hockey game was difficult, as the brightly dressed players left streaks of their own images against the white of the ice for seconds at a time. The patient also described the false perception of movement in stable objects, usually in his peripheral visual fields; halos around objects; and positive and negative afterimages. Other symptoms included mild depression, daily bitemporal headache, and a loss of concentration in the last year.

The visual syndrome had gradually emerged over the past 3 months, following experimentation with the hallucinogenic drug LSD-25 on three separate occasions in the preceding 3 months. He feared he had sustained some kind of "brain damage" from the drug experience. He denied use of any other agents, including amphetamines, phencyclidine, narcotics, or alcohol, to excess. He had smoked marijuana twice a week for a period of 7 months at age 17.

The patient had consulted two ophthalmologists, both of whom confirmed that the white pinpoint specks were not vitreous floaters (diagnostically insignificant particulate matter floating in the vitreous humor of the eye that can cause the perception of "specks"). A neurologist's examination also proved negative. A therapeutic trial of an anticonvulsant medication resulted in a 50% improvement in the patient's visual symptoms and remission of his depression.

Discussion of "A Man Who Saw the Air"

This young man is experiencing a variety of visual disturbances that are presumably similar to those that he experienced when he was intoxicated with the hallucinogen LSD. (For a description of the typical perceptual disturbances associated with LSD Intoxication, see "Dr. Hofmann," p. 536.) Mild and transient perceptual disturbances that occur long after cessation of use of a hallucinogen may be common. When the perceptual disturbance is severe enough to cause marked distress, as in this patient, it is called Hallucinogen Persisting Perception Disorder (Flashbacks) (DSM-IV-TR, p. 253). Usually such perceptual disturbances last for just a few seconds. More rarely, as in this patient, they are experienced throughout the day for long periods of time. The symptoms are often triggered by emergence from a dark environment or use of cannabis or of a phenothiazine. The symptoms can sometimes be reexperienced intentionally by the person.

LEATHER

A 35-year-old married writer sought consultation because he feared he might kill someone by acting upon sexually sadistic impulses.

The patient has been married for 15 years, and during the last year has had sexual intercourse with his wife approximately every other week. The patient's fantasy life is predominantly homosexual, however, and has been so since age 9. He has felt sexually attracted to males since childhood, but resisted acting on these impulses until mid-adulthood, long after he married. Before that, he felt sexually aroused by homosexual pornography (to which he was exposed from mid-adolescence), particularly by pornography with sadistic content. Although somewhat responsive to heterosexual pornography, his interest in it was much less than in homosexual pornography, and he was never excited by heterosexual pornography with sadistic content.

The patient had married for reasons of social propriety, and also because he consciously hoped that initiation into regular heterosexual activity would lead to diminution of his sadistic homosexual impulses. This was not the case, however. These impulses continued periodically to form the basis of the patient's masturbation fantasies. Typical masturbation fantasies were of a man bound, tortured, and killed. Sometimes the men in his fantasies were people he knew, such as colleagues or teachers, and sometimes movie stars or strangers. These fantasies were more intense at certain times than at others. The patient recalls, for example, that he was "wildly" aroused when he read about a homosexual lust murder as described in a detective magazine. Immediately following this, he masturbated many times a day, always with sadistic homosexual fantasies. After a few weeks, this period of intense arousal subsided, but the patient used the scenario of the events described in this magazine in subsequent masturbation fantasies.

About 8 years ago, the patient went to a gay bar with an associate from his office. At the time, he was under much pressure, and his work was being closely supervised by an aggressive, demanding male superior. The patient's associate was openly homosexual, and the patient allegedly went to the bar with him "as a lark." En route to the particular bar they visited, they passed other bars that, the patient's friend told him, were for "the leather crowd who like S and M [sadomasochism]." The patient had a brief homosexual encounter with someone he picked up in the bar they visited, following which he "put sex out of [his] mind."

Some months later, however, following a week of intense work at his office, the patient impulsively sought out one of the "S and M" bars he had previously walked past. There he met a man who was sexually aroused by being beaten, and the patient engaged in pleasurable sadistic activity with the understanding that the severity of the beating, administered with a belt, was under the control of his masochistic partner. That incident, occurring when he was age 28, was the first episode in a series of sexually sadistic activities, ultimately leading to his consultation. About once a month the patient would frequent a homosexual sadomasochistic bar. He would dress in a leather jacket and wear a leather cap. Once in the bar, he would seek out a masochistic partner and engage in a variety of activities, all of which the patient experienced as sexually exciting. The activities included binding the partner with ropes, whipping him, threatening to burn him with cigarettes, forcing him to drink urine and forcing him to "beg for mercy." The patient would experience orgasm during these activities, usually by "forcing" his partner to commit fellatio.

During the year before the consultation, the patient's wife had become progressively dissatisfied with their marriage. She was unaware of her husband's homosexual interest and of his sadistic tendencies. She felt, however, that his sexual involvement with her was desultory, and she wondered whether he had a mistress. She became confronting and also more hostile and demanding toward the patient. He realized that he "needed" his wife, and he did not wish the relationship to end, yet he felt unable to deal with her dissatisfactions directly. He avoided her as much as possible and argued with her when she insisted on talking to him. The patient's work pressures increased; he found, to his dismay, that the intensity of his sadistic impulses also increased.

On one occasion the patient convinced a partner to agree to being burned. Afterward, he felt guilty and ashamed. Just before the consultation, he bound a partner and cut the man's arm. At the sight of blood he experienced a powerful desire to kill his partner. He restrained himself and, alarmed that his sadistic impulses were out of control, sought psychiatric consultation.

Discussion of "Leather"

This man had first been aroused by sadistic homosexual fantasies in mid-adolescence. These intense sexually arousing fantasies persisted, and eventually he began to act on them. He married, hoping that marriage would be an antidote to his sadistic homosexual impulses, but found that this was not the case. He now enters treatment fearful that the sadistic impulses may become so strong that he will lose control and kill a sexual partner.

This is a fairly typical history of a person with severe Sexual Sadism (DSM-IV-TR, p. 574). This man was treated in 1978, before the AIDS epidemic. If he were seen now, one would certainly be concerned about his HIV status and whether his sexual activities were putting other people at risk for the infection.

NEW FACE

The patient, a single, unemployed 19-year-old male, was referred for psychiatric evaluation before undergoing surgery for a protruding mandible. The procedure was to create a new facial look and improve both function and aesthetics. The evaluation was requested to determine if there were any psychiatric contraindications to surgery.

The patient says that his jaw has been protruding since childhood; he feels it may have protruded because as a child he frequently stuck his tongue out, and "maybe this stretched my jaw." He knows his molars are in place, but the teeth on the sides are "pointed." His friends don't tease him about his jaw, but they do say, "You got a mug," and this upsets him. He describes himself as shy and feels it is partly from his self-consciousness about his jaw. He has difficulty talking and eating, as his teeth underbite and his tongue protrudes; thus, he cannot bite, but has to tear, his food. He has wanted to have his jaw fixed for a long time, but was "too shy" to ask about it. He says that, as a result, he hasn't seen a dentist for the last 4 years. He is aware that some teeth will have to be removed and that he will have his jaw wired for 6 weeks and will be on a liquid diet. He is uneasy about being unable to eat solid food. He hopes the surgery will correct his chewing problem and that he will feel better about his face and become more comfortable with other people.

The patient did well in school until he reached high school; then he started to cut classes and dropped out of the tenth grade. He worked for 2 years as a security guard. He is now unemployed, but wants to go back to school and become an auto mechanic.

The patient is the third in a family of eight children. His parents separated when he was 14. He lives with his mother and siblings. He argues with his siblings about doing household chores and, as a result, doesn't spend much time with his family; he just comes and goes and spends time with friends. He describes himself as quiet and shy. He restrains himself from telling his friends not to comment on his "mug," preferring to "keep it inside." He hopes that if the operation is successful, his friends will stop remarking on his looks.

When examined, the young man was noted to have mild acne and a very visibly protruding jaw with an underbite. His manner was somewhat awkward. There were no gross abnormalities of thinking, perception, or overt behavior. He denied ever having any problems with mood, sleeping, or eating, or in the use of alcohol or other drugs.

Discussion of "New Face"

The complaint of a defect in some aspect of one's physical appearance requires a clinical judgment about whether the complaint is out of proportion to any actual physical abnormality that may exist. A gross discrepancy suggests the possibility of Body Dysmorphic Disorder, or what has sometimes been referred to in the literature as "Dysmorphophobia." In this case, however, the interviewer notes the visibly protruding jaw and underbite, ruling out such a diagnosis.

The next question is whether or not the patient's reaction to his physical appearance is maladaptive, leading, for example, to marked social withdrawal, preoccupation, or depression. This does not appear to be the case. The young man is shy and sensitive to his friends' comments about his appearance, but this hardly indicates significant psychopathology.

On the basis of the limited information provided, there is no reason to suspect a mental disorder. Thus, the appropriate notations on Axes I and II are "No Diagnosis." His protruding jaw and underbite may be recorded on Axis III as relevant to understanding this young man, but the intent of Axis III is really to facilitate the recording of physical conditions relevant to a person with a mental disorder, which does not apply in this case.

GOODY TWO SHOES

Maryann West is an attractive, single 35-year-old woman, originally from San Diego, now working as a magazine editor and living by herself in a deteriorating Boston neighborhood. She was referred for psychotherapy by her female family doctor, who suggested she needed to work on problems in her relationships with men. Maryann resisted following through on the referral for a year, saying, "I don't like getting help. I like giving it."

When interviewed, Maryann appeared to be highly intelligent; she was affable and articulate and spoke in a breathy, girlish voice. She had metal-black hair, was dressed all in black—leather skirt and jacket and black top—and wore "punkish" glasses. She said, at the beginning of the interview, that she didn't want a male therapist because she was mistrustful of men, who, in her experience, wanted only to exploit women. However, with the exception of her family doctor, she had no close women friends.

Her story was that she had just extricated herself from a "destructive" relationship with a man, "my outlaw love," who was a heroin addict, and she was fighting her wish to return to him. Once, 4 years earlier, he had hit her and made her cry, but she told him that if he did that again, she'd leave, and it never recurred. She claimed she was not frightened of him and actually blamed herself for his attacking her. "I often tell him things he should know about himself, and he gets furious. I only do it to motivate him. I hit his soft spot."

Her lover's addiction persisted, and Maryann continued to support him financially whenever he needed help. She said she received many indications that this relationship could not make her happy. The man had gone out with other women while dating Maryann, served a brief jail sentence for selling drugs, and never wanted to engage in mutually entertaining activities, except sex, which was enjoyable. Maryann had gone to a university, but her lover had never completed high school. She felt that he was like a little child who needed mothering. He would tell her to get lost when she insisted he stop using drugs, but she continued to call him regularly in spite of his ungrateful behavior. She felt resentful and embittered because of all she had done for him, but she always helped him when he, typically, came back to her, late at night, asking for money or assistance. As a result, she said she felt "more like a Mother Teresa than a girlfriend."

Maryann is now seeing another "exciting" man, also a substance abuser. Although she considers herself "left-wing," her new friend is a collector of Nazi memorabilia. She knew that he treated his previous girlfriend cruelly by being unfaithful and abusive, but didn't think about whether this might happen to her. She has seen this man on and off for a year. He insisted he wanted a close relationship but did not tell her he was seeing one of her acquaintances on the side. When she found out about this, she was very upset, but continues to have an intense interest in him. A number of nicer men who had monogamous intentions have tried to date her, but she has avoided them because they were all "boring."

In her other relationships, Maryann always gives help, but never asks for it, even when she is in real need. Most of her friends and ex-boyfriends have been drug addicts or ex-addicts. She herself has never abused drugs. She often visits these people in jail and offers to help them; but when they are released, they hardly ever visit her.

At her job Maryann is hardworking and good at solving disputes, but she has sometimes gotten into trouble with her boss for arranging to use the magazine's resources to raise money for needy groups. She feels that her female colleagues "gang up on her" because of envy of her abilities and capacity for hard work, in spite of all the benefits that she has helped them obtain.

Maryann is the oldest of four children and often had to grudgingly care for her young siblings. She became a "goody two shoes," while her younger brothers were permitted to "act up." In church and school she did well and won many awards, until, in her teens, she rebelled and left home. Her parents predicted she would "go to hell." She went through a period of "sexual liberation" during which she had about 50 lovers, often in one-night stands, which she rarely enjoyed "because I didn't love those guys." As a young adult she was always involved in some worthy cause for the underprivileged, the poor, or the politically disadvantaged.

Discussion of "Goody Two Shoes"

Maryann seems to have gone through life playing the role of martyr. She has repeatedly been attracted to and chosen boyfriends who were inappropriate and mistreated her. She does not like to take help from others, and this has delayed her seeking treatment, even though she has realized for a long time that her relationships with people are harmful to her. She incites angry responses from others and then feels hurt when she is rejected (telling her boyfriend his failings). She is not interested in boyfriends who treat her well because they are "boring," and she engages in excessive self-sacrifice that is unsolicited by the recipients (visiting people in jail).

Behavior that appears to an outside observer as "self-defeating" may be observed when a person is in a situation in which he or she is afraid of being psychologically or physically abused, or when a person is depressed. In Maryann's case, however, it seems to be a pervasive personality pattern that expresses itself in many situations and relationships of her own choosing. This personality pattern has been called Masochistic Personality or Self-Defeating Personality Disorder. Many clinicians, particularly those who do psychodynamically oriented treatment of personality disorders, believe that this is a common and important diagnosis, which is nearly as common in males as in females. On the other hand, many clinicians, particularly those concerned with the potential for misuse of psychiatric diagnoses, have argued that the underlying construct of the disorder has no validity and that the diagnosis perpetuates blaming victims (primarily females) who have been abused. The category was included in an appendix of DSM-III-R after much controversy, but was eliminated entirely from DSM-IV. Such a case can still be diagnosed according to DSM-IV-TR as Personality Disorder Not Otherwise Specified (DSM-IV-TR, p. 729).

FLASHBACKS

A 23-year-old Vietnam veteran was admitted to the hospital 1 year after the end of the Vietnam War, at the request of his wife, after he began to experience depression, insomnia, and "flashbacks" of his wartime experiences. He had been honorably discharged 2 years previously, having spent nearly a year in combat. He had only minimal difficulties in returning to civilian life, resuming his college studies, and then marrying within 6 months after his return. His wife had noticed that he was reluctant to talk about his military experience, but she wrote it off as a natural reaction to unpleasant memories.

The patient's current symptoms began, however, at about the time of the fall of Saigon. He became preoccupied with watching TV news stories about this event. He then began to have difficulty sleeping and at times would awaken at night in the midst of a nightmare in which he was reliving his past war experiences. His wife became particularly concerned one day when he had a flashback while out in the backyard: as a plane flew overhead, flying somewhat lower than usual, the patient threw himself to the ground, seeking cover, thinking it was an attacking helicopter. The more he watched the news on TV, the more agitated and morose he became. Stories began to spill out of him about horrifying atrocities like those he had seen and experienced, and he began to feel guilty that he had survived when many of his friends had not. At times he also seemed angry and bitter, feeling that the sacrifices he and others had made were all wasted.

The veteran's wife expressed concern that his preoccupation with Vietnam had become so intense that he seemed uninterested in anything else and was emotionally distant from her. When she suggested that they try to plan their future, including having a family, he responded as if his life currently consisted completely of the world of events experienced two years earlier, as if he had no future.

Discussion of "Flashbacks"

This veteran has become totally preoccupied with his painful year in Vietnam. His combat experience obviously involved traumatic events in which he and others were threatened with death and that evoked feelings of fear and horror. He reexperienced this trauma through dreams and flashbacks. His responsiveness to his current environment became diminished (he was uninterested in things, emotionally distant from his wife, and had a sense of a foreshortened future). In addition, he had symptoms of increased arousal (disturbed sleep, outbursts of anger, and exaggerated startle response). This is the full picture of Posttraumatic Stress Disorder (DSM-IV-TR, p. 467). The disorder is further subclassified as Chronic, because the symptoms have been present for longer than 3 months, and With Delayed Onset, to indicate that the onset of the symptoms occurred at least 6 months after the trauma.

This patient displayed a common symptom seen in people who experience a life-threatening trauma shared with others: a sense of guilt that they have survived when others have not.

THE FAT MAN

Gregory, a 43-year-old theatrical manager, was evaluated at an eating disorders clinic in San Francisco. Although he had lost 58 pounds in the last 5 months, dropping from 250 to 192 pounds on a 6-foot, 1-inch frame, he was still terrified of getting fat.

Gregory first began to diet 5 months earlier when his wife told him he was "a fat slob" and implied that she might be considering a divorce. This terrified him and started him on a strict dietary regimen: an omelet and bran for breakfast, coffee for lunch, and salad and shrimp or chicken for dinner. His original goal was to lose about 50 pounds. When dieting did not result in sufficiently rapid loss of weight, he started sticking his finger down his throat to induce vomiting after meals.

Gregory is now "obsessed" with food. Before he goes to a restaurant, he worries about what he will order. He has done a study of what he eats in terms of what is easiest to purge, and he knows all the bathrooms in the areas he frequents. He cannot bear feeling full after eating and worries that his stomach is "fat." Three or four times a week he is unable to resist the urge to "binge." At those times he feels that his eating is out of control, and he may gobble down as much as three hamburgers, two orders of french fries, a pint of ice cream, and two packages of Oreo cookies. He always induces vomiting after a binge. He has never used laxatives, diuretics, or diet pills to lose weight.

Gregory is also preoccupied with being thin. He has progressively revised downward his original goal in dieting, first to 190, and then to 185 pounds. He has begun to exercise, walking at least an hour a day and, more recently, working out with weights several times a week. He believes that women look at him differently now: when he was heavy, they glanced at him casually; now their response is "admiring."

Gregory has always been somewhat heavy, turning to food in times of stress, but he never worried about his weight until his wife criticized his appearance. He can no longer enjoy any meals and feels he has lost control of this area of his life as he cannot stop dieting, even though his wife has told him he is now too thin. He therefore recently saw his internist, who found no physical problems and referred him for psychiatric evaluation.

Discussion of "The Fat Man"

Gregory's eating disorder began, as is often the case, with a reasonable attempt to lose some weight. He soon became preoccupied with losing weight and continued to view his body as "fat" even though others did not. This preoccupation with losing weight and distorted body image suggest Anorexia Nervosa, but this diagnosis is not made as Gregory has not let his weight go far below the normal minimum for his size.

Gregory's binges (recurrent eating of a large amount of food with a sense of loss of control), his recurrent inappropriate compensatory behavior in order to avoid weight gain (in his case, by self-induced vomiting), and the overconcern with weight and shape indicate Bulimia Nervosa (DSM-IV-TR, p. 594). As is usually the case in Bulimia Nervosa, the predominant method for avoiding weight gain is vomiting; hence the diagnosis is further qualified as Purging Type. Less common methods for avoiding weight gain are misuse of laxatives or diuretics (also considered as Purging Type), fasting, and excessive exercise (see "A Visit to Food Hell," p. 40).

This case is unusual in that Bulimia Nervosa, like Anorexia Nervosa, is far more common in women than in men.

FIRE SETTER

Mr. Rodriguez, a 52-year-old Cuban-born president of a successful family business in Miami, was brought to a hospital by his wife after he told her that he had suddenly remembered setting several major fires when he was a child and murdering a man 30 years ago.

Mr. Rodriguez tells the following story. He has been "on edge" recently because of a lot of financial problems in his business. A few weeks ago he became enraged with a long-time employee of whom he had been very fond, yelled at him for misspending a considerable amount of the firm's money, and almost threw an ashtray at him. He was stunned by the violence of his impulses and began to realize how angry and hateful he has always been, particularly in relation to his wife and children.

Later, at home, when thinking about the events of the day, "the curtains were opened and I was flooded with memories of acts that had previously been cut off from my conscious mind." He recalled having set fire to a woman's house while she was inside. This occurred when he was 5, at his father's urging. He also recalled having set fires in doctors' offices and libraries. In addition, he was convinced that, at 19, he had shot a man for having assaulted his wife. There were many other similar "memories" of violent acts, which he had never had before.

For 2 weeks Mr. Rodriguez stayed home from work. He sat, inactive, sometimes tearful about the damage he thought he had done, ruminating about what a terrible father he had been. Although his thoughts were painful, he actually "enjoyed the pleasure of knowing and discovering" and denied being persistently depressed. He also denied having experienced any change in weight, appetite, sleep, or psychomotor activity. He admitted to poor concentration, beginning about 1 month previously, when the financial pressures at work had begun to escalate. Sometimes he thought of killing himself.

The day before, he had had another sudden "revelation." He "remembered" for the first time that his father had beaten and sodomized him. He now understood that his destructiveness was caused by his father's abuse. With this realization, he no longer felt guilty about the terrible things that he had done. Nevertheless, he had agreed today to his wife's request that he come to the hospital.

Mr. Rodriguez is a tall, slender, neatly dressed man with a piercing gaze, poised demeanor, and polished manners. He smokes constantly throughout the session. He is quick-witted and playful, even when talking about the serious crimes he claims to have committed. He does well on tests of cognitive functioning. When told that his wife and others maintain that his memories cannot be accurate, he remarks, "Their facts do contradict my recollections. I can't explain the discrepancy. All I know is I set those fires." When asked to explain how he could have no police record, he replies that this is because he was so "quick and wily" that no one could catch him. He accounts for his wife's refusal to believe his stories by asserting that "she must have blocked the memories of the events because they are so upsetting to her."

On admission, physical examination of Mr. Rodriguez, including a neurological evaluation, revealed no abnormality. All laboratory tests were also negative.

Discussion of "Fire Setter"

There is no reason to believe that Mr. Rodriguez's "memories" are of actual events. We therefore conclude that he has many delusions about his past behavior. These delusions are not bizarre in that they involve situations that occur in real life, such as setting fires and committing violent crimes. Although Mr. Rodriguez was at first somewhat upset and depressed upon realizing what he had done, he does not have a full depressive syndrome, so the diagnosis of a psychotic Mood Disorder is ruled out. We therefore diagnose a Delusional Disorder (DSM-IV-TR, p. 329). The theme of Mr. Rodriguez's delusions, that he has done terrible things, is quite uncommon in Delusional Disorder and is not described by any of the specified types. Therefore, we would note Unspecified Type.

Follow-Up

Mr. Rodigruez was treated with an antipsychotic drug. Over the next few days the delusions became more and more vague. He said that he still felt as though he had set the fires, but acknowledged nonetheless that these events had never really taken place. Five days after medication was begun, he submitted a sign-out letter because he could "no longer stand the hospital." He did not appear to present any danger to himself or others, agreed to seek follow-up in Miami, and was discharged.

SEX IS A NASTY BUSINESS

Clara, a 33-year-old secretary, was referred by her gynecologist to a clinic specializing in sexual problems. The immediate reason for the referral was that he had been unable to conduct a pelvic examination because of extreme contractions of her paravaginal muscles.

At the first clinic visit, Clara was visibly uncomfortable as she discussed her sexual problems. Since the birth of her son, 2 years ago, she has been unable to have sexual intercourse because of vaginal spasms that are so extreme that neither her husband's nor her own little finger can be inserted into the vagina. She never looks forward to sexual contact with her husband and actively discourages his advances. Recently her husband has been pressuring her to become pregnant again. She would like to become pregnant both to please him and because she herself wants another child.

The onset of the paravaginal muscle spasms had been at an earlier time. A virgin at the time of her marriage, 8 years previously, Clara had not been able to allow vaginal penetration for the first year. After a year of an "unconsummated marriage," she and her husband had seen a marriage counselor, who had helped them considerably so that they were able to have intercourse, at least episodically, over the next 5 years. Clara had always had some anxiety about vaginal penetration and didn't really like it, although she could be orgasmic, albeit rarely, with appropriate sexual stimulation.

Clara was unable to get pregnant during the first 5 years of her marriage, apparently because of chronic endometriosis. When she finally gave birth, the baby was premature, weighing only 3 pounds, and was delivered about 11 weeks early. Clara felt guilty about having caused the premature birth, which she attributed to her having taken estrogen for the endometriosis. Since the birth, she has been extremely fearful of becoming pregnant again and possibly delivering another premature child.

Clara recalled the difficulty that her mother had in talking to her about menstruation and sex. Clara's religious upbringing precluded any discussion of premarital sex, birth control, and abortion, which were all considered sinful. She knew nothing about the use of a condom as a birth-control device. She acknowledged not knowing where her clitoris was and was unable to identify it on a model. She had never masturbated and indeed had learned about masturbation only recently. She expressed an aversion toward her husband's licking or sucking parts of her body, describing this as "yucky." She described a lifelong fear of bathtub water getting into her vagina and "infecting" her. She recalled dreams in which large and frightening objects penetrated her body.

Discussion of "Sex Is a Nasty Business"

Clara has a number of Sexual Dysfunctions, but her major difficulty at the present time is contraction of her paravaginal muscles, demonstrated, as it often is, during a pelvic examination. Recurrent or persistent involuntary spasm of the musculature of the outer third of the vagina that interferes with sexual intercourse is called Vaginismus and is classified as a Sexual Pain Disorder (DSM-IV-TR, p. 558).

Clara also has a lifelong aversion to anything connected with sex. Her avoidance of almost all genital sexual activity justifies the diagnosis of Sexual Aversion Disorder (DSM-IV-TR, p. 542). On the rare occasions when she does have sexual intercourse, she undoubtedly also has difficulty becoming sexually aroused and having an orgasm. However, diagnosing Female Sexual Arousal Disorder and Female Orgasmic Disorder (Inhibited Female Orgasm) would seem to be superfluous at the present time as she now so rarely has sexual intercourse.

Follow-Up

Treatment involved a combination of conjoint sessions to deal with the husband's frustration, anger, and impatience and to secure his cooperation in exercises that were designed to focus on sensual pleasure without intercourse (sensate focus exercises). Clara also had individual sessions and was given an antianxiety drug.

The main focus of treatment, however, was on vaginal dilatation, with Clara using her own fingers in a tub of warm water. Her progress with vaginal dilatation was slow and went through a series of gradual steps in which she could introduce the tip of one finger at the beginning and, gradually, two or three fingers. When the sensate focus exercises were added to the dilatation, she disliked her husband's sucking, licking, and kissing; she had to spend a great deal of time trying to achieve some comfort with her own body. This was later enhanced by group therapy for inorgasmic women.

Seen at first weekly, and then monthly, Clara slowly made progress, allowing penetration during intercourse to occur. She was still frightened of pregnancy, even when her husband used a condom, expressing marked fear that the condom would break or slip off. After several more months of therapy, her fear of pregnancy diminished, so that intercourse could take place without birth control.

TRACTION

The patient is a previously healthy 32-year-old carpenter from Nevada who was involved in a motor vehicle accident as he was returning from a 3-month trip to Mexico. He was found by the state police and taken to the hospital. On admission, he was revealed to have multiple fractures involving his pelvis, the toes of his right foot, and several ribs on his left side. He also sustained two small cuts on his head that required stitches. The patient reported that he had had a period of amnesia of about fifteen minutes and that he had lost consciousness during the accident, but this was not witnessed. He was alert and complained of severe back pain; he was not disoriented. He was treated with a narcotic, meperidine, 125 mg im tid; ahypnotic, secobarbital sodium, 100 mg po qhs; and a preanesthetic, promethazine, 25 mg im q3h. The following day his back pain was unimproved, and his pain medication was changed to morphine in addition to the promethazine.

Two days later he developed a fever and was sweaty and tremulous. Because a history of drinking five to six beers a day had been elicited, the diagnosis of Alcohol Withdrawal was considered, and a minor tranquilizer, diazepam, 5 mg po q6h, was added to his daily medication regimen, which at this time included Tylox (a combination of acetaminophen and oxycodone; an analgesic [narcotic]), 1 or 2 capsules po q3h–q4h, and secobarbital sodium, 100 mg qhs. The next day he was described as anxious, agitated, and constantly scratching. Two days later he was still febrile. Blood cultures, urinalysis, and chest X-ray were negative. Hydroxyzine, a tranquilizer, 25 mg po qid, was given to relieve itching.

The next day, 1 week after admission, the patient was noted to be disoriented. He complained that it took him some time to realize where he was upon awakening. His temperature was still elevated. He was receiving morphine, 3–10 mg q3h for pain; diazepam as a muscle relaxant, 5 mg po q6h; and flurazepam, a hypnotic, 30 mg po qhs. The next day, his pain medication was again changed, this time to percodan, a narcotic, 1–2 tablets q3h; and meperidine, 75 mg im q4h.

One day later the patient underwent an open reduction for a fractured left acetabulum. The surgery, done under general anesthesia, was tolerated well; but immediately following the procedure, the patient was disoriented to time and place and was noted to be picking at things in the air. His temperature was still elevated, and there was no documented source of infection. At this time the patient was taking meperidine, 75–100 mg im q4h; hydroxyzine, 75 mg q3h; and acetaminophen, 500 mg q4h.

Over the next few days the patient's mental status improved, although he was still disoriented at times and confessed, "You know, sometimes I can't pay attention to what you're saying." His temperature was still moderately elevated. Medication consisted of a synthetic opioid, hydromorphone, 2–4 mg q3h–q4h. The continuing periods of disorientation disturbed his doctors, and a psychiatric consultation was requested.

Upon initial interview, now 17 days after the accident, the patient was alert, fully oriented, and in good spirits. Results of mental status testing were normal. The patient admitted having had difficulties in thinking and "hallucinations" at times during the previous couple of weeks. He described them as "opiate dreams," caused by his pain medication.

Over the next few days, his condition was generally improved during the daytime hours, but at night he was frequently found to be taking his traction apparatus apart. When discovered, he would sometimes talk incoherently about the "traction thingamajig." If questioned the next day, he always denied having dismantled the equipment. At this time he was taking Tylox, two capsules q6h, for pain. He often complained of severe pain, many times arguing with his doctors in an attempt to persuade them to give him Tylox more often. The psychiatrist was called in again to help, and the Tylox dose was given more frequently. It was felt that his addiction potential was not very high at that time.

Several days later the patient was observed to be playing with fecal matter in his bed and once again dismantling his traction apparatus. When discovered, he admitted to these acts, was so upset that he could not sleep that night, and asked to see a psychiatrist. When interviewed, he appeared anxious and angry. He stated that he did not understand what was happening to him and was very upset about his behavior. He said he had not been sleeping more than 2–3 hours a night for at least 2 weeks. He was very frightened by the thought that his mind was doing things he was not aware of and could not control. He asked for a "game plan" to stop this behavior and even suggested stopping all pain medication if necessary. Over the next few days, pain medication was reduced. The patient now appeared alert and oriented, and there were no further episodes of disturbed behavior at night.

Discussion of "Traction"

Beginning with the second day of hospitalization and continuing for several weeks, this man intermittently had reduced ability to maintain attention to external stimuli ("I can't pay attention to what you are saying"), and disorganized thinking (he talked incoherently). He also had a reduced level of consciousness (it took him some time to realize where he was upon awakening), and visual hallucinations (he picked at things in the air and had "opiate dreams"). These are the characteristic features of a Delirium, and in this case there is no difficulty in identifying several physical factors that could have contributed to the development of the disturbance: infection, fever, and the large number of analgesics and sedatives that the patient received. (It is not clear from the case record why his medications were so often changed.) The diagnosis is therefore Delirium Due to Multiple Etiologies (DSM-IV-TR, p. 147). For coding purposes DSM-IV-TR requires that the specific codes for the different types of deliria (e.g., because of infection, being substance induced) be listed on Axis I. On Axis III the general medical conditions that we think caused or contributed to the Delirium would be noted.

FOOD FOR THOUGHT

Mr. Grim is a 46-year-old advertising salesman and writer for a small magazine. During 15 years of marriage, his wife had noticed loud snoring and episodes, lasting 10–15 seconds, during which he did not breathe. "Then he takes a giant breath, exhales, inhales one to four or five times, then he stops breathing for another one of these silences." During longer "not-breathing" periods, as she called them, "He is very restless. He can dish out quite a kick or punch if I haven't moved far enough out of the way." After nights full of such events, Mr. Grim groggily drags himself out of bed, finding he has a headache.

Mr. Grim is usually sleepy during the day, especially while driving the turnpikes around New England, which his work requires. To remain vigilant, he munches on coin-machine sandwiches, washed down by gallons of Coca Cola. Any alcoholic beverages make him want to fall asleep.

As a result of his snacks, Mr. Grim has 280 pounds packed onto his 5-foot, 8-inch frame. He is able to diet and lose weight only temporarily. Recently he has developed a hiatus hernia (associated with stomach pain and indigestion), mild diabetes, and high blood pressure, all complications of the obesity.

When he was a child, the patient's mother constantly berated him for being too fat, and he feared she would starve him. It was then that he developed a habit of stopping for food whenever he was out of the house.

Nasal stuffiness during the ragweed season worsened his snoring, the nocturnal "struggles," and the morning headaches. Just before his first interview about his sleep problems, he had cleaned out an old barn and attic, both full of dust and pigeon droppings, and had had a severe allergy attack. It was for this reason that he now came for help.

Physical examination disclosed a deviated nasal septum, enlargement and thickening of pharyngeal structures, and collapse of his pharyngeal walls into the airway upon taking a deep breath with his nose blocked.

A daytime continuous performance test was administered. The test involved his pushing a button whenever he saw certain letters presented at a rate of one per second. He scored 44% correct (compared with a normal rate of 66% to 78%), indicating moderate impairment in concentration, which was worse in the morning. Laboratory sleep monitoring revealed recurrent 15-second to 66-second periods of not breathing (sleep apnea), associated with decreased oxygen saturation (frequently below 50%) and decreased heart rate (50–55 beats per minute), followed by increased rates (to about 90 per minute). No normal periods of deep sleep were recorded on the polysomnograph. These findings indicated severe sleep apnea, which interfered with the quality of his nocturnal sleep and caused his daytime sleepiness and impaired daytime arousal. The clinician decided that Mr. Grim's obesity and the structural and functional impairment of his upper airway were the cause of the apnea.

Discussion of "Food for Thought"

Mr. Grim's primary problem is chronic excessive daytime sleepiness (hypersomnia), which is caused by recurrent periods of sleep apnea, which in turn result in sleep that is adequate in amount but not restful. On Axis I we note the sleep problem as Breathing-Related Sleep Disorder (DSM-IV-TR, p. 622). On Axis III we note the associated general medical conditions: sleep apnea associated with obesity, deviated nasal septum, and other upper airway obstructions. We also note the hypertension, hiatus hernia, and diabetes.

The cluster of symptoms that Mr. Grim has—loud snoring, respiratory pauses, upper airway problems, obesity, and hypertension—is commonly seen in people with the chief complaint of hypersomnia who present at sleep disorders centers.

Follow-Up

Treatment of the sleep apnea was by continuous positive airway pressure, a technique in which the pressure of the inspired air is increased by a machine connected to the patient with a tube and face mask at night, which helps overcome the airway obstruction. The patient's snoring and sleepiness were rapidly relieved, and he was now motivated, for the first time, to stay on a diet. Within 6 months he lost 80 pounds. He said he felt "like I have gotten my youth back."

Empty Shell

The patient is a 23-year-old veterinary assistant admitted for her first psychiatric hospitalization. She arrived late at night, referred by a local psychiatrist, saying, "I don't really need to be here."

Three months before admission, the patient learned that her mother had become pregnant. She began drinking heavily, ostensibly in order to sleep nights. While drinking she became involved in a series of "one-night stands." Two weeks before admission, she began feeling panicky and having experiences in which she felt as if she were removed from her body and in a trance. During one of these episodes, she was stopped by the police while wandering on a bridge late at night. The next day, in response to hearing a voice repeatedly telling her to jump off a bridge, she ran to her supervisor and asked for help. Her supervisor, seeing her distraught and also noting scars from a recent wrist slashing, referred her to a psychiatrist, who then arranged for her immediate hospitalization.

At the time of the hospitalization, the patient appeared as a disheveled and frail, but appealing, waif. She was cooperative, coherent, and frightened. Although she did not feel hospitalization was needed, she welcomed the prospect of relief from her anxiety and depersonalization. She acknowledged that she had had feelings of loneliness and inadequacy and brief periods of depressed mood and anxiety since adolescence. Recently she had been having fantasies that she was stabbing herself or a little baby with a knife. She complained that she was "just an empty shell that is transparent to everyone."

The patient's parents divorced when she was 3, and for the next 5 years she lived with her maternal grandmother and her mother, who had a severe drinking problem. The patient had night terrors during which she would frequently end up sleeping with her mother. At 6 she went to a special boarding school for a year and a half, after which she was withdrawn by her mother, against the advice of the school. When she was 8, her maternal grandmother died; and she recalls trying to conceal her grief about this from her mother. She spent most of the next 2 years living with various relatives, including a period with her father, whom she had not seen since the divorce. When she was 9, her mother was hospitalized with a diagnosis of Schizophrenia. From age 10 through college, the patient lived with an aunt and uncle but had ongoing and frequent contacts with her mother. Her school record was consistently good.

Since adolescence she has dated regularly, having an active, but rarely pleasurable, sex life. Her relationships with men usually end abruptly after she becomes angry with them when they disappoint her in some apparently minor way. She then concludes that they were "no good to begin with." She has had several roommates, but has had trouble establishing a stable living situation because of her jealousy about sharing her roommates with others and her manipulative efforts to keep them from seeing other people.

Since college she has worked steadily and well as a veterinary assistant. At the time of admission, she was working a night shift in a veterinary hospital and living alone.

Discussion of "Empty Shell"

This patient demonstrates the characteristic features of Borderline Personality Disorder (DSM-IV-TR, p. 710). She clearly has a pattern of unstable interpersonal relationships, self-image, affects, and control over impulses. Her relationships with men have been intense and unstable, ending when she becomes angry and devalues them. She reports that she is an "empty shell," evidence of chronic feelings of emptiness and a distorted self-image. Affective instability is suggested by the reference to her having brief periods of depressed mood and anxiety since adolescence. In addition, at least during the present episode, she demonstrates impulsivity (drinking and sex) and suicidal gestures or self-mutilating acts (slashing her wrists). It is quite likely that these characteristics have also been present during periods of stress in the past.

What about her recent symptoms? In the past 3 months, since hearing of her mother's pregnancy, this young woman has begun drinking heavily, has had several episodes of what appears to be depersonalization, and has been anxious, depressed, and suicidal. In addition, she briefly had auditory hallucinations telling her to kill herself. The diagnosis of a psychotic disorder, such as Psychotic Disorder Not Otherwise Specified, for the current episode is not warranted because the brief hallucination and her reaction to it as ego-dystonic are an example of the transient stress-related psychotic experiences that are often a feature of Borderline Personality Disorder. For the same reason, the diagnosis of Depersonalization Disorder to account for her recent symptoms of depersonalization is superfluous.

The patient's recent symptoms suggest other Axis I disorders, including Major Depressive Disorder, Alcohol Abuse, and Adjustment Disorder. Although she is depressed, there is no evidence of a sustained full depressive syndrome, which is required for the diagnosis of Major Depressive Disorder. We would add the diagnosis of Alcohol Abuse (DSM-IV-TR, p. 214) on Axis I to describe her significant recent problems with alcohol. Because the disturbance clearly represents an exacerbation of Borderline Personality Disorder, Adjustment Disorder would not be diagnosed.

Follow-Up

When she left the hospital, the patient resumed work and saw a woman therapist on a twice-weekly schedule. Her therapist felt that it was a tenuous relationship in which the patient sometimes seemed to seek nurturance or special favors and at other times was belligerent and viewed therapy as useless. After 3 months, the patient became involved with a new boyfriend and soon thereafter quit therapy, with the complaint that her therapist didn't really care or understand her.

FEAR OF FLYING

Lola, a 25-year-old laboratory technician, has been married to a 32-year-old cabdriver for 5 years. The couple has a 2-year-old son, and the marriage appears harmonious.

The presenting complaint is Lola's lifelong inability to experience orgasm. She has never achieved orgasm, although during sexual activity she has received what should have been sufficient stimulation. She has tried to masturbate, and on many occasions her husband has manually stimulated her patiently for lengthy periods of time. Although she does not reach climax, she is strongly attached to her husband, feels erotic pleasure during lovemaking, and lubricates copiously. According to both of them, the husband has no sexual difficulty.

Exploration of her thoughts as she nears orgasm reveals a vague sense of dread of some undefined disaster. More generally, she is anxious about losing control over her emotions, which she normally keeps closely in check. She is particularly uncomfortable about expressing any anger or hostility.

Physical examination revealed no abnormality.

Discussion of "Fear of Flying"

Lola's sexual difficulties are limited to the orgasm phase of the sexual response cycle (she has no difficulty in desiring sex or in becoming excited). During lovemaking there is what would ordinarily be an adequate amount of stimulation. The report of a "vague sense of dread of some undefined disaster" as she approaches orgasm is evidence that her inability to have orgasms represents a pathological inhibition. There is no suggestion of any other Axis I disorder or any physical disorder that could account for the disturbance. Thus, the diagnosis is Female Orgasmic Disorder Due to Psychological Factors, Lifelong Type, Generalized Type (DSM-IV-TR, p. 549).

If with treatment it became apparent that the fear of loss of control was a symptom of a Personality Disorder, such as Obsessive-Compulsive Personality Disorder, the diagnosis of a Sexual Dysfunction would still be made. However, if the sexual dysfunction occurred exclusively during the course of another Axis I disorder, such as Major Depressive Disorder, then the sexual disturbance would be assumed to be a symptom of the Axis I disorder and the diagnosis of a Sexual Dysfunction would not be made.

FALSE RUMORS

Bob, age 21, comes to the psychiatrist's office, accompanied by his parents, on the advice of his college counselor. He begins the interview by announcing that he has no problems. His parents are always overly con-

cerned about him, and it is only to get them "off my back" that he has
agreed to the evaluation. "I am dependent on them financially, but not
emotionally."

The psychiatrist is able to obtain the following story from Bob and
his parents. Bob had apparently spread malicious and false rumors about
several of the teachers who had given him poor grades, implying that
they were having homosexual affairs with students. This, as well as increasingly erratic attendance at his classes over the past term, following
the loss of a girlfriend, prompted the school counselor to suggest to Bob
and his parents that help was urgently needed. Bob claimed that his academic problems were exaggerated, his success in theatrical productions
was being overlooked, and he was in full control of the situation. He did
not deny that he spread the false rumors, but he showed no remorse or
apprehension about possible repercussions for himself.

Bob is a tall, stylishly dressed young man with a dramatic wave in his
hair. His manner is distant, but charming, and he obviously enjoys talking about a variety of intellectual subjects or current affairs. However, he
assumes a condescending, cynical, and bemused manner toward the
psychiatrist and the evaluation process. He conveys a sense of superior-
ity and control over the evaluation.

Accounts of Bob's development are complicated by his bland dis-
missal of its importance and by the conflicting accounts about it by his
parents. His mother was an extremely anxious, immaculately dressed,
outspoken woman. She described Bob as having been a beautiful, joyful
baby, who was gifted and brilliant. She recalled that after a miscarriage,
when Bob was age 1, she and her husband had become even more devoted to his care, giving him "the love for two." The father was a rug-
ged-looking, soft-spoken, successful man. He recalled a period in Bob's
early life when they had been very close, and he had even confided in
Bob about very personal matters and expressed deep feelings. He also
noted that Bob had become progressively more resentful with the births
of his two siblings. The father laughingly commented that Bob "would
have liked to have been the only child." He recalled a series of conflicts
between Bob and authority figures over rules and noted that Bob had expressed disdain for his peers at school and for his siblings.

In his early school years, Bob seemed to play and interact less with
other children than most others do. In fifth grade, after a change in teachers, he became arrogant and withdrawn and refused to participate in
class. Nevertheless, he maintained excellent grades. In high school he
had been involved in an episode similar to the one that led to the current

evaluation. At that time he had spread false rumors about a classmate whom he was competing against for a role in the school play.

In general, it became clear that Bob had never been "one of the boys." He liked dramatics and movies, but had never shown an interest in athletics. He always appeared to be a loner, though he did not complain of loneliness. When asked, he professed to take pride in "being different" from his peers. He also distanced himself from his parents and often responded with silence to their overtures for more communication. His parents felt that behind his guarded demeanor was a sad, alienated, lonely young man. Though he was well known to classmates, the relationships he had with them were generally under circumstances in which he was looked up to for his intellectual or dramatic talents.

Bob conceded that others viewed him as cold or insensitive. He readily acknowledged these qualities, and that he had no close friends, but he dismissed this as unimportant. This represented strength to him. He went on to note that when others complained about these qualities in him, it was largely because of their own weakness. In his view, they envied him and longed to have him care about them. He believed they sought to gain by having an association with him.

Bob had occasional dates, but no steady girlfriends. Although the exact history remains unclear, he acknowledged that the girl whose loss seemed to have led to his escalating school problems had been someone whom he cared about. She was the first person with whom he had had a sexual relationship. The relationship had apparently dissolved after she had expressed an increasing desire to spend more time with her girlfriends and to go to school social events.

Discussion of "False Rumors"

This case was supplied as an example of Narcissistic Personality Disorder (DSM-IV-TR, p. 717), and the reader will certainly be struck by Bob's grandiosity and insensitivity to others (lack of empathy). In addition, he is extremely jealous of his siblings, he spreads rumors about a student with whom he was competing, and he believes others envy him. In identifying behavior that justifies two additional criteria required for the disorder, we make some inference from the limited case material that is presented. For example, we assume that the reason Bob has had trouble with authorities about conforming to school rules is that he does not believe the rules should apply to him, and this behavior is an indication of entitlement. We interpret his spreading rumors about teachers and peers as evidence that he is interpersonally exploitative. His need for constant attention and admiration is suggested by his dramatic presentation.

THUNDERSTORMS

Sheila, a 28-year-old housewife, sought psychiatric treatment for a fear of storms that had become progressively more disturbing to her. Although she had been frightened of storms since she was a child, the fear seemed to abate somewhat during adolescence, but had been increasing in severity over the past few years. This gradual exacerbation of her anxiety, plus the fear that she might pass it on to her children, led her to seek treatment.

She is most frightened of lightning, but is uncertain about the reason for this. She is only vaguely aware of a fear of being struck by lightning and recognizes that this is an unlikely occurrence. When asked to elaborate on her fears, she imagines that lightning could strike a tree in her yard and the tree might fall and block her driveway, thus trapping her at home. This frightens her, but she is quite aware that her fear is irrational. She also recognizes the irrational nature of her fear of thunder. She begins to feel anxiety long before a storm arrives. A weather report predicting a storm later in the week can cause her anxiety to increase to the point where she worries for days before the storm. Although she does not express a fear of rain, her anxiety increases even when the sky becomes overcast because of the increased likelihood of a storm.

During a storm, she does several things to reduce her anxiety. Because being with another person reduces her fear, she often tries to make plans to visit friends or relatives or go to a store when a storm is threatening. Sometimes, when her husband is away on business, she stays overnight with a close relative if a storm is forecast. During a storm she covers her eyes or moves to a part of the house far from windows where she cannot see lightning should it occur.

Sheila has three young children. She describes her marriage as a happy one and states that her husband has been supportive of her when she is frightened and has encouraged her to seek psychiatric treatment. She is in good physical health, and at the time she entered treatment there were no unusually stressful situations in her life or other emotional difficulties. Her parents separated shortly after she began treatment. Although she found this distressing, she felt her personal supports were adequate and that this occurrence did not necessitate psychiatric attention.

She describes her personal history as generally unremarkable in terms of any obvious emotional problems, except for her fear of storms. She feels that she may have "learned" this fear from her grandmother, who also was frightened of storms. She denies panic attacks, or any other unusual or incapacitating fears.

Discussion of "Thunderstorms"

Many people feel uncomfortable during thunder and lightning storms, but Sheila's persistent fear of this circumscribed stimulus is clearly excessive, causes her considerable distress, and is acknowledged by her to be unreasonable. Furthermore, the fear and the avoidant behavior frequently interfere significantly with her normal routine. These features indicate the presence of a phobia. Although she is afraid of being alone during storms, there is apparently no fear of developing a panic attack or some other incapacitating or embarrassing symptom when alone or in public places away from home, as in Agoraphobia Without History of Panic Disorder. Her fear of storms does not involve a fear of humiliation or embarrassment in certain social situations, as in Social Phobia, and it is not related to the content of the obsessions of Obsessive-Compulsive Disorder. Therefore, by exclusion, the diagnosis is Specific Phobia, Natural Environment Type (DSM-IV-TR, p. 449).

VERTIGO

A 46-year-old housewife was referred by her husband's psychiatrist for consultation. In the course of discussing certain marital conflicts that he was having with his wife, the husband had described "attacks" of dizziness that his wife experienced that left her quite incapacitated.

In consultation, the wife described being overcome with feelings of extreme dizziness, accompanied by slight nausea, four or five nights a week. During these attacks, the room around her would take on a "shimmering" appearance, and she would have the feeling that she was "floating" and unable to keep her balance. Inexplicably, the attacks almost always occurred at about 4:00 P.M. She usually had to lie down on a couch and often did not feel better until 7:00 P.M. or 8:00 P.M. After recovering, she generally spent the rest of the evening watching TV; more often than not, she would fall asleep in the living room, not going to bed in the bedroom until 2:00 A.M. or 3:00 A.M.

The patient had been pronounced physically fit by her internist, a neurologist, and an ear-nose-throat specialist on more than one occasion. Hypoglycemia had been ruled out by glucose tolerance tests.

When asked about her marriage, the patient described her husband as a tyrant, frequently demanding and verbally abusive of her and their four children. She admitted that she dreaded his arrival home from work each day, knowing that he would comment that the house was a mess and the dinner, if prepared, not to his liking. Recently, since the onset of her attacks, when she was unable to make dinner he and the four kids would go to McDonald's or the local pizza parlor. After that, he would settle in to watch a ball game on TV in the bedroom, and their conversation was minimal. In spite of their troubles, the patient claimed that she loved and needed her husband very much.

Discussion of "Vertigo"

This woman complains of a variety of physical symptoms (dizziness, nausea, visual disturbances, loss of balance) that all suggest a physical disorder; but thorough examinations by a number of medical specialists have failed to detect a general medical condition that could account for the symptoms. Therefore, the differential diagnosis is between undiagnosed physical symptoms and a mental disorder.

The context in which these symptoms occur suggests the role of psychological factors in their development: they recur at virtually the same time each day, closely associated with the husband's arrival home from work; the husband's angry tirades and verbal abuse are undoubtedly very stressful. Because there is no evidence that the patient is conscious of intentionally producing the symptoms (e.g., taking a drug that would induce such symptoms, claiming to have the symptoms when they are not present), the diagnosis of a Factitious Disorder or Malingering is ruled out. Although the symptoms resemble those of a panic attack, there is no evidence that they occur unexpectedly, thus ruling out Panic Disorder. The disorder, therefore, is a Somatoform Disorder—a mental disorder with symptoms that suggest a neurological or general medical disorder.

Because the patient's complaints are not part of a long-standing polysymptomatic disturbance involving many organ systems, Somatization Disorder is excluded. The symptoms are limited to an alteration in sensory functioning; hence, the diagnosis is Conversion Disorder (DSM-IV-TR, p. 498).

STAY HEALTHY

Mr. Michaels, a 28-year-old computer programmer, seeks treatment because of fears that prevent him from visiting his terminally ill father-in-law in the hospital. He explains that he is afraid of any situation even remotely associated with bodily injury or illness. For example, he cannot bear to have his blood drawn, or to see or even hear about sick people. These fears are the reason he avoids consulting a doctor even when he is sick and avoids visiting sick friends or family members and even listening to descriptions of medical procedures, physical trauma, or illness. He became a vegetarian 5 years ago in order to avoid thoughts of animals being killed.

The patient dates the onset of these fears to a particular incident when he was 9 and his Sunday School teacher gave a detailed account of a leg operation she had undergone. As he listened, he began to feel anxious and dizzy, he sweated profusely, and finally he fainted. He recalls great difficulty receiving immunizations and being subjected to other routine medical procedures through the rest of his school years, as well as numerous fainting and near-fainting episodes throughout his teenage and adult years whenever he witnessed the slightest physical trauma, heard of an injury or illness, or saw a sick or disfigured person. When he recently saw someone in a store in a wheelchair, he started wondering if the person was in pain and became so distressed that he fainted and fell to the floor. He was greatly embarrassed, when he regained consciousness, by the crowd of people surrounding him.

Mr. Michaels denies any other emotional problems. He enjoys his work, seems to get along well with his wife, and has many friends.

Discussion of "Stay Healthy"

Mr. Michaels is afraid of thinking about or being near a situation involving bodily illness or injury. He recognizes that his fear is excessive and unreasonable, but nevertheless he avoids such situations. Although the fear and avoidance behavior apparently do not interfere with his normal routine or social activities, he is quite distressed about having the fear, which is the reason he now seeks treatment.

His fear is unrelated to Obsessive-Compulsive Disorder (e.g., an obsession involving being infected with germs) or to any trauma that might precede Posttraumatic Stress Disorder (e.g., having witnessed mutilation on the battlefield); therefore, neither of these diagnoses is made.

Mr. Michaels has a Specific Phobia (DSM-IV-TR, p. 449) called Blood-Injection-Injury Type. He feels faint in the presence of the phobic stimulus, as do many people with this type of phobia. Feeling faint is rarely seen in other Specific Phobias, such as fear of flying or of animals, or in Social Phobia or Agoraphobia.

PANTIES

A single, 32-year-old male free-lance photographer presented with the chief complaint of "abnormal sex drive." The patient related that although he was somewhat sexually attracted by women, he was far more attracted by "their panties."

To the best of the patient's memory, sexual excitement began at about age 7, when he came upon a pornographic magazine and felt stimulated by pictures of partially nude women wearing "panties." His first ejaculation occurred at 13 via masturbation to fantasies of women wearing panties. He masturbated into his older sister's panties, which he had stolen without her knowledge. Subsequently he stole panties from her friends and from other women he met socially. He found pretexts to "wander" into the bedrooms of women during social occasions, and would quickly rummage through their possessions until he found a pair of panties to his satisfaction. He later used these to masturbate into and then "saved them" in a "private cache." The pattern of masturbating into women's underwear had been his preferred method of achieving sexual excitement and orgasm from adolescence until the present consultation.

The patient first had sexual intercourse at 18. Since then he had had intercourse on many occasions, and his preferred partner was a prostitute paid to wear panties, with the crotch area cut away, during the act. On less common occasions when sexual activity was attempted with a partner who did not wear panties, his sexual excitement was sometimes weak.

The patient felt uncomfortable dating "nice women" as he felt that friendliness might lead to sexual intimacy and that they would not understand his sexual needs. He avoided socializing with friends who might introduce him to such women. He recognized that his appearance, social style, and profession all resulted in his being perceived as a highly desirable bachelor. He felt anxious and depressed because his social life was limited by his sexual preference.

The patient sought consultation shortly after his mother's sudden and unexpected death. Despite the fact that he complained of loneliness, he admitted that the pleasure he experienced from his unusual sexual activity made him unsure about whether or not he wished to give it up.

Discussion of "Panties"

This man's first remembered sexual arousal was in response to pictures of women wearing "panties." Ever since that time he has had recurrent, intense sexual urges and sexually arousing fantasies involving the use of nonliving objects by themselves (panties, alone or worn by a woman). Furthermore, the fantasies, urges, and behaviors cause him marked distress and impairment in social functioning. These are the features of Fetishism (DSM-IV-TR, p. 570).

Fetishism should not be confused with Transvestic Fetishism, in which a heterosexual male is sexually aroused by dressing like a woman. Whereas in Fetishism the nonliving object (in this case, a female garment) is sexually arousing in and of itself, in Transvestic Fetishism, the female garment is sexually stimulating not by itself but by virtue of the person's having the experience of cross-dressing.

As is generally the case with the Paraphilias, the deviant sexual act itself gives only pleasure, and it is the secondary consequences (humiliation, fear of exposure, or criminal prosecution) that cause the person to seek treatment.

SITTING BY THE FIRE

Paddy O'Brien is a 26-year-old bachelor, living with his mother and two older brothers on the family farm in the west of Ireland. He is interviewed as part of a family study of mental disorders in Ireland.

Paddy is described by his mother as having been a "normal" youngster up until 14. He was average to slightly below average in his schoolwork. He had friends he played with after school, and he helped his brothers and father with the chores around the farm. When he was 14, he began to "lose interest" in his schoolwork. His teacher noted that he was "staring into space" while in class and rarely followed the work. Soon thereafter, his mother noticed that he no longer played with his friends after school but would just come home and sit in front of the turf fire. It also became harder and harder to get him to do the farm chores. Sometimes he would come in and say the work was finished. Only hours later would they notice that only some of the cows had been milked, or only some of the eggs collected.

When he was 16, because his condition had become progressively worse, Paddy was withdrawn from school and was admitted to the county psychiatric hospital. The hospital records indicate that he was socially withdrawn and had a flat affect. It was not possible to interest him in ward activities. No psychotic symptoms could be elicited.

Paddy has been in psychiatric care intermittently ever since that time. For the last year and a half, Paddy has been attending a day-care center 2 days a week.

When interviewed by the research team, Paddy is observed to be an obese, rather disheveled young man. He replies to most questions with a yes, no, or "could be." He denies any psychotic symptoms, feelings of depression or elation, or difficulty with appetite or energy. He does, however, admit to unspecified problems with his "nerves" and problems in sleeping. On probing, he admits to feeling uncomfortable around "people," except his family. Eye contact is poor; he looks at the floor during most of the interview. His affect is flat. Despite all attempts, the interviewer is unable to establish rapport with him.

According to Paddy's family, when he is not at the day-care center, he sits all day in front of the fire at home. Occasionally he can be encouraged to help with a farm chore, but he usually stops after about 15 minutes and returns to his chair by the fire. Unless prompted, he will not wash or change his clothes. He refuses to attend any social functions, and his childhood friends have long ago stopped calling at the house for him.

At the day-care center, Paddy sometimes works for brief periods of time at simple tasks in occupational therapy, but then soon quits and goes to sit by himself in the day room. Both the family and staff note that he is quite aware of what is going on around him, as reflected by an occasional perceptive comment. Neither his family nor any of the psychiatric staff who care for Paddy has ever been able to elicit any psychotic symptoms.

Discussion of "Sitting by the Fire"

Paddy has a pervasive pattern of social and interpersonal deficits marked by discomfort with and reduced capacity for close relationships. He also has cognitive and perceptual distortions and eccentricities of behavior. He is socially anxious and odd in appearance and has no friends or confidants. His speech is odd, and his affect is constricted. These are all characteristic of Schizotypal Personality Disorder. However, his clinical picture is so typical of the residual symptoms of chronic Schizophrenia, the negative symptoms and social impairment are so profound, and the deterioration from a previous level of functioning is so clear that his illness is not what is ordinarily thought of as a "personality disorder."

The definition of Schizophrenia in DSM-IV-TR does not permit the diagnosis in cases in which there have been only the "negative" symptoms of schizophrenia, such as affective flattening or marked apathy (avolition). However, Paddy's illness corresponds to the traditional Bleulerian concept of Simple Schizophrenia in that the primary symptoms of autism, loose associations or other "thought disorder," and affective blunting are present in the absence of any secondary psychotic symptoms (delusions or hallucinations), and the disturbance represents a marked deterioration from a previous level of functioning.

According to DSM-IV-TR, we would have to diagnose Schizotypal Personality Disorder, Severe (DSM-IV-TR, p. 701), although the marked change in functioning that Paddy experienced when he was about age 14 is certainly not characteristic of personality disorders. The diagnostic concept of Simple Schizophrenia (Simple Deteriorative Disorder) is included in Appendix B of DSM-IV-TR (p. 771) for criteria sets provided for further study.

MR. AND MS. B.

Mr. and Ms. B. have been married for 14 years and have three children, ages 8 through 12. They are both bright and well educated. Both are from Scotland, from which they moved 10 years ago because of Mr. B.'s work as an industrial consultant. They present with the complaint that Ms. B. has been able to participate passively in sex "as a duty," but has never enjoyed it since they have been married.

Before their marriage, although they had intercourse only twice, Ms. B. had been highly aroused by kissing and petting and felt she used her attractiveness to "seduce" her husband into marriage. She did, however, feel intense guilt about their two episodes of premarital intercourse; during their honeymoon, she began to think of sex as a chore that could not be pleasing. Although she periodically passively complied with intercourse, she had almost no spontaneous desire for sex. She never masturbated, had never reached orgasm, thought of all variations such as oral sex as completely repulsive, and was preoccupied with a fantasy of how disapproving her family would be if she ever engaged in any of these activities.

Ms. B. is almost totally certain that no woman she respects in any older generation has enjoyed sex and that despite the "new vogue" of sexuality, only sleazy, crude women let themselves act like "animals." These beliefs have led to a pattern of regular, but infrequent, sex that at best is accommodating and gives little or no pleasure to her or her husband. Whenever Ms. B. comes close to having a feeling of sexual arousal, numerous negative thoughts come into her mind, such as "What am I, a tramp?" "If I like this, he'll just want it more often" or "How could I look at myself in the mirror after something like this?" These thoughts almost inevitably are accompanied by a cold feeling and an insensitivity to sensual pleasure. As a result, sex is invariably an unhappy experience. Almost any excuse, such as fatigue or being busy, is sufficient for her to rationalize avoiding intercourse.

Yet, intellectually Ms. B. wonders, "Is something wrong with me?" She is seeking help to find out whether she is normal or not. Her husband, although extraordinarily tolerant of the situation, is in fact very unhappy about their sex life and is very hopeful that help may be forthcoming.

Discussion of "Mr. and Ms. B."

This couple seeks help for the wife's long-standing sexual problem. Clearly this woman's sexual difficulties stem from her many negative attitudes toward sexuality and cannot be accounted for by a nonsexual Axis I disorder, such as Major Depressive Disorder. The diagnosis of Sexual Aversion Disorder needs to be considered. Although she certainly has a persistent extreme aversion to genital sexual contact and might like to avoid sexual activity, she does, in fact, have regular though infrequent intercourse. The persistent absence of sexual fantasies and desire for sexual activity justify the diagnosis of Hypoactive Sexual Desire Disorder, Due to Psychological Factors, Lifelong Type, Generalized Type (DSM-IV-TR, p. 541). When she does have sexual intercourse, she probably does not become sexually excited, so the additional diagnosis of Female Sexual Arousal Disorder (DSM-IV-TR, p. 544) should be considered. The diagnosis of Female Orgasmic Disorder would be added only if there were many occasions when during sexual activity she failed to have an orgasm, but had no disturbance in sexual excitement—extremely unlikely in this case.

The absence of any significant complaint on the part of the husband is reflected in the notation No Diagnosis or Condition on Axis I for him.

BEASTS

A white man in his mid-30s, in prison for molesting prepubescent girls, volunteered for an interview with a sex researcher. He had been reared in a rural area by lower-middle-class parents with a grammar-school education. His mother, who was extremely prudish, frightened her son with tales of venereal disease and the dire consequences of masturbation and impressed upon him that all sexual activity was nasty and that men were "beasts." He therefore felt guilty about his heterosexual urges and his preadolescent heterosexual play and with puberty at age 12 ceased all heterosexual activity. Masturbation had begun a year before puberty and ceased a year after puberty, evidently because of the maternal warnings. During adolescence he was shy and fearful of females, although he desired them. Girls accused him of being "tied to his mother's apron strings."

He had always been sexually aroused by the sight of stallions and mares copulating and sometimes fantasized about animal contact while masturbating. He had heard of animal contact from his peer group, and, as a substitute for masturbation, he engaged in coitus with cows almost daily from age 13 to age 18. Some affectional component developed, such as one might have for a pet animal. However, he never found the idea of sexual activity with an animal as exciting as the idea of sexual activity with a girl.

When he was 18, an epidemic of brucellosis appeared among the farm animals in the region, and the young man associated this mentally with venereal disease—concerning which he had a deep horror, instilled by his mother. He therefore terminated his animal contacts. Lacking any adult heterosexual activity, and afraid to masturbate or engage in animal contacts, the young man reverted to his preadolescent pattern (which had been very gratifying) and began seeking contact with prepubescent girls. This led to his arrest and imprisonment.

Discussion of "Beasts"

The Institute for Sex Research at Indiana University, founded by Alfred C. Kinsey, was asked to submit a case for this book of Zoophilia, a specific Paraphilia Not Otherwise Specified that is recognized by DSM-IV-TR. A computer search of their extensive files of thousands of people interviewed between 1938 and 1963 revealed 96 cases involving intensive sexual activity with animals, but in not a single case was the animal contact or the fantasy of contact with animals the preferred source of achieving sexual excitement. Unlike the other Paraphilias, sexual activity with animals may always be a second choice, as it was in this case. Apparently there are no cases in which the idea of sexual activity with an animal is more exciting than the idea of sexual activity with a human.

The behavior that led to this young man's incarceration involved sexual activity with prepubescent girls. Therefore, the most likely diagnosis at the time of his arrest is Pedophilia, Sexually Attracted to Females (DSM-IV-TR, p. 572), with a history of Paraphilia Not Otherwise Specified (Zoophilia) (DSM-IV-TR, p. 576). When he was younger he apparently was attracted to adolescent girls. Therefore, we would also specify Nonexclusive Type to indicate that his sexual attraction was not limited to children.

BURT TATE

The patient is a 42-year-old white male who was brought to the emergency room by the police. He was involved in an argument and fight at the diner where he is employed. When the police arrived and began to question the patient, he gave his name as Burt Tate, but had no identification. Burt had drifted into town several weeks earlier and begun working as a short-order cook at the diner. He could not recall where he had worked or lived before his arrival in this town. There were no charges against him, but the police convinced him to come to the emergency room for an examination.

When questioned in the emergency room, Burt knew what town he was in and the current date. He admitted that it was somewhat unusual that he could not recall the details of his past life, but he did not appear very upset about this. There was no evidence of alcohol or drug abuse, and a physical examination revealed no head trauma or any other physical abnormalities. He was kept overnight for observation.

When the police ran a description check on the patient, they found that he fit the description of a missing person, Gene Saunders, who had disappeared a month before from a city 200 miles away. A visit by Mrs. Saunders confirmed the identity of the patient as Gene Saunders. Mrs. Saunders explained that for 18 months before his disappearance, her husband, who was a middle-level manager at a large manufacturing company, had been having considerable difficulty at work. He had been passed over for a promotion, and his supervisor had been very critical of his work. Several of his staff had left the company for other jobs, and the patient found it impossible to meet production goals. Work stress made him very difficult to live with at home. Previously an easygoing, gregarious person, he became withdrawn and critical of his wife and children. Immediately preceding his disappearance, he had had a violent argument with his 18-year-old son. The son had called him a "failure" and stormed out of the house to live with some friends who had an apartment. It was 2 days after this argument that the patient disappeared.

When brought into the room where his wife was waiting, the patient stated that he did not recognize her. He appeared noticeably anxious.

Discussion of "Burt Tate"

The police brought this man to the emergency room because of his amnesia concerning where he had previously lived and worked. This impairment in memory suggests a Cognitive Disorder, such as Delirium, Dementia, or Amnestic Disorder. However, ordinarily in such a disorder the disturbance in memory is more marked for recent than for remote events and there is often a disturbance in consciousness or orientation, which is not present in this case.

In addition to having amnesia, Mr. Saunders has assumed a new identity as Mr. Tate. Because there is no suggestion that the two distinct identities or personality states are alternating in recurrently taking control of this man's behavior, Dissociative Identity Disorder (Multiple Personality Disorder) is ruled out.

The critical role of psychological factors in the patient's amnesia becomes more apparent when we learn that just before the development of his symptoms, on top of increasing difficulties at work, he had a violent argument with his son. The additional feature of sudden, unexpected travel away from his home justifies the diagnosis of Dissociative Fugue (DSM-IV-TR, p. 526).

EGGS

Kevin is a 19-year-old white male who, until admission, was working in a mailroom and planning to apply to college. The onset of his illness is not clear. According to him, he has not been "the same" since his mother died of a cerebral hemorrhage 9 months before his admission. According to his father, however, he exhibited a normal mourning response to his mother's death and changed only 3 months earlier.

At that time, shortly after his girlfriend had rejected him for another man, he began to think that male co-workers were making homosexual advances toward him. He began to fear that he was homosexual and that his friends believed he was homosexual. He finally developed the conviction that he had a disorder of the reproductive system, that he had one normal testicle that produced sperm and that his other testicle was actually an ovary that produced eggs. He thought that this was evidence that a "woman's body resides inside my man's body." He began to gamble, and was convinced that he had won $400,000 and was not paid by his bookie and that he was sought after by talk show hosts to be a guest on their shows and tell his unusual story (all not true). He claimed that he had a heightened awareness, an "extra sense," and that sounds were unusually loud. He had difficulty sleeping at night, but no appetite disturbance.

On admission, Kevin's speech was somewhat rapid, and he jumped from topic to topic. His affect was neither irritable, euphoric, nor expansive. He said he was now seeking treatment because "there is a war between my testicles, and I prefer to be male."

When he was 10, his pediatrician became concerned that he had an undersized penis. This led to a complete endocrine workup and examinations of his genitals every 4 months for the next 4 years. At that time it was concluded that there were no significant abnormalities.

During high school Kevin had been a poor student with poor attendance. He claims always to have had many friends. He has never received psychiatric treatment. He admits to occasional marijuana and cocaine use in the past, but denies any use of hallucinogens.

Kevin is the oldest child in a family of six children. His parents met when they were both patients in a psychiatric hospital.

Discussion of "Eggs"

The significant features of Kevin's illness include bizarre somatic delusions, grandiose delusions, and disorganization in his speech (he jumped from topic to topic). Although the grandiose delusions and pressured speech suggest the possibility of a Manic Episode, this is ruled out by the absence of an elevated, expansive, or irritable mood.

When did his illness begin? Although he says he has not been the same since his mother died 9 months ago, he does not describe any change in himself that is out of keeping with normal bereavement. Furthermore, his father claims that his abnormal behavior began only 3 months ago. Giving the patient the benefit of the doubt, we date the onset of the illness at 3 months before admission. The presence of the characteristic symptoms of Schizophrenia in an illness of at least 1, but less than 6, months' duration, in the absence of a mood disorder or a substance use or general medical condition responsible for the disturbance, indicates Schizophreniform Disorder (DSM-IV-TR, p. 319). Kevin's affect is not blunted or flat. However, because it is unclear whether the onset of the illness was within 4 weeks of the first noticeable change in his usual behavior (he and his father give different accounts), we are unable to subtype the disorder in terms of its prognosis.

Follow-Up

Kevin was treated in the hospital with lithium and chlorpromazine and was soon well enough to go home. He entered college the following fall and finished the first semester with A's and B's. The following year he stopped taking his medication and again became very disturbed. He was irritable, loud, angry, and verbally abusive. He talked incessantly, did not sleep, and ran naked into the street. He expressed bizarre ideas about "time running backward" and again believed that he had an ovary. There were several such episodes requiring hospitalization over a period of 3 years. Finally, he became convinced that he could avoid such episodes only if he kept taking medication. For the past year, he has been taking lithium alone and has been well. He has his own apartment and an active social life and has just passed a licensing examination to become a plumber.

The clinical picture of Manic Episodes subsequent to his first hospitalization certainly suggests the need to change the diagnosis to Bipolar Disorder with Mood-Incongruent Psychotic Features. In retrospect, there was a suggestion of expansive mood during his initial presentation, but it was not marked enough to warrant the diagnosis of a Manic Episode at that time.

THE FASHION PLATE

Mr. A., a 65-year-old security guard, formerly a fishing-boat captain, is distressed about his wife's objections to his wearing a nightgown at home in the evening, now that his youngest child has left home. His appearance and demeanor, except when he is dressing in women's clothes, are always appropriately masculine, and he is exclusively heterosexual. Occasionally, over the past 5 years, he has worn an inconspicuous item of female clothing even when dressed as a man, sometimes a pair of panties, sometimes an ambiguous pinkie ring. He always carries a photograph of himself dressed as a woman.

His first recollection of an interest in female clothing was putting on his sister's bloomers at age 12, an act accompanied by sexual excitement. He continued periodically to put on women's underpants—an activity that invariably resulted in an erection, sometimes a spontaneous emission, and sometimes masturbation, but was never accompanied by fantasy. Although he occasionally wished to be a girl, he never fantasized himself as one. He was competitive and aggressive with other boys and always acted "masculine." During his single years he was always attracted to girls, but was shy about sex. Following his marriage at age 22, he had his first heterosexual intercourse.

His involvement with female clothes was of the same intensity even after his marriage. Beginning at age 45, after a chance exposure to a magazine called *Transvestia,* he began to increase his cross-dressing activity. He learned there were other men like himself, and he became more and more preoccupied with female clothing in fantasy and progressed to periodically dressing completely as a woman. More recently he has become involved in a transvestite network, writing to other transvestites contacted through the magazine and occasionally attending transvestite parties. Cross-dressing at these parties has been the only situation in which he has cross-dressed outside his home.

Although still committed to his marriage, sex with his wife has dwindled over the past 20 years as his waking thoughts and activities have become increasingly centered on cross-dressing. Over time this activity has become less eroticized and more an end in itself, but it still is a source of some sexual excitement. He always has an increased urge to dress as a woman when under stress; it has a tranquilizing effect. If particular circumstances prevent him from cross-dressing, he feels extremely frustrated.

The patient's parents belonged to different faiths, a fact of some importance to him. He was the eldest of three children, extremely close to his mother, whom he idolized, and angry at his "whoremaster, alcoholic" father. The parents fought constantly. He is tearful, even now at age 65, when he describes his mother's death when he was 10. He was the one who found her dead (of pleurisy), and he says he has been "not the same from that day . . . always [having] the feeling something's not right." The siblings were reared by three separate branches of the family until the father remarried. When the patient was 20, his father died, a presumed suicide; but Mr. A believes he may have been murdered, as he could not figure out a suicide motive. His brother also died traumatically, drowned in his teens.

Because of the disruptions in his early life, the patient has always treasured the steadfastness of his wife and the order of his home. He told his wife about his cross-dressing practice when they were married, and she was accepting so long as he kept it to himself. Nevertheless, he felt guilty, particularly after he began complete cross-dressing, and periodically he attempted to renounce the practice, throwing out all his female clothes and makeup. His children served as a barrier to his giving free rein to his impulses. Following his retirement from fishing, and in the absence of his children, he finds himself more drawn to cross-dressing, more in conflict with his wife, and more depressed.

Discussion of "The Fashion Plate"

This man demonstrates the characteristic development and course of Transvestic Fetishism (DSM-IV-TR, p. 575). Over a long period of time, Mr. A., a heterosexual male, has acted upon recurrent intense sexual urges and sexually arousing fantasies involving cross-dressing. However, until recently, he would not have qualified for a diagnosis, since his urges and behaviors did not cause significant distress or impairment. Now that the behavior is affecting his marriage, he does qualify for the diagnosis. Since he is never in doubt about his gender identity as a male, the diagnosis Gender Identity Disorder does not apply.

Characteristically, his urge to cross-dress increases under stress, and the cross-dressing has a calming effect. If the behavior is prevented, he feels intensely frustrated. Frequently, as in this case, as the person becomes more involved in cross-dressing, the practice becomes less eroticized and more an end in itself. If the cross-dressing is no longer a source of any sexual excitement and there is a persistent sense of inappropriateness about being a male, the diagnosis should be changed to Gender Identity Disorder, Adult.

Three Voices

A 23-year-old man was admitted to the hospital. He was almost totally mute. His parents reported that he had been apparently well until about 4 years previously, when he broke off with his girlfriend. Since then he had been living at home, spending much time by himself, holding various odd jobs, and unable to pursue any long-term goals. About 4 months before his hospital admission, he decided to go to California to find a new job and change his environment. However, shortly after he arrived there, his parents received a telephone call from him in which he "sounded bad." His father flew to California and found him vigilant, paranoid, and frightened, having seemingly not eaten for several days. The father brought his son home, where he saw a neurologist and was found to be essentially normal neurologically. Shortly thereafter he saw a psychologist, who recommended admission to a psychiatric hospital.

On admission the patient was sleeping 10–12 hours a night, had little appetite, and had lost perhaps 20 pounds in weight over the last couple of months. He reported a profound loss of energy and did not speak except to give occasional monosyllabic answers to the interviewer's questions. During his first few days in the hospital, the patient showed virtually no interest or pleasure in any activities and spent most of the time sitting on his bed and staring into space. On questioning he did not complain of any specific feelings of worthlessness, self-reproach, or guilt, nor did he mention thoughts of death or suicide, although it was difficult to be certain about any of these points because of his paucity of speech.

In the hospital the patient was seen daily by a medical student who took a great interest in him and gradually gained his trust. Eventually the patient revealed to the student that he was hearing three distinct voices: the voice of a child, the voice of a woman, and the voice of a man impersonating a woman. The three voices talked among themselves and sometimes talked to him directly. At times they spoke about him in the third person, and on some occasions they seemed to echo his thoughts. The voices spoke about many different subjects and did not focus on any specific depressive themes, such as guilt, sin, or death.

On the second day after admission to the hospital, the patient was started on a regimen of antipsychotic and antidepressant medication. For the first 2 weeks there was virtually no improvement. By the second week he displayed some increased restlessness. The dosage of antipsychotic medication was reduced and was eventually stopped entirely by about the third week. On the twenty-third hospital day, the patient began to experience a marked improvement in his energy level; by the end of the fourth week, he was smiling, talkative, sleeping and eating well, and able to reminisce about the hallucinations, which he stated had now completely disappeared. A week later he was discharged home on a maintenance dose of an antidepressant, but no other psychotropic medication.

Approximately 8 months after his discharge, the patient ran out of his medication and did not obtain more from his pharmacy. His symptoms reappeared rapidly over the course of a few days. After a phone call from his parents to his doctor, the antidepressant treatment was hastily resumed, and the patient again reverted essentially to normal after another week or so.

The patient's mother had had a postpartum depressive episode of about a year's duration that had gradually remitted spontaneously without treatment. In addition, the mother's sister had had a "nervous breakdown" when she was in her 40s that had required her to be hospitalized; she had received a course of 12 electroconvulsive treatments. Since that time the aunt had had a complete remission and was described as functioning normally.

Discussion of "Three Voices"

This young man apparently had a 4-year period during which he had some nonspecific difficulties (social withdrawal and inability to pursue long-term goals), followed by an episode of illness with paranoid behavior, bizarre auditory hallucinations, loss of interest and pleasure, anorexia and a 20-pound weight loss, hypersomnia, loss of energy, and psychomotor retardation (paucity of speech and spending most of his time sitting on the bed staring into space).

In the past this might well have been diagnosed as Schizophrenia, the 4-year period being viewed as prodromal to the acute psychotic phase. The loss of interest and pleasure and the other nonpsychotic symptoms would have been considered merely associated features. According to DSM-IV-TR, the loss of interest and pleasure and other nonpsychotic symptoms actually constitute a full

Major Depressive Episode. Because the psychotic symptoms apparently have been present only when the patient had a Major Depressive Episode, they are considered a psychotic feature of a Major Depressive Episode. This is true in spite of the fact that the content of the delusions and hallucinations is not consistent with such usual depressive themes as personal inadequacy, guilt, or deserved punishment. Thus, on admission the diagnosis would be Major Depressive Disorder, Single Episode, Severe With Mood-Incongruent Psychotic Features (DSM-IV-TR, p. 375), a diagnosis that is certainly supported by the good response to an antidepressant and the family history of a mood disorder.

What are we to make of the 4-year period reported by his parents? Did this represent mild depressive symptoms or identity problems? Either would be consistent with our recommended diagnosis. If mild depressive symptoms were present for more than 2 years, the additional diagnosis of Dysthymic Disorder would be made. On the other hand, if closer examination revealed more malignant symptoms, such as ideas of reference or bizarre behavior that preceded the depressive symptoms, this would seem to indicate that the psychotic disturbance was not just a feature of Major Depressive Disorder and would suggest the eventual diagnosis of a primary psychotic disorder such as Schizoaffective Disorder or Schizophrenia.

Another question raised by this case is the appropriate subclassification of Major Depressive Disorder at the time of the reappearance of the depressive syndrome when medication was discontinued. Should this be regarded as Major Depressive Disorder, Recurrent, or as the continuation of the Major Depressive Disorder, Single Episode, the symptoms of which had been suppressed by medication? DSM-IV-TR considers a 2-month period in which the criteria are no longer met for a Major Depressive Episode the minimal amount of time needed to consider a recurrence a different episode. Because this patient's symptoms reappeared after 8 months, this resurgence of depressive symptomatology would appear to indicate a recurrent episode. However, given the brief duration (perhaps 10 days at the most), the episode fails to meet the duration criteria for a Major Depressive Episode. Thus, we would note Single Episode, In Partial Remission, to indicate that although some symptoms are present during the current period, they do not meet the full criteria.

THUNDERBIRD

A 43-year-old divorced carpenter is examined in the hospital emergency room because for the last few days he has been confused and unable to take care of himself. The patient's sister is available to provide some information. The sister reports that the patient has consumed large quantities of cheap wine daily for over 5 years. He had a reasonably stable home life and job record until his wife left him for another man 5 years previously. The sister indicates that the patient drinks more than a fifth of wine a day and that this has been an unvarying pattern since the divorce. He often has had blackouts from drinking and has missed work; consequently, he has been fired from several jobs. Fortunately for him, carpenters are in great demand, and he has been able to provide marginally for himself during these years. However, 3 days ago he ran out of money and wine and had to beg on the street to buy a meal. The patient has been poorly nourished, eating perhaps one meal a day and evidently relying on the wine as his prime source of nourishment.

The morning after his last day of drinking (3 days earlier), he felt increasingly tremulous, his hands shaking so grossly that it was difficult for him to light a cigarette. Accompanying this was an increasing sense of inner panic, which had made him virtually unable to sleep. A neighbor became concerned about the patient when he seemed not to be making sense and clearly was unable to take care of himself. The neighbor contacted the sister, who brought him to the hospital.

On examination, the patient alternates between apprehension and chatty, superficial warmth. He is quite keyed up and talks almost constantly in a rambling and unfocused manner. At times he recognizes the doctor, but at other times he gets confused and thinks the doctor is his older brother. Twice during the examination he calls the doctor by his older brother's name and asks when he arrived, evidently having lost track entirely of the interview up to that point. He has a gross hand tremor at rest, and there are periods when he picks at "bugs" he sees on the bed sheets. He is disoriented to time and thinks that he is in a supermarket parking lot rather than in a hospital. He indicates that he feels he is fighting against a terrifying sense that the world is ending in a holocaust. He is startled every few minutes by sounds and scenes of fiery car crashes (evidently provoked by the sound of rolling carts in the hall). Efforts at testing memory and calculation fail because his attention shifts too rapidly. An electroencephalogram indicates a pattern of diffuse encephalopathy.

Discussion of "Thunderbird"

This carpenter, with a long history of heavy alcohol use, develops severe withdrawal symptoms after he stops drinking. He has the characteristic symptoms of a Delirium: difficulty sustaining attention and other cognitive deficits including disorganized thinking (rambling), perceptual disturbances (he sees scenes of car crashes provoked by the sound of rolling carts in the hall), and disorientation to place and person (mistakes the doctor for his brother and the hospital for a parking lot). The appearance of a Delirium with marked autonomic hyperactivity (hand tremors) shortly after cessation or reduction of heavy alcohol ingestion indicates Alcohol Withdrawal Delirium (DSM-IV-TR, p. 146).

Although the treatment will initially be directed at the Alcohol Withdrawal Delirium, the additional diagnosis of Alcohol Dependence (DSM-IV-TR, p. 213) can be assumed from the information that he has been a heavy daily user of alcohol for more than 5 years, has lost jobs because of his alcohol use, and has been poorly nourished. The Alcohol Dependence is noted as Severe because he almost certainly has many of the symptoms of dependence and they interfere markedly with his occupational and social functioning.

BETTER LIVING THROUGH CHEMISTRY

Ray, age 22, brings his brother Danny, age 17, to the emergency room at 3:00 A.M. on a Sunday morning. Upon returning home from a date, Ray found Danny stumbling about their parents' basement den crying and mumbling, "Everything is blurry and double." Ray says that his brother cursed him out on the way to the hospital. He says that Danny drinks alcohol and smokes both tobacco and marijuana, but he doesn't know of any other drug use.

The examining physician notes that Danny is wearing an earring and a T-shirt that bears the inscription "Better Living Through Chemistry." Around his neck on a chain is a coke spoon hanging outside his shirt. His breath has an odor suggestive of an organic solvent. There is a symmetrical erythematous rash about his mouth and nose. His pupils are symmetrical and responsive to light although the whites of his eyes are markedly inflamed. Close inspection reveals transparent viscous material just inside both nostrils.

On questioning Danny, the doctor notes that he has an extremely short attention span. His manner at one moment is apathetic and disinterested, and at the next, belligerent and abusive. Neurological examination reveals no localized signs. Danny appears intoxicated, with slurred speech and unsteady, staggering gait. Reflexes are bilaterally depressed, his muscular strength is generally diminished, and there is an intentional tremor (a tremor of the hand when it is extended) and horizontal and vertical nystagmus (involuntary rapid movements of the eyeballs). Examination of the oral and pharyngeal mucosa reveals diffuse irritation. Several times during the examination, Danny attempts to leave, and once he takes the reflex hammer and starts testing the doctor. The physical examination is otherwise unremarkable.

Over the 45-minute course of the examination, Danny comments that the blurring of his vision and double vision have disappeared. Over the same period, it was observed that his reflexes had become more vigorous. Despite these changes, Danny's affect continues to vacillate between apathy and hostility.

A urine specimen is collected for a drug toxicology screening, and Danny is placed in a holding area while a psychiatric consultant is called. Danny waits a short while and then, against medical advice, leaves the hospital. All attempts to reach his parents are unsuccessful. Subsequently, the urine drug toxicology screen reveals aromatic inhalants.

Discussion of "Better Living Through Chemistry"

Ray says that his brother uses only marijuana and alcohol, but the doctor smells an organic solvent on his breath, notices a rash around his nose and mouth, and therefore wonders whether he may be intoxicated from inhaling a volatile substance such as gasoline, glue, paint, or paint thinner. The doctor's suspicion of Inhalant Intoxication (DSM-IV-TR, p. 260) is confirmed by the urine drug test.

Aromatic substances are inhaled sometimes by soaking a rag with the substance, which is then applied to the mouth and nose and the vapors breathed in. Alternatively, the substance may be inhaled directly from containers or from aerosols. The inhalants quickly reach the lungs and bloodstream and cause an acute intoxication state. Danny's visual symptoms, slurred speech, unsteady gait, lethargy, depressed reflexes, tremor, and muscle weakness are characteristic of Inhalant Intoxication. The diagnosis is made when these symptoms are accompanied by maladaptive behavioral changes, such as, in this case, belligerence alternating with apathy.

We assume that this is not the first time that Danny has used an inhalant. Therefore, we make a provisional diagnosis of Inhalant Abuse (DSM-IV-TR, p. 259).

The most serious complication of recurrent Inhalant Intoxication is brain damage, which, when severe, takes the form of a Dementia. Because the patient's current symptoms of cognitive impairment result from the acute effects of the drug intoxication, it is not possible to know whether some of these symptoms represent an incipient Dementia.

MR. AND MS. ALBERT

Mr. and Ms. Albert are an attractive, gregarious couple, married for 15 years, who present in the midst of a crisis over their sexual problems. Mr. Albert, a successful restaurateur, is 38. Ms. Albert, who since marriage has devoted herself to child rearing and managing the home, is 35. She reports that throughout their marriage she has been extremely frustrated because sex has "always been hopeless for us." She is now seriously considering leaving her husband.

The difficulty is the husband's rapid ejaculation. Whenever any lovemaking is attempted, Mr. Albert becomes anxious, moves quickly toward intercourse, and reaches orgasm either immediately upon entering his wife's vagina or within one or two strokes. He then feels humiliated and recognizes his wife's dissatisfaction, and they both lapse into silent suffering. He has severe feelings of inadequacy and guilt, and she experiences a mixture of frustration and resentment toward his "ineptness and lack of concern." Recently, they have developed a pattern of avoiding sex, which leaves them both frustrated, but which keeps overt hostility to a minimum.

Mr. Albert has always been a perfectionist, priding himself on his ability to succeed at anything he sets his mind to. As a child he was a "good boy," in a vain effort to please his demanding father. His inability to control his ejaculation is a source of intense shame, and he finds himself unable to talk to his wife about his sexual "failures." Ms. Albert is highly sexual and easily aroused by foreplay but has always felt that intercourse is the only "acceptable" way to reach orgasm. Intercourse with her husband has always been unsatisfying, and she holds him completely responsible for her sexual frustration. Because she cannot discuss the subject without feeling rage, she usually avoids talking about it. As a result, they have never developed other sexual techniques for pleasing each other, and sex has always been a disaster.

In other areas of their marriage, including rearing of their two children, managing the family restaurant, and socializing with friends, the Alberts are highly compatible. Despite these strong points, however, they are near separation because of the tension produced by their mutual sexual disappointment.

Discussion of "Mr. and Ms. Albert"

This couple presents with a sexual problem that is threatening their marriage. Because DSM-IV-TR includes a classification of disturbed dyadic units, the clinician could note the V code Partner Relational Problem (DSM-IV-TR, p. 737) to indicate that this couple, as a unit, was the focus of clinical attention. However, it is also important to consider the diagnosis of each marital partner separately.

The husband's sexual difficulty is that he lacks a reasonable degree of voluntary control over ejaculation, so that he invariably ejaculates almost immediately upon penetration during intercourse. As a result, his wife is never sexually satisfied, and he feels extremely inadequate. Because the lack of control is not limited to novel situations and does not occur only after long periods of abstinence, the Axis I diagnosis of Premature Ejaculation (DSM-IV-TR, p. 554) is made. Because the husband's "perfectionism" is mentioned, and this might be related to either the development or the perpetuation of the sexual problem, obsessive-compulsive personality traits could be noted on Axis II.

There is little information about the wife's difficulties, other than that she clearly has a relationship problem. With this limited information, the V code Partner Relational Problem is appropriate; it should be understood, however, that with more information it may need to be changed to, for example, a Personality Disorder.

Some clinicians might consider the diagnosis of Adjustment Disorder for either the husband or the wife, or both. In the husband's case, the diagnosis would not be made because the distress he is experiencing seems to be an associated feature of the Premature Ejaculation rather than a separate illness. In the wife's case, an Adjustment Disorder diagnosis would imply that her reaction to her husband's sexual problem (her rage and threatening separation) is excessive and indicates significant psychopathology. This might be the case, but such a judgment would require more information than is available.

EMBARRASSED

A 46-year-old married male was referred to a psychiatrist for evaluation in 1966 because of unremitting tics. At age 13 he had developed a persistent eye blink, soon followed by lip smacking, head shaking, and barking-like noises. Despite these symptoms, he functioned well academically and eventually graduated from high school with honors. He was drafted during World War II. While in the army his tics subsided significantly, but were still troublesome and eventually resulted in a medical discharge. He married, had two children, and worked as a semiskilled laborer and foreman. By age 30 his symptoms included tics of the head, neck, and shoulders; hitting his forehead with his hand and various objects; repeated throat clearing; spitting; and shouting out "Hey, hey, hey; la, la, la." Six years later, noisy coprolalia started: he would emit a string of profanities, such as "Fuck you, you cocksucking bastard," in the middle of a sentence and then resume his conversation.

From 1951 to 1957, various treatments, all without benefit, were tried: insulin shock therapy, electroconvulsive therapy, and administration of various phenothiazines and antidepressants. The patient's social life became increasingly constricted because of his symptoms. He was unable to go to church or to the movies because of the cursing and noises. He worked at night to avoid social embarrassment. His family and friends became increasingly intolerant of his symptoms, and his daughters refused to bring friends home. He was depressed because of his enforced isolation and the seeming hopelessness of finding effective treatment. At 46, he sought a prefrontal lobotomy; but after psychiatric evaluation, his request was denied. This led to the 1966 referral. After completing the evaluation, the psychiatrist decided to try a new experimental drug, haloperidol.

Discussion of "Embarrassed"

This patient has the characteristic features of Tourette's Disorder (DSM-IV-TR, p. 114): onset before age 21; multiple motor and one or more vocal tics (involuntary cursing or shouting); the tics occurring many times a day (usually in bouts), nearly every day, or intermittently throughout a period of more than 1 year; and changes over time in the anatomic location, number, frequency, complexity, and severity of the tics.

When the patient was evaluated, he was described as being "depressed over his enforced isolation and the seeming hopelessness of finding effective treatment." This raises the question of Adjustment Disorder With Depressed Mood or of a Major Depressive Disorder. The concept of Adjustment Disorder generally does not include situations in which the patient is distressed because of the consequences of the symptoms of, or the reaction of others to, his or her mental disorder. Such distress is commonplace in chronic illnesses and is better thought of as an associated feature of the illness rather than as Adjustment Disorder. On the other hand, if the depression were so severe as to meet the criteria for a Major Depressive Episode, then the additional diagnosis of Major Depressive Disorder would be appropriate. In this case there is no information about the other features of a depressive syndrome that would be necessary to make such a diagnosis.

When the disorder was first studied, the coprolalia and other bizarre symptoms were thought to represent conversion symptoms expressing conflicts arising during the pregenital phase of psycho-sexual development. Now most investigators believe that whatever psychological disturbance may be present is best understood as a reaction to the chronic, incapacitating symptoms, which have a biological etiology. In this case, when the symptoms of Tourette's Disorder were brought under control (see below), the patient was no longer depressed.

Follow-Up

The haloperidol had a dramatic effect in that it eliminated 99% of his symptoms. He resumed a normal social life and was no longer depressed. When last seen, many years later, he continued to do well on the same maintenance dosage of haloperidol.

Foggy Student

A 20-year-old male college student sought psychiatric consultation be-cause he was worried that he might be going insane. For the past 2 years he had experienced increasingly frequent episodes of feeling "outside" himself. These episodes were accompanied by a sense of deadness in his body. In addition, during these periods he was uncertain of his balance and frequently stumbled into furniture; this was more apt to occur in public, especially if he was somewhat anxious. During these episodes he felt a lack of easy, natural control of his body and his thoughts seemed "foggy" as well, in a way that reminded him of having received intravenous anesthetic agents for an appendectomy some 5 years previously.

The patient's subjective sense of lack of control was especially troublesome, and he would fight it by shaking his head and saying "stop" to himself. This would momentarily clear his mind and restore his sense of autonomy, but only temporarily, as the feelings of deadness and of being outside himself would return. Gradually, over a period of several hours, the unpleasant experiences would fade. The patient was anxious, how-ever, about their return, as he found them increasing in both frequency and duration.

At the time the patient came for treatment, he was experiencing these symptoms about twice a week, and each incident lasted from 3 to

4 hours. On several occasions the episodes had occurred while he was driving his car and was alone; worried that he might have an accident, he had stopped driving unless someone accompanied him. Increasingly he had begun to discuss this problem with his girlfriend; eventually she had become less affectionate toward him, complaining that he had lost his sense of humor and was totally self-preoccupied. She threatened to break off with him unless he changed, and she began to date other men.

The patient's college grades remained unimpaired; they had, in fact, improved over the past 6 months, as he was spending more time studying than had previously been the case. Although discouraged by his symptoms, he slept well at night, had noted no change in appetite, and had experienced no impairment in concentration. He was neither fatigued nor physically "edgy" because of his worry.

Because a cousin had been hospitalized for many years with severe mental illness, the patient had begun to wonder if a similar fate might befall him, and sought direct reassurance on the matter.

Discussion of "Foggy Student"

Depersonalization—that is, the experience of feeling detached from, and as if one is an outside observer of, one's mental processes or body—can be a symptom of a variety of mental disorders, such as Schizophrenic, Anxiety, Mood, Personality, and Cognitive Disorders. Mild depersonalization, without functional impairment, occurs at some time in a large proportion of young adults and does not by itself warrant diagnosis as a mental disorder. When, as in this case, the symptom of depersonalization occurs in the absence of a more pervasive disorder and is sufficiently severe and persistent to cause marked distress, the diagnosis Depersonalization Disorder is made (DSM-IV-TR, p. 532).

DISABLED VET

The patient is a 32-year-old man who admits himself to a mental hospital in 1982 after attempting suicide by taking sleeping pills. He says that nothing in particular prompted this attempt, but that he has been very depressed, with only minor fluctuations, ever since he returned from Vietnam 10 years earlier.

He describes a reasonably normal childhood and adolescence. "I never in my life felt like this before I got to Nam." He had friends throughout high school, always got at least average grades, and never was in trouble with the law or other authorities. He has had many girlfriends, but has never married. After high school, he went to technical school, was trained as an electrician, and was working in this occupation when he was drafted for military service in Vietnam. He loathed the violence there; but on one occasion, evidently swept away by the group spirit, he killed a civilian "for the fun of it." This seems to him totally out of keeping with his character. The memory of this incident continues to haunt him, and he is racked with guilt. He was honorably discharged from the army and has never worked since, except for 3 weeks when an uncle hired him. He has been living on various forms of government assistance.

In the army the patient began to drink heavily and to use whatever drugs he could get his hands on, abusing most of them; but in the past few years, he has turned to alcohol almost exclusively. He has been drinking very heavily and nearly continually for the past 10 years, with blackouts, frequent arrests for public intoxication, and injuries in barroom brawls. He has acquaintances, but no friends. Whenever he "dries out," he feels terribly depressed (as he also does when he drinks); he has made four suicide attempts in the past 7 years. For the month before his latest suicide attempt, he had been living in an alcohol-treatment residence, the longest dry period he can remember, all previous attempts at cutting down on his drinking having failed.

The patient presents as a very sad, thoughtful, introspective man with a dignified bearing, and in informal conversation appears to be of at least average intelligence. He is not interested in anything and confides that when he sees others enjoying themselves, he is so jealous he wants to hit them; this urge is never evident from his unfailingly courteous behavior. There is no evidence of delusions and no history of hallucinations except during several bouts of Alcohol Withdrawal Delirium in the past. His appetite is normal, as is his sex drive, "but I don't enjoy it." He has trouble falling asleep or staying asleep without medication. He is not psychomotorically slow. He complains of "absentmindedness."

After 2 weeks, the patient still has trouble finding his way around the ward. He seems very well motivated to cooperate with neuropsychological testing and is extremely distressed by his disabilities. Testing reveals impaired immediate and long-term memory, apraxias, agnosias, peripheral neuropathy, and constructional difficulties; his IQ is measured as 66.

The patient has not responded to antidepressant medication. He is sorry that his suicide attempt did not succeed, and he says that if things aren't going to get any better, he definitely wants to die.

Discussion of "Disabled Vet"

What occasioned this patient's hospital admission was a suicide attempt, a symptom of his long-standing depression. A 10-year period of depressed mood and anhedonia, with associated symptoms such as sleep difficulties and recurrent suicidal acts, suggests a chronic Major Depressive Episode. Because one more symptom is required for the diagnosis and we are unsure whether his "absent-mindedness" is a symptom of depression or of dementia, we make a provisional diagnosis of Major Depressive Disorder (DSM-IV-TR, p. 375). Although the depression has been persistent for 10 years, because there is no evidence of a period without significant symptoms of depression, we note Single Episode. Because the episode has lasted 2 years without a period of 2 months or longer of a full remission, we also add Chronic. Finally, because the symptoms and functional impairment are between mild and severe, we note the severity as Moderate.

There is a long history of heavy drinking, unsuccessful efforts to cut down on alcohol use, reduced involvement in social, occupational, and recreational activities because of alcohol use, and continued drinking despite knowledge of recurrent problems caused by alcohol use (blackouts, frequent arrests, and injuries in barroom brawls). These, together with the history of episodes of withdrawal (Alcohol Withdrawal Delirium), indicate the presence of Alcohol Dependence (DSM-IV-TR, p. 213). Because the patient has not been drinking for the past month, the course is noted as Early Full Remission, as with such a brief period of remission, the likelihood of relapse is extremely high. If he continued to show no evidence of abuse of or dependence on alcohol for a full year, the course would be changed to Sustained Full Remission.

Furthermore, the patient has severe memory loss and evidence of impairment of higher cortical functioning (apraxias, agnosias, and constructional difficulties) and a decrement in intellectual abilities (IQ of 66) that interferes with functioning. Because this apparently results from the patient's long history of Alcoholism and is not limited to memory loss (as in Alcohol-Induced Persisting Amnestic Disorder), the diagnosis of Alcohol-Induced Persisting Dementia (DSM-IV-TR, p. 170) is given. Because this diagnosis is more relevant to his current condition than the Alcohol Dependence, in Early Full Remission, it is listed as the second diagnosis.

MIRIAM AND ESTHER

Miriam was hospitalized after her mother called the police because she feared Miriam might hurt both of them. Miriam claimed she was age 56 and lived with her 76-year-old "assumed" or "estranged" mother, Esther, and her 12-year-old daughter, Alice. She described Esther as a family friend who had given her and her daughter a room some years ago, but who had increasingly angered her by acting as a mother and a grandmother, invading her privacy, attacking her in her sleep, and jealously turning Alice against her.

According to the patient, domestic squabbling had threatened to become violent on the night of admission, causing Esther to send her to the hospital "for hygiene." The patient expected to leave as soon as the ward social worker could relocate her and Alice in a "condominium or other suitable environment in which to rear my own child, who is coming of age as a young lady." She admitted to a recent sense of confusion, but denied sleep and appetite changes, mood disturbance, and hallucinations. However, she did describe a "whooshing" sound in her "cranium" intermittently over the past several years, which she felt resulted from fluid in her ear; at other times she had felt "very aware" of her own thoughts, but she denied hearing voices.

Miriam gave a vague but complex history, as follows: She was born 56 years ago in Italy. Her "biologic parents" (as she put it), Louise and William, were wealthy from oil. They took her to their country house in Mt. Vernon, New York, where she spent her childhood. Esther, a family friend, visited often. Miriam recalled people driving Packards and Rolls Royces. She stated she later lived in Europe and North Africa and was present in Hiroshima when the atom bomb was dropped. This event left her with a steel plate in her head and an "atom brain." She lived with Louise and William from 1957 to 1968. She said that she had had three husbands and seven children. Her youngest, Alice, fathered by her last husband, was born in 1968, 4 years after his death. When asked how this could be, she explained that a "tubal infection" had delayed the baby's conception in a "technical way."

According to Miriam, after the birth of Alice she moved in with Esther and enrolled at Hunter College in a special program for middle-aged students, where she excelled in Romance languages. She became an alcoholic, consuming up to a pint of whiskey daily. Once when she didn't drink, she became shaky and broke into a sweat. Following the death in 1973 of her "biologic mother," Louise, Miriam became depressed and lost weight. A "nervous breakdown" landed her in a state mental hospital for 3 months, where she stopped drinking and improved with medication. For several years thereafter, a local "mental hygiene" clinic gave her medication for "stability," including Prolixin (an antipsychotic), which made her hair fall out. Since then she had worked steadily, first for the Board of Education and then as a home health aide. For the past year she had remained home to care for her child.

Miriam's mother, Esther, related a quite different history, corroborated by family members and clinic staff. Miriam is actually 30. Esther is 56 and is, in fact, her biological mother. When Miriam was 7, her father walked out on the family. The next year she and her older sister were sent, probably for financial reasons, to Mt. Vernon to live with Esther's middle-class Aunt Louise and Uncle William. Esther visited on weekends.

Miriam was a good student, but had few friends and kept to herself. In 1968, at 17, she became pregnant by a cousin from Trinidad, whom she never saw again. She finished high school but, ashamed, returned to her mother's home to have the baby. Esther cared for them both and took responsibility for rearing her granddaughter, Alice. Miriam attended night classes in business skills for 2 years at Hunter College, but did poorly. She then worked for a year as a home health aide, but quit because she thought people were against her. She began to hear voices that commented about her actions and was finally admitted to a state hospital in 1973, where she improved with medication. The voices ceased several months after discharge. She lived at home and worked occasionally as a secretary, but failed a stenography and typing course.

In 1977 her mother paid for Miriam to have her own apartment. Miriam mismanaged her money and was evicted after a year. The stress apparently caused her to become psychotic again (details are not known). She moved back to her mother's and improved greatly on antipsychotics. She worked inconsistently for a year, again as a home health aide, but then stopped her medication and quit work. She began to call her mother Esther rather than Mother and began to say she was not her real mother. Friction developed because of Esther's disappointment in Miriam and Miriam's jealousy of the continued mothering role taken by Esther toward Miriam's child. The child clearly preferred Esther.

Miriam spent more time alone in her room, friendless, venturing out only for shopping trips, during which she would spend her disability check on expensive clothes. Relatives say she was often belligerent when talking about her mother. She became unkempt and unable to help with the household chores. She began yelling at imaginary people to leave her alone and not touch her. On several occasions, by the time police had been summoned, Miriam had calmed down. However, the night of admission she was out of control, threatening to throw herself and her mother out the window, and was forcibly handcuffed and brought to the hospital.

Miriam's mental status in numerous interviews was characterized by calm, socially appropriate behavior. She was obese and homely, but tastefully dressed. Speech and movement were of normal tempo and quantity. Her affect was constricted, although at times she seemed pedantic and slightly haughty. Contained anger and sarcasm were apparent during a joint interview with her mother. Thought processes were slightly loose, vague, and circumstantial. Most striking was her odd language, ranging from idiosyncratic usage—"my assumed mother," "my estranged mother"—to neologisms ("Medicine makes me incognizant. . . . I am not correlative enough. . . . My mother does not accreditize me. . . . The hospital will have my records if they are consortive. . . . My cousin was a devasive schizoid").

When confronted with inconsistencies in her account of her life, Miriam only smiled or giggled. While hospitalized she admitted neither to currently hearing the "whooshing" sound nor to any hallucinations.

Nurses reported that when unknowingly observed, she acted as if she were aware of nonexistent beings.

Discussion of "Miriam and Esther"

This woman clearly has an illness with prominent psychotic features, the most notable being a delusion that the woman who claims to be her mother is actually only a family friend. (This delusion seems to be a variant of Capgras syndrome, in which the person believes that one or more people in his or her environment are actually impostors who look exactly or almost exactly like the people whose roles they have assumed.) Other bizarre delusions include the beliefs that the conception of her child was delayed several years beyond the death of the biological father and that she was in Hiroshima when the atom bomb was dropped, leaving her with a steel plate in her head.

Although she denies hallucinations, the sound in her head probably is an auditory hallucination; her mother claims that she has heard voices in the past.

The absence of a general medical condition or the use of a substance that could account for the symptoms, the deterioration in functioning over several years, and the bizarre delusions and hallucinations clearly establish the diagnosis as Schizophrenia (DSM-IV-TR, p. 312). Preoccupation with one or more delusions and the absence of such features as disorganized speech and flat or inappropriate affect indicate the Paranoid Type (DSM-IV-TR, p. 314). The course of her illness is characterized as "Episodic With Interepisode Residual Symptoms" (e.g., inability to work, social isolation).

An unusual feature of this case is what is sometimes referred to as *pseudologia fantastica,* the presentation of fantastic and elaborate details about oneself that are completely false, but that the patient appears to believe. In Miriam's case this is illustrated by her account of her personal history—being born in Italy, growing up with wealthy parents, later living in Europe and North Africa—and her claim of having had a serious alcohol problem (which her family denied).

THE MEN'S ROOM

Nick, a single 26-year-old grocery clerk complained: "I have a problem with shit." He was referred to a mental health clinic by a pastoral counselor who had been seeing him for the past 6 months for interpersonal problems.

Over the past 3–4 years, during periods of low sexual activity, Nick has become sexually frustrated and gone to public rest rooms, where he turns off the water to the toilets and then waits for a man whom he finds sexually attractive to enter. He waits until this person uses a toilet and then "retrieves" the feces and takes them home in a plastic bag. He warms the feces by placing the bag in boiling water and subsequently plays with the feces, which sexually excites him. He then masturbates to orgasm. This behavior has occurred about once a month. He admits to a great deal of guilt and concern over his habit because "it is not socially acceptable."

Nick is homosexual, but is extremely reluctant to frequent "gay" bars. When he does, he stays only a short time; if he is not approached within the first 15–20 minutes, he leaves. He shares an apartment with a roommate but is not emotionally involved with him. He has a limited circle of friends.

He has had an attraction for rest rooms since early adolescence. Some of his earliest sexual contacts occurred in rest rooms. Once he was excited by urine; however, this is not currently the case.

Nick recalls having been a "loner" throughout his childhood. At an early age he realized that this sexual attraction to other boys made him different from his peers. This led him to be socially isolated. His first sexual activity occurred at age 10 with group masturbation. At age 11 Nick began engaging in homosexual activity. This has continued throughout his life, and he has had no history of heterosexual arousal or activity.

Nick is short, stocky, rather masculine, and meticulously dressed and groomed. During the interview he is tense and stiff, especially when describing his sexual behavior. His affect is constricted. He complains of feeling depressed but has no associated symptoms of depression. His speech is overinclusive and circumstantial. There is no evidence of psychotic symptoms.

Discussion of "The Men's Room"

How should the use of feces for achieving sexual excitement be classified? In DSM-IV-TR, Coprophilia is given as an example of Paraphilia Not Otherwise Specified. In Coprophilia, the person is excited by observing the act of defecation or by being defecated upon. In this case, however, it is the feces themselves that serve as the stimulus. Therefore, it seems to us no different from the use of other nonliving objects by themselves, such as female undergarments, for sexual excitement and as such should be classified as Fetishism (DSM-IV-TR, p. 570). (We cannot claim that classifying this disorder as Fetishism rather than as a Paraphilia Not Otherwise Specified has profound treatment implications.)

In view of the history of social isolation and inability to initiate relationships with people, it seems reasonable to give an Axis II diagnosis of Personality Disorder Not Otherwise Specified (DSM-IV-TR, p. 729), Provisional, Rule Out Schizoid Personality Disorder. (Note: This case was submitted before the acquired immunodeficiency syndrome epidemic, and no follow-up information is available.)

SEX PROBLEM

Ms. B. is a 43-year-old housewife who entered the hospital in 1968 with a chief complaint of being concerned about her "sex problem"; she stated that she needed hypnotism to find out what was wrong with her sexual drive. Her husband supplied the history: he complained that she had had many extramarital affairs, with many different men, all through their married life. He insisted that in one 2-week period she had had as many as a hundred different sexual experiences with men outside the marriage. The patient herself agreed with this assessment of her behavior, but would not speak of the experiences, saying that she "blocks" the memories out. She denied any particular interest in sexuality, but said that apparently she felt a compulsive drive to go out and seek sexual activity despite her lack of interest.

The patient had been married to her husband for over 20 years. He was clearly the dominant partner in the marriage. The patient was fearful of his frequent jealous rages, and apparently it was he who suggested that she enter the hospital in order to receive hypnosis. The patient maintained that she could not explain why she sought out other men, that she really did not want to do this. Her husband stated that on occasion he had tracked her down, and when he had found her, she acted as if she did not know him. She confirmed this and believed it was because the episodes of her sexual promiscuity were blotted out by "amnesia."

When the physician indicated that he questioned the reality of the wife's sexual adventures, the husband became furious and accused the doctor and a ward attendant of having sexual relations with her.

Neither an amytal interview nor considerable psychotherapy with Ms. B. was able to clear the "blocked out" memory of periods of sexual activities. The patient did admit to a memory of having had 2 extramarital relationships in the past: one 20 years before the time of admission and the other just a year before admission. She stated that the last one had actually been planned by her husband and that he was in the same house at the time. She continued to believe that she had actually had countless extramarital sexual experiences, though she remembered only two of them.

Discussion of "Sex Problem"

One's first impression is that an amnestic syndrome should be considered, either dissociative or resulting from a general medical condition or substance use. However, the plot thickens as evidence accumulates that the husband, the chief informant, has delusional jealousy, believing that his wife is repeatedly unfaithful to him. Apparently under his influence, his wife has accepted this delusional belief, explaining her lack of memory of the events by believing that she has "amnesia." It would seem that she has adopted his delusional system and does not really have any kind of "amnesia." Before the onset of her delusions, there was no indication of any preexisting psychotic disorder, nor did she have any of the prodromal symptoms of Schizophrenia. Because her delusional system developed as a result of a close relationship with another person who had an already established delusion (i.e., her husband) and because her delusions are similar in content to his delusions, the diagnosis is Shared Psychotic Disorder (DSM-IV-TR, p. 334), traditionally known as *folie à deux*. An interesting twist to this case is that it is the patient who, by virtue of her alleged extramarital activity, is the source of the husband's distress. It is more common in a Shared Psychotic Disorder for the person who has adopted the other's delusional system to believe that he or she is also being harmed.

THE HEAVENLY VISION[*]

An obese 34-year-old woman was brought to a local hospital by the police. She had removed her clothing and, standing naked beside her car in a gas station, had ostentatiously engaged in fellatio with her 5-month-old son. She later claimed that she did this in response to a vision: "I felt I had been instructed to step out of the car, remove my clothes as a sort of shocking, attention-getting episode depicting the stripping that this nation is going to be going through soon." She explained that the depiction of oral sex was in order to draw attention to the abuse of children in vile ways in this country, as in prostitution and pornography. She described her own behavior as a "bizarre act" and understood that it was viewed as evidence of a "mental aberration." But, in her own words, "There's method to my madness."

The patient had apparently, for the past 20 years, been having "different levels of visionary states" during which she both saw and heard God. Recently she had been receiving religious and political messages from God and believed that "The Communist Party and the Nazi Party have joined hands and will be occupying the country . . . the strike of the invasion point will come over Canada down through the Midwest to the point of St. Louis."

The patient's description of her visionary experiences and her history was coherent and articulate and delivered in a matter-of-fact manner, although with many vivid and startling details.

Records from a previous hospitalization noted that the patient had a completely positive review of physical symptoms. Her presenting complaint at the time was migraine headaches; but as each physician exam-

---

[*]Adapted from Spitzer RL, Gibbon M, Skodol A, et al.: "The Heavenly Vision of a Poor Woman: A Down-to-Earth Discussion of the DSM-III Differential Diagnosis." *Journal of Operational Psychiatry* 11:169–172, 1980.

ined her, the symptom list grew longer and longer. Records from a psychiatric outpatient evaluation 9 years before the current admission noted that she complained of extreme shakiness, which had gone on for a number of years; of a painful "knot" growing at the lower part of the back of her head; and of blackout spells. After these spells she said she frequently went into a deep sleep. Several electroencephalograms were negative. A neurologist who examined her did not think she had epilepsy and recommended that she see a psychiatrist.

During her current hospitalization, the patient had some physical complaints, particularly back pain, which she attributed to a fall at age 18 and to arthritis of the lower spine. She had difficulty walking and had consulted many doctors about this. She had a 100% disability rating for "nerves and arthritis."

On physical examination the patient was noted to be overweight. She had several small lipomas on her back and arm. Palpation of her abdomen revealed a poorly localized right quadrant tenderness. She complained of polymenorrhea. A Pap smear and endometrial biopsy were normal. An electrocardiogram showed a right bundle branch block and left ventricular hypertrophy. Radiological examination of her skull revealed microcephaly (greater than two standard deviations below the lower limits of normal) and osteosclerosis. A rheumatology consultant diagnosed mechanical low back pain exacerbated by obesity.

Her personal history was obtained from the patient alone. She reported that her father was a fundamentalist Christian minister, and she had been deeply involved in the church from an early age. She was baptized at age 12 and was "speaking in tongues." At that age she "felt a call to the ministry." She completed high school with above-average grades. At age 18, after a broken engagement (which she describes very dramatically, as she does every event in her history), she joined the Women's Army Corps (WACs), against her parents' wishes; she has been alienated from her family ever since. She claims to have been raped while in the service, and later to have fallen down, hit her head on concrete, and been "unconscious for 9 days," after which she was "very weak" and had "bouts of amnesia." She left the WACs after 13 months and married a man who turned out to be a bigamist. She lived with him for 12 years, had four children, and separated from him when she discovered that he had molested her daughters. She has worked sporadically since then.

After her marital separation, the patient left town with her children because she was being "harassed" by gossiping neighbors. She moved to another town, but the harassment continued. At one point she took the children to Israel, with no money and no plans other than to settle there, claiming that she had traced a "Jewish bloodline" in her ancestry. She gives the impression of having been "on the road" a good deal of the time since her separation (4 years ago). For at least part of that time, she placed her children in state foster homes.

Fourteen months before admission, she had slept with a stranger in a motel. She claims that this was her only sexual contact in 4 years; it resulted in the birth of her son 5 months ago.

During her hospital stay the patient was quite verbal, and the staff noted her to be "hostile and histrionic." She held firmly to her religious beliefs and referred to many prophecies that, she claimed, had come true. She produced tape cassettes from various people throughout the country who shared her religious beliefs. In these tapes she was generally praised for her steadfast faith and her gift of prophecy. In some tapes "speaking in tongues" was prominent. The staff had the impression that she experienced brief "psychotic episodes," which centered on feelings of persecution by the government.

The patient was discharged after a month. She refused any follow-up care and told a few people that she was heading west in the hope of matriculating in an evangelist training school. Her children remained in the custody of the appropriate state social service agency. Several days after her discharge, she was sought by law-enforcement officials because she had allegedly written about $650 in bad checks and had apparently stolen the car she had been driving before admission.

Discussion of "The Heavenly Vision"

The central question in the differential diagnosis in this case is whether or not the visions, voices, unusual beliefs, and bizarre behavior are symptoms of a true psychotic disorder—a disorder in which there is gross impairment in reality testing. By definition, a delusion is a belief that is not ordinarily accepted by other members of the person's culture or subculture. This patient has a long history of association with fundamentalist religious sects in which such experiences as speaking in tongues and having visions of God are not uncommon. Can this woman's unusual perceptual experiences and strange notions be entirely accounted for by her religious beliefs? We think not. It is true that receiving messages from God and instructions to do various things to carry out God's will are common among such groups. However, this patient's elaborate notions of a combined invasion by Communist and Nazi forces and her instructions to reveal the sexual depravity of this country seem to us well beyond the range of even extreme fundamentalist beliefs. Thus, we doubt that this woman's behavior is merely the reflection of a culture-bound pattern of beliefs and behavior and without psychopathological significance.

Having ruled out subcultural identifications as an explanation for her "symptoms," we must ask whether the symptoms are genuine (i.e., true delusions and hallucinations) or in some way intentionally produced, or whether they are on a point along a genuine–fake continuum. There is some evidence that at least some of the symptoms, particularly the bizarre behavior that occasioned her admission to the psychiatric hospital, were produced for dramatic effect. The patient seemed particularly aware of the likely reactions to what she was saying and doing. Such awareness is generally not seen in a person who is currently in a psychotic state.

In the interview itself, the patient described events in her life that strained credulity and suggested that many of them might be at least consciously exaggerated or outright fabrications (*pseudologia fantastica*). Was she unconscious for 9 days? Did she trace her lineage back to a Jewish ancestor? Did she conceive during a single occasion of intercourse?

Further evidence suggesting that this woman's "psychotic" symptoms may not be genuine is the long history of physical complaints that appear not to be symptomatic of genuine physical illness. The patient has had episodes of amnesia with blackout "spells," yet her electroencephalograms were negative. She has been noted to have a completely positive review of physical symptoms, many of which presumably cannot be traced to organic pathology. Finally, both the interviewer and the ward staff are apparently impressed with her histrionic manner and presentation.

The DSM-IV-TR concept of Factitious Disorder is meant to encompass the murky area between the act of Malingering, motivated by external incentives (e.g., feigning illness to avoid military duty), and a genuinely psychotic experience over which the person has no control whatever. The two critical judgments involved in making a diagnosis of a Factitious Disorder are that the "symptoms" are intentionally produced and that the motivation is not an external incentive. Because the sense of intentionally producing a symptom is subjective and can only be inferred by an outside observer, what circumstances would favor such a judgment? Examples would include the "patient" who appears to be hallucinating only when he believes that he is being observed or the "patient" who claims to have a cluster of symptoms that generally do not coexist (e.g., a severe Dementia with systematized persecutory delusions).

The judgment that the motivation is not for an external incentive is based on the assumption that in a Factitious Disorder the "patient" is motivated to achieve some benefit that is subsumed within the concept of the patient role. This might be the obvious benefit of treatment and being taken care of in a hospital or the less obvious benefit of being absolved of certain responsibilities that are normally a part of adult life, such as having to work for a living, even though it means being a "patient" for life.

What evidence do we have that this patient's crazy behavior is motivated by the desire to assume some benefits of the patient role? There is the possibility that she realized that her sexual behavior with her infant son would result in her being hospitalized in a mental hospital. Furthermore, whether or not she deliberately sought to have her children removed from her care, this did occur, divesting her of the responsibility for their care and making it possible for her to take off more easily on her own pursuits. We regard this "evidence" as equivocal.

If one accepts the authenticity of the delusions and hallucinations in this case, then the following specific DSM-IV-TR categories need to be considered: Schizophrenia (or Schizophreniform Disorder), Brief Psychotic Disorder, Bipolar Disorder, and Delusional Disorder. Schizophrenia and Schizophreniform Disorder require marked impairment in functioning in areas such as work, social relations, and self-care that is markedly below the highest level achieved before onset of the disturbance. There is no evidence of this in our patient. Furthermore, such common features of Schizophrenia as flat affect and disorganized speech are not present. A Delusional Disorder is ruled out by hallucinations lasting more than a few hours.

Although the patient is grandiose and expansive, none of the other characteristic symptoms of the manic syndrome were noted by either the interviewer or the ward staff; therefore, the diagnosis of Bipolar Disorder seems unlikely.

In DSM-IV-TR the diagnosis of Brief Psychotic Disorder may be used when the clinician judges that the patient has an episode of psychosis that lasts for at least 1 day but no more than 1 month, with eventual full return to premorbid functioning. Thus, in this case, if we accept the staff's impression that her periods of genuine psychosis were brief, then the diagnosis of Brief Psychotic Disorder (DSM-IV-TR, p. 332) would seem to be appropriate. We would also note the need to rule out Factitious Disorder With Predominantly Psychological Signs and Symptoms (DSM-IV-TR, p. 517).

Although this woman has real physical illness, it is unlikely that this accounts for her amnesia, menstrual symptoms, and probable conversion seizures, reported during a previous hospitalization. This suggests the need to rule out Somatization Disorder, an illness characterized by recurrent and multiple somatic complaints that apparently do not result from any physical disorder, but for which medical attention is sought. In this case we are told about the characteristic pseudoneurological symptoms (shakiness, blackout spells, difficulty walking) and sexual symptoms (polymenorrhea), but only three of the four required pain symptoms (headache, lower back pain, right quadrant tenderness) and none of the required gastrointestinal symptoms. However, we make the diagnosis of Somatization Disorder (DSM-IV-TR, p. 490) at a provisional level because we strongly suspect that the other required symptoms have been present.

In view of the long history of disturbed interpersonal relationships, a diagnosis of a Personality Disorder would certainly seem appropriate. The patient's history reveals prominent histrionic features and a suggestion of significant antisocial traits (car theft, passing bad checks, possible abandonment of children). In the absence of more information, a diagnosis of Personality Disorder Not Otherwise Specified (DSM-IV-TR, p. 729) With Histrionic and Antisocial Traits seems appropriate.

INHIBITED

A 24-year-old woman was referred by her psychiatrist to a sexual dysfunction clinic because she was no longer able to achieve orgasm. She has been married for 5 years and previously was able to reach orgasm and enjoyed a regular, sexually satisfying relationship with her husband.

Two years ago she had a classic Major Depressive Disorder with melancholic and psychotic features, which was successfully treated with antidepressant drugs, imipramine and tranylcypromine. She now has no associated symptoms of the depressive syndrome, such as loss of appetite or trouble sleeping, yet she still feels "down" and does not think she has fully recovered her normal, healthy ebullience. For this reason her psychiatrist has continued to prescribe the tranylcypromine.

The patient often initiates sexual encounters, finds pleasure in sexual activities, and claims her husband is a "good and satisfactory lover." However, she has to use a lubricant as she finds she does not lubricate enough for him to penetrate without causing her discomfort; and, more disturbingly, she has been unable to have an orgasm since her depression. She has tried to masturbate herself to orgasm without success.

Discussion of "Inhibited"

According to the history, this woman had a Major Depressive Episode from which she has recovered, but not entirely. The issue is whether her difficulty with sexual excitement (not lubricating enough) and orgasm should be regarded as residual symptoms of the Major Depressive Episode or side effects from her medication. Because monoamine oxidase inhibitors, such as tranylcypromine, and the selective serotonin reuptake inhibitors are known to cause both impairment in sexual arousal and, more commonly, difficulty in orgasm, it is more practical to regard these symptoms first as drug side effects (noted on Axis III), as reducing the dose sometimes alleviates the sexual symptoms. Intoxication or withdrawal from alcohol and other substances of abuse can also cause similar disturbances in sexual functioning. Had this woman, for example, developed problems with orgasm that apparently stemmed from intoxication or withdrawal during the course of Alcohol Abuse or Alcohol Dependence, the diagnosis would be Alcohol-Induced Sexual Dysfunction.

On Axis I we would diagnose Major Depressive Disorder, Single Episode, In Partial Remission (DSM-IV-TR, p. 375), as there are still some residual symptoms of the disturbance (still feels "down" and is not her normal, healthy, ebullient self).

MASTERS AND JOHNSON

A 33-year-old stockbroker sought treatment because of "impotence." Five months previously, a close male friend had died of a coronary occlusion, and within the following week the patient developed anxiety about his own cardiac status. Whenever his heart beat fast because of exertion, he became anxious that he was about to have a heart attack. He had disturbing dreams from which he would awaken anxious and unable to get back to sleep. He stopped playing tennis and running.

The patient began to avoid sexual intercourse, presumably because of his anxiety about physical exertion. This caused difficulties with his wife, who felt that he was deliberately depriving her of sexual outlets and was also preventing her from becoming pregnant, which she very much desired. In the past month, although no longer worried about his heart, the patient had avoided sexual intercourse entirely. He claimed to still have some desire for sex, but when the situation arose, he could not bring himself to do it. He became so upset about his sexual difficulties that he began to have trouble concentrating at work. He felt himself to be a failure both as a husband and as a man.

Before his marriage, the patient had had no sexual experience and had masturbated by rubbing his penis against the bedclothes, without ever manually touching it. Four years previously, at 29 and after 3 years of marriage, he had presented himself for treatment with the complaint that he had never attempted to have sexual intercourse with his wife. Sexual activity consisted of his obtaining an erection without either his wife or himself touching his penis, and ejaculation occurred by rubbing his penis on his wife's abdomen. He was unable to touch his wife's genitalia with his hands or allow his penis to be placed anywhere near his wife's genitalia.

Treatment had consisted of 2 weeks of intensive couples therapy, using the techniques developed by Masters and Johnson, with dramatic success. Sexual activity became frequent, with vaginal penetration and ejaculation. The husband began to display flirtatious sexuality toward other females, which led to some embarrassing social situations, but not to promiscuity. His wife's anxiety about her own sexuality and the adoption of a more passive role led her to seek treatment in her own right. After 1 year of psychotherapy, her anxieties were allayed; sexual intercourse and interpersonal relations between the patient and his wife had been at a satisfactory level until the present problem arose.

Discussion of "Masters and Johnson"

This man's reaction to the death of his friend 5 months previously involved severe anxiety and restriction in his physical activities because of fear that he might have a heart attack; had he been evaluated at that time, an appropriate diagnosis would have been Adjustment Disorder With Anxious Mood. What then happened was that his anxiety affected his sexual functioning, and it is the sexual difficulties that have persisted and occasioned this evaluation.

His current sexual problem is a recurrence of the problem that caused him to seek sex therapy 4 years ago: avoidance of sexual intercourse because of the anxiety associated with it. Although he refers to his problem as "impotence," the diagnosis of Male Erectile Disorder presumes that there is sexual activity during which a man fails to attain or maintain an erection until completion of the sexual activity. However, what this man demonstrates is avoidance of sexual intercourse. Persistent or recurrent extreme aversion to, and avoidance of, all or almost all genital sexual contact with a partner is diagnosed as Sexual Aversion Disorder, Due to Psychological Factors, Acquired Type (DSM-IV-TR, p. 542).

WASH BEFORE WEARING

A 41-year-old man was referred to a community mental health center's activities program for help in improving his social skills. He had a lifelong pattern of social isolation, with no real friends, and spent long hours worrying that his angry thoughts about his older brother would cause his brother harm. He had previously worked as a clerk in civil service, but had lost his job because of poor attendance and low productivity.

On interview the patient was distant and somewhat distrustful. He described in elaborate and often irrelevant detail his rather uneventful and routine daily life. He told the interviewer that he had spent an hour and a half in a pet store deciding which of two brands of fish food to buy and explained their relative merits. For 2 days he had studied the washing instructions on a new pair of jeans—Did "Wash before wearing" mean that the jeans were to be washed before wearing the first time, or did they need, for some reason, to be washed each time before they were worn? He did not regard concerns such as these as senseless, though he acknowledged that the amount of time spent thinking about them might be excessive. He described how he often would buy several different brands of the same item, such as different kinds of can openers, and then would keep them in their original bags in his closet, expecting that at some future time he would find them useful. He was, however, usually very reluctant to spend money on things that he actually needed, although he had a substantial bank account. He could recite from memory his most recent monthly bank statement, including the amount of every check and the running balance as each check was written. He knew his balance on any particular day, but sometimes got anxious if he considered whether a certain check or deposit had actually cleared.

He asked the interviewer whether, if he joined the program, he would be required to participate in groups. He said that groups made him very nervous because he felt that if he revealed too much personal information, such as the amount of money that he had in the bank, people would take advantage of him or manipulate him for their own benefit.

Discussion of "Wash Before Wearing"

This man's long-standing maladaptive pattern of behavior indicates a Personality Disorder. Prominent symptoms include the absence of close friends or confidants, magical thinking (worrying that his angry thoughts would cause his brother harm), constricted affect (observed to be "distant" in the interview), odd speech (providing elaborate and often irrelevant details), and social anxiety associated with paranoid fears. These features are characteristic of Schizotypal Personality Disorder (DSM-IV-TR, p. 701).

Although the absence of close friends or confidants is also characteristic of Schizoid Personality Disorder, this patient's eccentricities of thought and speech preclude that diagnosis. There are many similarities between Schizotypal Personality Disorder and the symptoms seen in the Residual Type of Schizophrenia, but the absence of a history of overt psychotic symptoms rules out that diagnosis.

The patient's concerns with choosing the best brand of fish food and understanding the instructions for washing his jeans suggest obsessions, but the ego-syntonic nature of the concerns indicates that they are not true obsessions, but rather examples of perfectionism. He is also preoccupied with organizing his financial affairs and is miserly with his money. Because these are traits of Obsessive-Compulsive Personality Disorder (DSM-IV-TR, p. 729), we should also note them, but the full criteria for the disorder do not seem to be met.

FOSTER MOTHER

Cheryl Jones, a 44-year-old mother of three teenagers, is hospitalized for treatment of depression. She gives the following history.

One year previously, after an argument that ended her relationship with her lover, she became acutely psychotic. She was frightened that people were going to kill her and heard voices of friends and strangers talking about killing her, sometimes talking to each other. She heard her own thoughts broadcast aloud and was afraid that others could also hear what she was thinking. Over a 3-week period she stayed in her apartment, had new locks put on the doors, kept the shades down, and avoided everyone but her immediate family. She was unable to sleep at night because the voices kept her awake, and unable to eat because of a constant "lump" in her throat. In retrospect, she cannot say whether she was depressed, denies being elated or overactive, and remembers only that she was terrified of what would happen to her. The family persuaded her to enter a hospital, where, after 6 weeks of treatment with an antipsychotic drug, the voices stopped. She remembers feeling "back to normal" for 1–2 weeks, but then she seemed to lose her energy and motivation to do anything. She became increasingly depressed, lost her appetite, and woke at 4:00 A.M. or 5:00 A.M. every morning and was unable to get back to sleep. She could no longer read a newspaper or watch TV because she couldn't concentrate.

Ms. Jones's condition has persisted for 9 months. She has done very little except sit in her apartment, staring at the walls. Her children have managed most of the cooking, shopping, bill paying, and so on. She has continued in outpatient treatment, and was maintained on the antipsychotic drug until 3 months before this admission. There has been no recurrence of the psychotic symptoms since the medication was discontinued; but her depression, with all the accompanying symptoms, has persisted.

In discussing her history, Ms. Jones is rather guarded. There is, however, no evidence of a diagnosable illness before last year. She apparently is a shy, emotionally constricted person who has "never broken any rules." She has been separated from her husband for 10 years, but in that time has had two enduring relationships with boyfriends. In addition to rearing three apparently healthy and very likable children, she cared for a succession of foster children full-time in the 4 years before her illness. She enjoyed this and was highly valued by the agency she worked for. She has maintained close relationships with a few girlfriends and with her extended family.

Discussion of "Foster Mother"

During her initial period of illness, this patient demonstrated such characteristic schizophrenic symptoms as bizarre delusions (people could hear what she was thinking) accompanied by auditory hallucinations (voices of friends and strangers talking to each other). There was deterioration in functioning to the point that she was unable to take care of her house. With treatment, after about 9 weeks the psychotic symptoms remitted, but she remembers being "back to normal" for only about a week. She then developed the characteristic symptoms of a Major Depressive Episode, with depressed mood, poor appetite, insomnia, lack of energy, loss of interest, and poor concentration. The depressive period has lasted for about 9 months.

Are the two periods of illness two separate disorders or a single illness? If they represent two separate disorders, they could be characterized as either Schizophreniform Disorder (because the duration is greater than 1 month but less than 6 months) followed by Major Depressive Disorder, or Schizophrenia (the period after the psychotic phase being considered a residual phase of Schizophrenia) with a superimposed depression (for the second period of illness). If there is a single disorder, it is hard to know what diagnosis would subsume all of the features of the separate episodes of psychosis and depression.

This case would seem to be an example of an instance in which it is difficult to make a differential diagnosis with any degree of certainty between a Mood Disorder and Schizophrenia or Schizophreniform Disorder. Many clinicians would want to call it Schizoaffective Disorder. This diagnosis, according to DSM-IV-TR criteria, cannot be made because there is apparently no temporal overlap of the patient's psychotic symptoms and her depression. Therefore, we would diagnose Schizophreniform Disorder (DSM-IV-TR, p. 319) for the psychotic period, and Major Depressive Disorder, Single Episode, for the depressive period (DSM-IV-TR, p. 375).

Follow-Up

Ms. Jones was treated with an antidepressant and a stimulant. She recovered within a few months, went back to school to get her general equivalency diploma, and began working as a homemaker for the welfare department. A year later she returned to the hospital, depressed and anxious and with psychotic symptoms. She was treated with a combination of antidepressant and antipsychotic drugs, and she recovered within a few months.

With this follow-up information, indicating an episode in which psychotic and depressive symptoms co-occurred, the diagnosis for the second episode would seem to be Major Depressive Disorder, Recurrent, Severe With Psychotic Features (DSM-IV-TR, p. 376).

SLEEPY

A 55-year-old businessman had had excessive sleepiness since age 21, which he had described to his new family physician, who then referred him to a sleep specialist. Typically, he slept regularly from 10:15 P.M. to 6:30 A.M. He also took ½-hour to ¾-hour naps between 9:00 A.M. and 10:15 A.M., and 1:30 P.M. and 2:00 P.M., and napped irregularly between 4:30 P.M. and 8:30 P.M. When napping at work, on his office floor, he deferred all calls. He awoke temporarily refreshed. Delaying his naps caused overwhelming fatigue. He had no sudden loss of muscle tone (as in cataplexy) or other symptoms suggesting narcolepsy and neither snored nor had any other symptoms suggesting a Breathing-Related Sleep Disorder.

The patient owned a television station in Birmingham, Alabama. He was spared obligatory hard work as his staff could run the operation. Nevertheless, he was an organized, motivated person. He was in good health and jogged 4–5 miles daily. He lived with his wife and youngest son. He enjoyed socializing with his married children and their families and dabbling in local politics. He would take a longer afternoon nap in anticipation of any evening activity, which he always left early in favor of his regular bedtime.

His father had taken a nap daily after lunch, and his paternal grandfather had been excessively sleepy. During childhood the patient had had some nightmares, but no other sleep problem. He had been athletic and spontaneously ran along his paper route.

The patient drank about two beers a week, but avoided additional alcohol, caffeine, and other drugs. Previous physical exams had revealed good health, with a resting heart rate maintained in the 50s, blood pressures that ran around 110/70 to 105/70 mm Hg, normal thyroid function, and normal fasting blood sugar.

When interviewed, the patient was friendly, informative, and self-assured. He denied depressed mood or loss of interest or pleasure. He regarded his sleepiness as a difficulty with which he had come to terms, but would be grateful for further relief.

Tests of daytime vigilance indicated impaired arousal. He had an average interval to sleep onset of 11 minutes during five polygraphically recorded naps, which is within the normal range. During a nighttime polygraphic recording, he had normal-appearing sleep that continued uninterrupted for 9½ hours until he had to be awakened.

Discussion of "Sleepy"

In most patients with a chief complaint of excessive daytime sleepiness (hypersomnia) sufficiently severe to cause the person to seek help at a sleep disorders center, either a general medical condition or use of a substance or medication is found to cause the disturbance. This case illustrates the relatively uncommon situation in which neither of these factors nor another mental disorder (such as Major Depressive Disorder) can account for the disturbance. The diagnosis is therefore Primary Hypersomnia (DSM-IV-TR, p. 609). Primary Hypersomnia is usually associated, as in this case, with normal sleep latency and patterns as measured by the polysomnograph.

Follow-Up

Treatment with a long-acting stimulant caused severe headaches. Amphetamines and caffeine-containing beverages did not help, as their initial stimulation was followed by increased sleepiness.

Because the patient speculated that psychotherapy might shed light on his problem and pose fewer disadvantages, he began a course of weekly sessions. However, after 2 years of this treatment with a psychoanalyst, his sleep pattern was unchanged, and he continued to manage his sleepiness with regular naps.

THE REPORTER

Michael Dodge, a 29-year-old newspaper reporter, had been a heavy drinker for 10 years. One evening after work, having finished a feature article, he started drinking with friends and continued to drink through the evening. He fell asleep in the early morning hours. Upon awakening he had a strong desire to drink again and decided not to go to work. Food did not appeal to him, and instead he had several Bloody Marys. Later he went to a local tavern and drank beer throughout the afternoon. He met some friends and continued drinking into the evening.

The pattern of drinking throughout the day persisted for the next 7 days. On the eighth morning, Michael tried to drink a cup of coffee and found his hands were shaking so violently he could not get the cup to his mouth. He managed to pour some whiskey into a glass and drank as much as he could. His hands became less shaky, but now he was nauseated and began having "dry heaves." He tried repeatedly to drink, but could not keep alcohol down. He felt ill and intensely anxious and decided to call a doctor friend. The doctor recommended hospitalization.

When evaluated on admission, Michael is alert; he has a marked resting and intention tremor of the hands, and his tongue and eyelids are tremulous. He has feelings of "internal" tremulousness. Lying in the hospital bed, he finds the noises outside his window unbearably loud and begins seeing "visions" of animals and, on one occasion, a dead relative. He is terrified and calls a nurse, who gives him a tranquilizer. He becomes quieter, and his tremor becomes less pronounced. At all times he realizes that the visual phenomena are "imaginary." He always knows where he is and is otherwise oriented. He has no memory impairment. After a few days the tremor disappears, and Michael no longer hallucinates. He still has trouble sleeping, but otherwise feels normal. He vows never to drink again.

When questioned further about his history of drinking, Michael claims that although during the last 10 years he has developed the habit of drinking several scotches each day, his drinking has never interfered with his work or relations with colleagues or friends. He denies having aftereffects of drinking other than occasional mild hangovers, ever going on binges before this one, and needing to drink every day in order to function adequately. He admits, however, that he has never tried to reduce or stop drinking.

Discussion of "The Reporter"

This heavy drinker markedly increases his amount of drinking for a week and then stops drinking as he becomes sick with nausea and vomiting. He then develops visual hallucinations; tremor of the hands, tongue, and eyelids; and anxiety. Significantly, he has intact reality testing in that he realizes that the hallucinations are imaginary and he remains alert, fully oriented, and without memory impairment. These symptoms, associated with the reduction in heavy alcohol use, indicate Alcohol Withdrawal (DSM-IV-TR, p. 216). Furthermore, the specifier With Perceptual Disturbances is noted to indicate the presence of hallucinations occurring with intact reality testing.

Many clinicians might conclude that this was Alcohol Withdrawal Delirium (delirium tremens) because of the visual hallucinations. Delirium, however, requires reduced ability to maintain attention to external stimuli, disorganized thinking, and other symptoms such as disorientation and memory impairment, in addition to whatever perceptual disturbances may be present. The visual hallucinations with intact reality testing that Michael experienced are rather common in Alcohol Withdrawal.

Does the presence of Alcohol Withdrawal invariably indicate the presence of Alcohol Dependence? The DSM-IV-TR criteria for Substance Dependence require more than mere physiological signs of dependence (i.e., tolerance or withdrawal) that might develop after heavy recreational use of alcohol. The criteria for dependence require evidence of impaired control or harmful consequences from drug use. In this case the patient denies impaired control of his drinking and claims that his drinking does not interfere with his work or social relations. If this is actually true (we doubt it), he would not have the additional diagnosis of Alcohol Dependence (or even Abuse). We would note the need to rule out this diagnosis and are skeptical about Michael's ability to stop drinking, as he has vowed to do.

COUGH MEDICINE

A 42-year-old executive in a public relations firm was referred for psychiatric consultation by his surgeon, who discovered him sneaking large quantities of a codeine-containing cough medicine into the hospital. The patient had been a heavy cigarette smoker for 20 years and had a chronic, hacking cough. He had come into the hospital for a hernia repair and found the pain from the incision unbearable when he coughed.

An operation on his back 5 years previously had led his doctor to prescribe codeine to help relieve the incisional pain at that time. Over the intervening 5 years, however, the patient had continued to use codeine-containing tablets and had increased his intake to 60–90 5-mg tablets daily. He stated that he often "just took them by the handful—not to feel good, you understand, just to get by." He had spent considerable time and effort developing a circle of physicians and pharmacists to whom he would "make the rounds" at least three times a week to obtain new supplies of pills. He had tried several times to stop using codeine, but had failed. During this period he lost two jobs because of lax work habits and was divorced by his wife of 11 years.

Discussion of "Cough Medicine"

Spending a great deal of time obtaining a supply of a substance, repeated unsuccessful efforts to cut down use, tolerance (markedly increased amounts are needed to achieve the desired effect: his taking 60–90 tablets a day), and use of the substance to avoid withdrawal symptoms all indicate Psychoactive Substance Dependence. The diagnosis is coded as Opioid Dependence (DSM-IV-TR, p. 270), because codeine is classified as an opioid. However, the name of the specific substance, codeine, rather than the class of substance, opioid, is recorded. The diagnosis can be further specified as With Physiological Dependence because he has evidence of both tolerance and withdrawal.

Although the criteria for Psychoactive Substance Abuse are also met in this case (a maladaptive pattern of use indicated by continued use despite knowledge of consequent social and occupational impairment), the diagnosis of Psychoactive Substance Dependence takes precedence.

EDGY ELECTRICIAN

A 27-year-old married electrician complains of dizziness, sweating palms, heart palpitations, and ringing of the ears of more than 18 months' duration. He has also experienced dry mouth and throat, periods of extreme muscle tension, and a constant "edgy" and watchful feeling that has often interfered with his ability to concentrate. These feelings have been present most of the time over the previous 2 years; they have not been limited to discrete periods. Although these symptoms sometimes make him feel "discouraged," he denies feeling depressed and continues to enjoy activities with his family.

Because of these symptoms the patient had seen a family practitioner, a neurologist, a neurosurgeon, a chiropractor, and an ear-nose-throat specialist. He had been placed on a hypoglycemic diet, received physiotherapy for a pinched nerve, and been told he might have "an inner ear problem."

He also has many worries. He constantly worries about the health of his parents. His father, in fact, had a myocardial infarction 2 years previously, but is now feeling well. He also worries about whether he is "a good father," whether his wife will ever leave him (there is no indication that she is dissatisfied with the marriage), and whether he is liked by co-workers on the job. Although he recognizes that his worries are often unfounded, he can't stop worrying.

For the past 2 years the patient has had few social contacts because of his nervous symptoms. Although he has sometimes had to leave work when the symptoms became intolerable, he continues to work for the same company he joined for his apprenticeship following high-school graduation. He tends to hide his symptoms from his wife and children, to whom he wants to appear "perfect," and reports few problems with them as a result of his nervousness.

Discussion of "Edgy Electrician"

This man has consulted numerous physicians for his symptoms, but the absence of preoccupation with fears of having a specific physical disease precludes a diagnosis of Hypochondriasis. He recognizes that his worries are often excessive, but they do not have the intrusive and inappropriate quality that characterizes the obsessions of Obsessive-Compulsive Disorder.

His predominant symptom is excessive and uncontrollable anxiety and worry for most of the time over the past 2 years. This suggests the diagnosis of Generalized Anxiety Disorder. He also has the characteristic associated symptoms of feeling on edge, difficulty concentrating, and muscle tension. His worries cause him significant distress and impair his social functioning. The diagnosis of Generalized Anxiety Disorder (DSM-IV-TR, p. 476) is made in this case because the worries are not confined to the features of another Axis I disorder (e.g., worrying about having a panic attack, as in Panic Disorder, or being embarrassed in public, as in Social Phobia), the symptoms do not occur only during the course of a Mood or Psychotic Disorder, they are not the direct effects of a substance (e.g., drugs of abuse or medication) or a general medical condition (e.g., hyperthyroidism), and the disturbance has persisted for more than 6 months.

The diagnosis of Generalized Anxiety Disorder first appeared in DSM-III when Panic Disorder was separated out of what previously had been called Anxiety Neurosis. Since that time there has been controversy as to how best to define the condition. The current definition emphasizes the cognitive component of excessive worry and deemphasizes autonomic symptoms. However, many patients, particularly in medical settings, present with primarily somatic symptoms of anxiety and deny excessive worry. It is not at all clear that these patients, who are not eligible for this diagnosis, have a different disorder.

THE BOARDS

A married 29-year-old woman was presented as the neurology patient at the examination of a young psychiatrist for his specialty certification in psychiatry. Four months previously she had been riding in a car, driven by her husband, that was involved in a minor traffic accident. She was thrown forward, but was kept from hitting the window or dashboard by her seat belt. Three days later she began to complain of a stiff neck and sharp pains radiating down both arms, her spine to the small of her back, and both legs. Because an orthopedic consultation failed to uncover the cause of the pain, she was referred to the neurology clinic.

The patient was an attractive, statuesque woman in obvious distress who described her injury and her symptoms in vivid detail, tracing the course of her pains down her arms and legs with her hands. She smiled frequently at the young psychiatrist and at the two examiners who were observing him. She performed each test of neurological function with precision and appeared to relish the attention. The neurological examination findings were totally normal.

The psychiatrist inquired into the patient's personal history and present life. There was no previous history of emotional disturbance. The patient currently worked as a computer programmer. She had been married 4 years and had no children. Until recently her marriage had been smooth, except that her husband sometimes complained that they were "mismatched" sexually. He seemed considerably more interested in frequent and "imaginative" sex, whereas she seemed satisfied with weekly intercourse without variation or much foreplay.

Two weeks before the accident, the patient had discovered a woman's phone number in her husband's wallet. When she confronted him with it, he admitted that he had seen several women over the preceding year, mainly for "sexual release." The patient was bitterly hurt and disappointed for several days, then began to get angry and attacked him for his "hang-ups." At the time of the accident, they had been arguing in the car on the way to a friend's house for dinner. After the accident they decided to try harder to please each other in their marriage, including sexually; but because of the pains that the patient was experiencing, they had not been able to have any sexual contact.

The young psychiatrist passed the exam.

Discussion of "The Boards"

The predominant focus of this woman's clinical presentation is pain in several anatomical sites. The absence of physical findings and the apparent genuineness of the symptoms rule out a physical disorder, Malingering, and a Factitious Disorder. The pain is of sufficient severity to cause her to seek treatment, and it impairs her functioning.

It is difficult to escape the conclusion that this woman's pain serves the function of enabling her to avoid an activity that is noxious to her: having to deal with both her husband's increasing sexual demands and their apparent sexual incompatibility. Further positive evidence of the role of psychological factors is the temporal relationship between the onset of the symptoms and the discovery of and argument about the husband's extramarital sexual activity. When psychological factors are judged to have an important role in the onset, severity, exacerbation, or maintenance of pain, and no general medical condition is judged to have an important role, the DSM-IV-TR diagnosis is Pain Disorder Associated With Psychological Factors (DSM-IV-TR, p. 503). We would specify Acute, as the duration of the symptoms is less than 6 months.

THE HIKER

A 61-year-old high-school science department head who was an experienced and enthusiastic camper and hiker became extremely fearful while on a trek in the mountains. Gradually, over the next few months, he lost interest in his usual hobbies. Formerly a voracious reader, he stopped reading. He had difficulty doing computations and made gross errors in home financial management. On several occasions he became lost while driving in areas that were formerly familiar to him. He began to write notes to himself so that he would not forget to do errands. Very abruptly, and in uncharacteristic fashion, he decided to retire from work, without discussing his plans with his wife. Intellectual deterioration gradually progressed. He spent most of the day piling miscellaneous objects in one place and then transporting them to another spot in the house. He became stubborn and querulous. Eventually he required assistance in shaving and dressing.

When examined 6 years after the first symptoms had developed, the patient was alert and cooperative. He was disoriented with respect to place and time. He could not recall the names of four or five objects after a 5-minute interval of distraction. He could not remember the names of his college and graduate school or the subject in which he had majored. He could describe his job by title only. In 1978 he thought that Kennedy was president of the United States. He did not know Stalin's nationality. His speech was fluent and well articulated, but he had considerable difficulty finding words and used many long, essentially meaningless phrases. He called a cup a vase and identified the rims of glasses as "the holders." He did simple calculations poorly. He could not copy a cube or draw a house. His interpretation of proverbs was concrete, and he had no insight into the nature of his disturbance.

An elementary neurological examination revealed nothing abnormal, and routine laboratory tests were also negative. A computed tomography scan, however, showed marked cortical atrophy.

Discussion of "The Hiker"

This patient has memory impairment, impairment in abstract thinking (concrete interpretation of proverbs), and other disturbances in higher cortical functioning (aphasia). These signs of global cognitive impairment, severe enough to interfere significantly with work and social activities and not occurring exclusively during the course of Delirium, indicate a Dementia. There is an insidious onset, beginning before age 65, with a generally progressive, deteriorating course and no specific cause. Thus the diagnosis is Dementia of the Alzheimer Type's, With Early Onset (DSM-IV-TR, p. 157). Because of the absence of clinically significant behavioral problems (most of the patient's problems are related to the cognitive impairment), we note the subtype to be Without Behavioral Disturbance.

Given that some degree of supervision is necessary, the severity of the Dementia is noted as Moderate. We note the presence of the neurological disease, Alzheimer's disease, on Axis III.

Follow-Up

This man's condition progressed, and he required admission to the hospital within a year of his initial assessment. Over the next year, he became essentially mute, and mental status testing was virtually impossible. He had a tendency to pace back and forth constantly in the ward; on one occasion he managed to get out of the locked ward and was found some miles from the hospital. (Note that at this point in the course, the subtype With Behavioral Disturbance would have been warranted.)

His retained physical appearance was in striking contrast to his devastated intellectual capacities for a long time, but eventually he began to lose weight, took to his bed, and developed contractures (permanent muscular contractions).

He died at age 72 of pneumonia. Autopsy revealed cerebral atrophy and, microscopically, the plaques and tangles diagnostic of Alzheimer's disease.

END TIMES

Mr. P., a 25-year-old man from Arkansas indicted for the murder of an 8-year-old girl, was interviewed by a forensic psychiatrist on court order to determine his sanity at the time of the crime. The following is excerpted from the psychiatrist's report.

The defendant says that on the day of the crime, he smoked his usual six to seven pipe bowls of marijuana. He used no alcohol or other drugs that day. During the day he watched television. His mood was normal. His girlfriend was around all day until she left for her father's birthday party at about 6:30 P.M. or 7:00 P.M.; she returned about 9:30 P.M.

After his girlfriend left the house, Mr. P. went to sit on the porch. About half an hour later, he saw some neighborhood children running around the house. Three youngsters, including the victim, asked if they could see his pet tarantula. He said they must come in one at a time. The girl's younger brother and another boy left. She then asked if she could come in to see the spider. She looked at the spider and started to walk back out of the house. No one else was around. The defendant grabbed her around her chest. He said he made up his mind to "do it" as she was walking out since, he thought, this was a possible chance to obtain a dead body.

The defendant reports that he ran into the bathroom with the victim, and turned on the bathtub water. "She just stood there and looked like she didn't know what was going on." Once he had sufficient water in the tub to submerge her face, he did so. She kicked and struggled, and screamed briefly. He never said a word to her. He was panicky and nervous. "I didn't believe I was actually doing it." After holding her face under water for 3 or 4 minutes, he pulled her up. She tried to catch her breath, and he realized that he had "pulled her up too quickly." He was fearful that her brother might come looking for her, so he ran with her to a large crawl space under a floor board in a closet on the first floor. He was fearful that if her brother came back, he would tell their parents and they would "catch us," and then he would be unable to fulfill his fantasy of having sex with her dead body.

In the crawl space he hit her on the head with a brick he found there. She appeared to lose consciousness after the first blow. He struck her head many more times with the brick. He claims that he was crying and that it was "horrible, much harder than the drowning." He then put her body under a piece of plastic, closed off the crawl space, and straightened up the things he had knocked over. He turned on the television set.

A short time later, the victim's brother, who was about 5 years old, walked in the door and asked if his sister was there. Mr. P. said, "No." He instructed the boy to get out, and the youngster left. About half an hour later, the police came and asked to see his spider and permission to look around. Mr. P. was nervous, but he did not think they would find the crawl space. They did not in their first 15-minute search.

The next morning, after his girlfriend went to work, police detectives came again, and this time found the crawl space, but didn't notice the body in the dark. He felt that they would be unlikely to search the house again. Later that morning, he went back into the crawl space and took the clothes off the victim's body. He put Vaseline on her anus and inserted his penis, while he placed his finger in her vagina. He was so scared that he had only a partial erection, but he did ejaculate. He felt he had to do it because otherwise "it all would have been for nothing." He wrapped the body in the plastic, put it farther back against a slope in the crawl space, and pushed dirt over it. He hoped he would be able to go back for additional sexual activity with the corpse, but at that point was more concerned about not being detected.

The police returned the next day, used a better light to search the crawl space, and found the body. Mr. P. was down there with them. He felt terror and could not stop sweating. "I was more or less in shock." He said, "That's her" when they found the body. At that point he felt the "jig was up": there was no way that he could say he didn't kill the child.

In response to my questions, Mr. P. stated that when he grabbed the victim, it was for the purpose of carrying out his sexual fantasy. He was willing to take an "allowable minor risk" of getting caught if the risk was very small. He reports that his urge to grab her was sufficient to outweigh a small risk, but not sufficient to outweigh a substantial risk of getting caught. "Once I started, I felt I couldn't stop. All I was thinking about was carrying out my fantasy." He says he knew his actions were "wrong in the eyes of the law." The only justification he felt was that "It was in my destiny, something I needed to experience. It was for the purpose of knowing what all kinds of sex were like." When I asked for clarification of the issue of his "destiny," he indicated that his destiny was "to have sex with a dead body, not necessarily to kill." The decision to kill rather than steal a dead body was his own. In his fantasy, however, he reports there was the "killing part" because of his inability to obtain an already dead body.

Past history revealed bed-wetting until age 6 and cruelty to animals as a child. As an adolescent, Mr. P. cut the legs off frogs and put firecrackers in their mouths. He put a small dog on top of the refrigerator and watched it fall off.

His sexual history indicated that when he was 4 years old, an adult man in the neighborhood had him perform oral sex and performed oral sex on him. Between the ages of 12 and 14, he had homosexual relationships with two boys his age. Although Mr. P. had a regular girlfriend from age 16 on, he also commonly had sex with prostitutes and masturbated frequently, usually with the fantasy that he was having anal sex with a woman. He says that he was preoccupied with sex; it was the strongest of all his feelings.

When he was 18, he became interested in more unusual sexual objects, including women's underwear and sexual devices, such as a rubber penis, a rubber vagina, and a blow-up doll, with which he had all varieties of intercourse. He performed fellatio on a dog and trained it to insert its penis into his anus. He killed another dog and then performed sex on it. He became interested sexually in the urine and feces of attractive women and finally got the idea of having sex with a dead human female body. Before the incident that led to his arrest, the fantasy of having sex with a dead body occurred to him every time he masturbated.

His necrophiliac fantasy became more clearly defined over time. It involved drowning a woman, taking her to the crawl space in his house, undressing her, and then doing "all kinds of mutilation." The fantasy included "eating her feces, drinking urine, anal sex, biting her ear," and "scratching her back with my nails." He also had thoughts of "licking eyeballs, opening the abdomen" and putting his hand in. He thought of removing the uterus and inserting it in his anus. He thought of "chewing on an ear, nose or tongue while raping the body." Fantasies included eating various body parts, such as the "breasts, vulva, nose, and tongue." He thought of eating the clitoris and labia raw, or after cooking them. While masturbating with these fantasies, he took pleasure in fantasizing about both mutilating the body and using the body parts. His fantasies were more like an "explosion of ideas" than methodical plans. He took pleasure in the idea that any thought he had at the time he would actually be able to carry out. All the fantasies were sexually exciting. The most exciting involved the anus of the dead body. He thought of putting his hand in the anus and eating the anus, either raw or cooked.

As a teenager Mr. P. became interested in Satan. He enjoyed reading both the Old and New Testaments, particularly the books "Revelation" and "The Prophets." He felt that he could relate passages in the Bible to current events and concluded that we were living in the "end times." He reports that while a teenager, at times he felt he was "the Antichrist." He believed that he would eventually rise to power and rule things in the "end times." He felt he knew things that others did not know. By referring to passages in the Bible, he thought he could understand some events going on now and in the future. He reports he was able to convince many people that they were living in the "end times" and that Armageddon would be here by the year 2000.

Mr. P. made predictions about comets, the Israeli invasion of Lebanon, and certain natural disasters before they occurred. He felt he had a gift for prediction. He used the writings of Nostradamus for his predictions.

When he was 15, Mr. P. was unsure about whether he was the prophet Elijah or the Antichrist. He looked at his eyes in a mirror and felt that they looked strange, especially when he was on drugs. He felt he should know something he had not yet been told, that he was on the verge of acquiring new knowledge. He reports that the uncertainty as to whether he was a prophet or the Antichrist persisted until the killing. He felt that if he were the prophet, he could predict things; if he were the Antichrist, he would do things to increase his power so that he would eventually be able to rule the world. He usually preferred to be the prophet, but at other times being the Antichrist was more appealing. When he was close to people he knew, he wanted to do good; when he was alone, he wanted to do bad sexual things.

I questioned Mr. P. closely to try and clarify the length and degree of certainty he felt regarding his ideas of being an Antichrist. He repeated that since he had begun to have the idea at age 15, he alternated in believing that he was either the Antichrist or the prophet Elijah. He was certain that he was going to be "something big religiously." When he engaged in perverse sexual activity, it would be as the Antichrist. When he spoke with friends about religion, it would be as a prophet. Once he was arrested after the body had been found, he immediately gave up the idea that he would be something great religiously because he thought that a criminal record would preclude success as a religious person. When I questioned the likelihood of his becoming a great prophet, in view of his work and school attainment, he replied that Hitler and Einstein had done poorly in school. When I asked whether he had prepared himself for exercising great power by taking courses in political science, he replied that he had not.

Discussion of "End Times"

Running through the story of Mr. P.'s life are three themes: extremely intense uncontrollable sexual impulses, violent fantasies, and a tenuous relationship to reality. The sexual impulses have been paraphiliac, first involving nonhuman objects and body parts (female undergarments, sexual toys, dogs, urine, feces) and later focusing on anal intercourse with a dead body. As a child, he tortured animals; when he was an adolescent, his violent impulses became intertwined with overpowering sexual impulses.

Since adolescence Mr. P. has had two opposing grandiose fantasies: either he is the Antichrist (bad, violent, and sexual) or the prophet Elijah (a powerful religious leader). His grandiosity has apparently never been of delusional intensity; rather, he has entertained the possibility that he might be either of these figures.

There is no doubt about the diagnosis of Mr. P.'s deviant sexual behavior. Like many people with paraphiliac disorders, his choice of deviant sexual stimuli has changed over time. He has a history of Fetishism (nonhuman objects), and his current diagnosis is the rare disorder Necrophilia (erotic attraction to corpses), classified as a Paraphilia Not Otherwise Specified (DSM-IV-TR, p. 576).

The diagnosis of Mr. P.'s long-term problems in perceiving, relating to, and thinking about the environment and himself is more difficult. His odd beliefs about himself and his magical thinking (that he can foretell the future) suggest Schizotypal Personality Disorder, but the case material does not describe other features of the disorder. He tortured animals as a child but has none of the other features of either Antisocial Personality Disorder or the DSM-III-R appendix diagnosis of Sadistic Personality Disorder. Because his personality is so obviously pathological, we use the residual and not very descriptive diagnosis of Personality Disorder Not Otherwise Specified (DSM-IV-TR, p. 729).

Follow-Up

The defense lawyers planned to argue for an insanity defense by presenting expert psychiatric testimony that Mr. P. had a Schizotypal Personality Disorder (DSM-IV-TR, p. 701) and, because of that, was unable to refrain from the homicide. The prosecution expert who prepared this case concurred in the diagnosis of Schizotypal Personality Disorder, but did not believe that this qualified for an insanity defense. At some point in his trial Mr. P. accepted a plea bargain in order to avoid the possibility of a death sentence. He is now serving a life term.

Chapter 2

Mental Disorders in Children and Adolescents

DAYDREAMER

Mark is an 11-year-old boy who is brought for a psychiatric consultation by his parents for problems he has had "since he was born." He is described as socially immature and has always had trouble making friends. His mother sees him as unhappy; his father, as unfocused and lazy. This school year has been particularly hard. He is picked on and seems always to do and say the wrong thing.

Mark was a "demanding" baby. He never seemed to sleep, and he cried a lot. His developmental milestones were within normal limits. As a toddler he was "on the quiet side."

In first grade he had trouble waiting in line and became attached to certain toys, preferring to play the same games repeatedly. He has always had difficulty with change and transitions (e.g., changing the seating arrangement for dinner can throw him into a tizzy).

Academically, elementary school was uneventful. Mark maintained a B average, but his grades dropped in seventh grade. His father was very demanding and felt that Mark constantly wasted time when studying, daydreaming instead of focusing on homework. His absent-minded behavior was evident when he became a member of the traveling basketball team in sixth grade. His father was an assistant coach and observed that Mark "got lost on the court" and was socially less mature than the others. He had poor eye contact and lacked social skills. He missed out on jokes and didn't join in the team comradery.

Mark's mother says he usually starts school off on a positive note, but as the work becomes more difficult and complex, he gets disorganized. At meals Mark has trouble following the conversation. During the summer he has less trouble, as he is a good athlete and spends a lot of time in sports activities. However, in day camp he made only one friend; and since starting sleep-away camp at age 8, he has never developed a social network. The camp director reported that Mark was inflexible, said silly things, and had difficulty following instructions.

Mark's mother, age 40, has a master's degree in audiology. His father, age 41, has an MBA from an Ivy League school and is a successful investment banker. The marriage is described as excellent, and Mark seems to be the only focus of conflict. His father is disappointed and irritated with Mark, and his mother is protective and worried. There are two younger brothers, ages 9 and 7, who are without any emotional problems.

Mark had to be coerced by his mother to attend the evaluation. He says he has trouble making friends and he doesn't do as well in school as he should. His favorite subjects are math and English, even though he does poorly in both. He says he fights with his parents and that his father's criticism can make him cry. He is afraid that coming to see a psychiatrist must mean that he is crazy. He says he has no problem sleeping, his appetite is excellent, and he loves to watch TV for hours, especially sports events. He has no friends and spends his weekends alone. He can't understand why people don't like him. He acknowledges trouble keeping his attention on his work in school and admits that his mind wanders while the teacher talks. At camp things are okay when he's playing sports, but he has no close friends. He prefers tennis to team sports because "it's easier to pay attention when you know the ball is always coming to you." He wishes that it would be easier to keep friends, that he and his father would stop fighting, and that he could eventually become a professional basketball player.

School reports consistently state that Mark has poor organizational skills. He is able to sit for 10 or 15 minutes, but frequently gets drinks of water or makes bathroom trips. He has poor concentration. When being tutored one-to-one, he can accomplish a lot, and he is evaluated as bright by his tutor. No disciplinary problems are reported in school.

The Teacher's version of the Conners Teacher Rating Scale (1990), which assesses hyperactivity, impulsivity, and attention, was completed by several of his teachers. They indicated that he had a short attention span, was easily distracted, daydreamed much of the time, and consistently failed to finish things he started. The neuropsychological testing data indicated problems with attention and processing speed. He did poorly on a spatial relations test, a timed, complex task requiring rapid processing of information. He also did poorly on following oral directions that required attention to both visual and verbal detail. On a test of memory and learning, he did well on memory tasks that are meaningful, but poorly on memory tests of randomly connected information.

Discussion of "Daydreamer"

Mark's problems seem to fall into two general categories: he has trouble focusing and paying attention, and socially, he is immature and unable to make friends. It is likely that his problems with focusing and paying attention contribute to the social difficulties that he experiences. In any case, his social problems are not severe enough to consider a Pervasive Developmental Disorder, and there is no evidence of a Social Phobia.

Mark's problems with focusing and paying attention have been apparent since he began school. Over the years he has displayed difficulty paying attention to details, sustaining attention to particular tasks, listening to instructions, and finishing what he has begun. In addition, he appears to be easily distracted. These are the attentional symptoms that are required for the diagnosis of Attention-Deficit/Hyperactivity Disorder (DSM-IV-TR, p. 92). (The diagnosis would not be made if the disorder were better accounted for by another mental disorder, such as a Pervasive Developmental Disorder.) This disorder usually involves symptoms of hyperactivity and impulsivity (see "Into Everything," p. 351). Mark has few, if any, of these symptoms; hence, the diagnosis would be further specified as Predominantly Inattentive Type.

Follow-Up

Two months after the evaluation, at the beginning of the school term, Mark was started on methylphenidate, a stimulant that paradoxically has a calming effect on children with Attention-Deficit/Hyperactivity Disorder. His academic performance during eighth grade improved dramatically. He received all A's and B's, except for a C in social studies. The Conners Teacher Rating Scale scores showed significant improvement on measures of inattention.

His relationship with his parents improved, his mother claiming that everyone was getting along better. Mark reported making two new friends from the basketball program, and his mother reports that classmates have called him to set up dates. Blood pressure, pulse, height, and weight were monitored. No adverse side effects to the medication were reported.

Reference

Conners CK: Manual for Conners Rating Scales. North Tonawanda, NY, Multi Health Systems, 1990

BOTTLE BABY

Six-month-old Robert was admitted to a hospital for evaluation of his failure to gain weight when, at 15 pounds, he fell below the fifteenth percentile for weight for his age. He was the second of two children born to working-class parents following an unplanned but normal pregnancy. He weighed almost 9 pounds at birth.

Although this first son was the apple of his father's eye, Robert's mother has had continual difficulties with the infant. He was bottle fed, and his mother reported that he had severe colic. His pediatrician made several formula changes and suggested other treatments for colic, but Robert continued to fail to gain weight.

In the hospital, the nurses watched his mother attempt to feed him. There was poor synchrony between the mother and baby around feeding, in that she often did not seem to know when he was hungry, when he needed to be burped, and when he had finished eating. Consequently, feeding was a distressing experience for both parties. However, the nurses and aides were able to feed Robert without any difficulty. Various medical investigations failed to disclose any specific medical condition that might account for the baby's difficulties. Discussion with the mother gradually revealed that she had been depressed throughout the pregnancy and resented the demands of the baby. Treatment of her depression and the underlying marital problems and focused instruction on feeding facilitated the mother's adjustment. With this, Robert's feeding difficulties gradually diminished markedly, and within a few weeks he gained several pounds.

Discussion of "Bottle Baby"

Feeding Disorder of Infancy or Early Childhood (DSM-IV-TR, p. 108) is diagnosed if a child fails to eat adequately and to gain weight or suffers a significant weight loss over at least 1 month and if the condition, as in this case, cannot be better accounted for by a medical condition (e.g., gastroesophageal reflux), by simple absence of available food, or by Rumination Disorder. In Rumination Disorder, weight loss is sometimes observed but is accompanied by characteristic regurgitation and rechewing of food (see "Baby Susan," p. 374).

In this case, chronic marital stress and maternal depression probably contributed to the mother's difficulties in feeding her child.

THE PRETZEL

Victor, a legally blind 14-year-old boy with severe mental retardation, was evaluated when he transferred to a new residential school for children with multiple disabilities. Observed in his classroom, he was noted to be a small boy who appeared younger than his age. He held his hands in his pockets and spun around in place. Periodically he approached his teacher, kissed her, positioned himself to receive a return kiss, and clearly enjoyed the contact with her. When offered a toy (which had to be held very close to his eyes), he took it and manipulated it for a while. When he was prompted to engage in various tasks that required that he take his hands out of his pockets, he began hitting his head with his hands. If his hands were held by the teacher, he hit his head with his knees. He was very adept in contorting himself, so he could hit or kick himself in almost any position, even while walking. Soon his face and forehead were covered with black-and-blue marks.

Only sketchy personal history was available. He was a premature baby, with birth weight of 2 pounds. Retinopathy of prematurity and severe mental retardation were diagnosed early in life. His development was delayed in all spheres, and he never developed language. Comprehensive studies did not disclose the etiology of Victor's developmental disabilities other than prematurity. He lived at home and attended a special educational program. His self-injurious behaviors developed early in life, and when his parents tried to stop him, he became aggressive. Gradually he became too difficult for them to manage, and at age 3 he was placed in a special school. The self-abusive and self-restraining (i.e., holding his hands in his pockets) behavior was present throughout his stay there, and virtually all the time he was on one antipsychotic medication or another. He carried a diagnosis of "cerebral dysfunction." Although the psychiatrist's notes mentioned improvement in his self-injurious behavior, other notes described it as continuing and fluctuating. He was transferred to the new school because of lack of progress and difficulties in managing him as he became bigger and stronger. His intellectual functioning was within the 34–40 IQ range. His adaptive skills were poor. He required full assistance in self-care, could not provide even for his own simple needs, and required constant supervision for his safety.

In a few months Victor settled into the routine in his new school. His self-injurious behavior fluctuated. It was reduced or even absent when he restrained himself by holding his hands in his pockets or inside his shirt, or even by manipulating some object with his hands. If left to himself, he could contort himself, while holding his hands inside his shirt, to such degree that he was nicknamed "Pretzel." Because the stereotypic self-injurious and self-restraining behavior interfered with his daily activities and education, it became a primary focus of a behavior modification program. For a few months he did well, especially when he developed a good relationship with a new teacher, who was firm, consistent, and nurturing. With him, Victor could engage in some school tasks. When the teacher left, Victor regressed. To prevent injuries, the staff started blocking his self-hitting with a pillow. He was offered activities he liked and could engage in without resorting to self-injury. After several months his antipsychotic medication was slowly discontinued, over a period of 11 months, without any behavioral deterioration.

Discussion of "The Pretzel"

This unfortunate youngster apparently suffered brain injury because of premature birth, which was complicated by retinopathy. The criteria for Severe Mental Retardation (DSM-IV-TR, p. 49) are met by virtue of his significantly low intellectual and adaptive functioning and onset of the disturbance prior to age 18. He has exhibited for many years repetitive, driven, nonconstructive, inappropriate behaviors, which have resulted in tissue damage. Self-restraint, frequently seen in cases with self-injurious behavior, is present as well. The self-injurious and self-restraining behaviors are the main obstacles to Victor's habilitation, and a major focus of treatment.

Because of his lack of communicative language, it is not possible to ascertain whether the motivation for these behaviors is in response to obsessions, as one would expect in Obsessive-Compulsive Disorder. However, when self-injurious behavior occurs in Obsessive-Compulsive Disorder (e.g., severe hand-washing), the goal is not the self-injury, as it appears to be in this case. The presence of self-stimulating behaviors, such as body spinning and object manipulation, and lack of language might at first glance suggest Pervasive Developmental Disorder; but unlike people with this disorder, Victor has an ability to relate to his caregivers and form basic attachments (within the limits of his mental retardation). This leaves us with the relatively nonspecific diagnosis of Stereotypic Movement Disorder (formerly Stereotypy/Habit Disorder) With Self-Injurious Behavior (DSM-IV-TR, p. 134).

QUIET KEVIN

Kevin is a playful, attractive 6-year-old child who is in first grade in a suburban school. His mother brought him for an evaluation, saying, "He won't speak in school or in any social situations." During the evaluation he whispers to his mother, but won't speak to the interviewer. His mood seems good, his affect very broad, with exuberance, some apprehensiveness when he's expected to speak, but no sadness. He agrees with his mother that not speaking is a real problem, and he wants to overcome it.

Kevin's mother reports that he has been reluctant to speak to people outside of his home setting since he was about 2. He never answered a greeting, and there are very few people he will talk to if he is outside his home. He did not speak in kindergarten at all. He likes going to parties and playing with others—laughing, running around, singing—but will not converse. He doesn't avoid social situations or strangers. He takes piano lessons and will play in front of others, but he won't speak. He enjoys going shopping and will sing out loud in the supermarket, but when people speak to him, he becomes mute. At home he can amuse himself with games and puzzles, as well as play happily with other children.

There is no history of medical problems. His mother describes him as a low-key kid, always easy to get along with, and quite verbal when he's alone with the family. He has always been very bright and has done well academically.

In kindergarten he was referred for "play therapy" with a private psychologist, but several months of treatment did not result in any change in his symptom.

Discussion of "Quiet Kevin"

Kevin appears to be normal in all respects except for his refusal to talk to any people other than his immediate family. This dramatic symptom can hardly be ignored. When, as in Kevin's case, it does not result from lack of familiarity with the language spoken in school, or from a Communication Disorder, such as severe Stuttering, the symptom is given diagnostic status and is called Selective Mutism (DSM-IV-TR, p. 127).

The disorder most commonly appears when the child first enters the school system, but, as in Kevin's case, there often are some mild signs of the disorder earlier. Typically, the child is unable to explain why he or she will not talk, but looks frightened, suggesting that it is some kind of anxiety disorder. Consistent with this is the frequent association of Specific Phobias, such as fear of animals, and Separation Anxiety Disorder. Some children who develop Selective Mutism have mild Communication Disorders or physical disorders that interfere with articulation.

Selective Mutism (formerly called Elective Mutism in DSM-III-R) has been recognized in child psychiatry for a long time because of the dramatic nature of the disturbance. It is unclear whether such cases are not merely one example of the more general category of Social Phobia and whether such children, as adults, often have other manifestations of social anxiety that would warrant the diagnosis of Social Phobia, Generalized Type.

Follow-Up

Kevin was first treated with 4 weeks of behavioral therapy. When this produced no improvement, he was treated with an antidepressant. By the end of the 9 weeks he was talking a little bit in school and talking to his grandparents on the phone. Over the summer he began to speak to his psychiatrist and to peers in day camp. After 22 weeks, the medication was slowly decreased; and over the next few weeks, Kevin's mutism returned with all but his immediate family and his psychiatrist. His mood was less exuberant and more subdued, and behavior was more oppositional at home.

At the beginning of the next school term, Kevin initially refused to take medication; but after 10 days—during which he was speaking to peers and teachers in school—he went back on the medication for a month. He returned to his former state of feeling comfortable and exuberant and was speaking in school and all social settings. By the end of the school year he was a happy, comfortable, talkative second-grader who was voted president of his class. He was now speaking to everyone—except those teachers who knew him as a mute kindergartner.

GRANDMA'S CHILD

Tanya, age 4, was seen for assessment in a child psychiatry clinic at the request of her grandparents. Tanya was the only child of parents who were longtime heroin users. Several months ago, not having seen Tanya or her parents for several years, the grandparents were called by the child protection agency in another state and informed that Tanya's parents had been arrested and she had been placed in foster care.

Soon thereafter, when Tanya came to live with them, the grandparents noticed that she did not have the verbal skills of a normal 4-year-old child, and she had marked problems with social interaction. She often seemed oblivious to ordinary invitations to hug or play with her grandparents and other relatives. She also exhibited a rapidly alternating mixture of responses in which sometimes she seemed to want to get very close to people and at other times would push them away. The grandparents later learned that, since she was an infant, Tanya had often been left with various friends of her parents, many of whom were themselves heavy drug users, and they were often only minimally attentive to her.

On examination Tanya was found to have mild language delays and marked problems in social interaction. She tended to avoid interaction, or, when it could not be avoided, become very anxious and disorganized. After several months of consistent care in her grandparents' home, her use of language became much more appropriate for a 4-year-old child, but she still had some difficulties in social interaction.

Discussion of "Grandma's Child"

This patient displays the characteristic features of Reactive Attachment Disorder (DSM-IV-TR, p. 130): persistent failure to interact socially in a developmentally appropriate manner as a result of a noxious psychosocial environment (e.g., one that is neglectful of the child's basic needs for continuity of care, stimulation, and affection). This may also arise, as in this case, when repeated changes in primary caretaker prevent formation of stable attachments. The inappropriate social behavior may be a pattern either of inhibition (avoidance and lack of attachments, as in this case) or of disinhibition (overly diffuse relationships with a lack of selective attachments).

The reversal, at least in part, of the syndrome with institution of an appropriate environment is consistent with the diagnosis. The major differential diagnosis is a Pervasive Developmental Disorder, in which disturbances in social relationships arise, apparently on a neurobiological basis, but are accompanied by characteristic disturbances in communication, social interaction, and stereotyped patterns of behavior.

REGGIE'S REGRESSION

Reggie was 4 when he was evaluated by a child psychiatrist because of alarming changes in his behavior over the past 2 months. He is the first child born to professional parents. According to them, he was a normally sociable baby whose early development was entirely within normal limits—he was walking and saying single words by his first birthday and spoke in sentences before age 2. He was enrolled in nursery school at age 3 and was toilet trained at that time. The parents said they had videotapes showing that his development up to that point was entirely normal.

Two months ago, shortly following the birth of his sibling, Reggie appeared to become nonspecifically anxious and agitated. Over the course of several weeks, his behavior regressed markedly in multiple areas: he was no longer toilet trained, no longer engaged in age-appropriate self-care activities, and became entirely mute. He similarly regressed markedly in his social skills, and his parents observed that he now spent hours rocking back and forth.

The psychiatric evaluation indicated that, although age 4, he was now functioning at the 1-year level in terms of his cognitive and communicative abilities. From direct observation and descriptions of his behavior by his parents, he exhibited many behavioral features suggestive of autism (e.g., lack of social responsivity, difficulties with transitions, stereotyped movements, and so forth). Review of the videotapes of his early development confirmed the history of normal development provided by the parents.

The psychiatrist arranged for extensive medical evaluations, including an electroencephalogram, a magnetic resonance imaging scan, and various laboratory studies. However, they failed to discover any specific medical condition that might account for his disturbance.

Discussion of "Reggie's Regression"

Because of severe impairment in language and social reciprocity and the presence of stereotyped patterns of behavior, one immediately thinks of Autistic Disorder. However, the normal development in Reggie's first few years indicates Childhood Disintegrative Disorder (DSM-IV-TR, p. 79).

Childhood Disintegrative Disorder is apparently much less common than Autistic Disorder, but the condition has probably been underrecognized. The two conditions are quite similar except for age at onset and prognosis. Whereas in Autistic Disorder there is evidence before age 3 of abnormal social interaction, communicative language, and symbolic or imaginative play, in Childhood Disintegrative Disorder development is normal during the first few years, and the prognosis is even worse than it is for Autistic Disorder. As in Autistic Disorder, a neurological condition that might account for the disturbance is identified in rare cases. Although parents commonly report an association of the condition with some psychosocial event (e.g., the birth of a sibling), it seems likely that these are chance associations reflecting the frequency of certain life changes in preschool children.

Follow-Up

Seen 2 years later at age 6, Reggie was enrolled in a special education program in which he was provided with a full-time aide and special educational supports in a mainstream class. Unfortunately, he had made few, if any, developmental gains and remained almost entirely mute.

SAIGON PETE FROM GROSSE POINT

On the day before Pete's 16th birthday, he was admitted to the psychiatric unit of a general hospital in the wealthy Detroit suburb in which he lives. He had slashed his wrist with a butcher knife, severing nerves and tendons in his left hand, and drifted in and out of consciousness during the night, finally calling a friend's mother for help in the morning.

Pete is the son of a Vietnamese mother and an American serviceman. He lived with his mother in Saigon until he was 2, when he came to the United States to be adopted by an American family through an agency specializing in adoption of Vietnamese children. He was apparently abused (burned and beaten) in this family, removed to a foster home for a brief period, and, at age 2½, placed with his current adoptive parents.

Although always somewhat reserved and uncommunicative with his adoptive parents, Pete initially did well in his new surroundings. He was a bright and quite beautiful little boy who was sought out by other children from the time he started school. He always got along well with his friends, but his relationship with his parents was stormy, and they describe him as the most difficult of the four children they have adopted.

By the time he was in junior high, Pete was hanging out with a group of long-haired, counterculture kids who skipped school to smoke marijuana, considered nihilism a philosophy of life, shoplifted beer from the local supermarket, and disparaged the values of their parents and teachers. His grades dropped, and he got into trouble for shooting at squirrels with his BB gun, blowing up mailboxes with firecrackers, and fighting with the "jocks" from his school.

When Pete was 14, his parents separated; he elected to stay with his father rather than move with his mother and siblings to another state. His misdemeanors escalated. He and his friends were picked up for "borrowing" the car of a vacationing neighbor to go joyriding. By 15 he was truant more days than he was in school and was using any drug he and his friends could get hold of—mostly LSD, mescaline, glue, and marijuana. His parents sent him away to military school, but he had been expelled the month before his admission to the hospital because he never attended classes.

On admission Pete is described as an immensely appealing, waiflike young man who was immediately adored by every adolescent girl on the ward. He says that he did not intend to kill himself when he slashed his wrist. When pressed, he finally tells the following story: He was dropping acid with some friends. After they left, he thought he heard a police siren. Thinking to save himself from being arrested, he slashed his wrist and then lost consciousness. He denies being depressed, but says his life is pointless and it makes no difference whether he lives or dies.

Discussion of "Saigon Pete From Grosse Point"

Although Pete's ticket of admission to a psychiatric hospital seemed to be a suicide attempt, he later tells us that it was a clever way of avoiding being arrested. Whether or not he was also depressed and did intend to kill himself, there does not seem to be evidence of a full Major Depressive Episode that would justify that diagnosis; nor do we have enough information to make a positive diagnosis of Dysthymic Disorder, although his feeling that life is pointless suggests that this is likely. The diagnosis that best accounts for the current admission is Adjustment Disorder, With Depressed Mood (DSM-IV-TR, p. 683), as the depressed mood and suicide attempt seem to have been triggered by the stress of what he believed was an impending arrest.

There can be little doubt that Pete has a history of a chronic pattern of antisocial behavior in which the basic rights of others and age-appropriate societal norms are violated. He has stolen, been truant, broken into someone's car, been cruel to animals, and initiated physical fights. This warrants the diagnosis of Conduct Disorder (DSM-IV-TR, p. 98). Because the onset of the conduct disturbance was in adolescence, we specify Adolescent-Onset Type. Because Pete does not cause considerable harm to others or engage in extensive vandalism or theft, we note the severity as Moderate.

Pete certainly has abused various drugs. We do not have sufficient information to know whether he was ever dependent on any of them. Given that his suicide attempt was related to his use of LSD, it appears that his use of hallucinogens is certainly having negative consequences, justifying the diagnosis of LSD Abuse (DSM-IV-TR, p. 252). Similarly, the extensive use of marijuana, leading to repeated absences from school, would justify the diagnosis of Cannabis Abuse (DSM-IV-TR, p. 236). We realize that careful questioning would probably reveal abuse of other drugs.

DON'T WORRY

A worried psychiatrist and his wife were referred to a speech therapist for a consultation on their 3-year-old son, Aaron. The psychiatrist explained that he and his wife had first noticed several months previously that at times Aaron was "stuttering." When this happened, he would get stuck on words or initial syllables, often repeating them many times until he was finally able to finish the sentence. Sometimes he was unable to finish the sentence and just gave up. Initially these periods were rare; but in the last few weeks, they had become much more frequent, and now Aaron was visibly upset when they occurred. A few days earlier he had become so frustrated that he began striking his head with his fist in an effort to get the words out.

Aaron's parents knew that transient stuttering, particularly among boys, was common. However, they now wondered if something needed to be done to make sure that the problem did not become chronic. They had consulted their pediatrician, who tried to reassure them; but the pediatrician's own slight but noticeable stuttering was disconcerting, to say the least.

The speech therapist told the parents that it was important to maintain their own composure during Aaron's episodes of distress and not to complete his sentences for him. She sympathized with their concern, but said that most likely the stuttering would go away and would not leave any permanent emotional scars.

Discussion of "Don't Worry"

Although Aaron's father was a psychiatrist, any layperson would have had little trouble making the diagnosis. Stuttering (DSM-IV-TR, p. 69) is a marked impairment in the normal fluency and time patterning of speech that is inappropriate for the child's age. In Aaron's case, as in most cases, it was manifested by prolongations and repetitions of sounds and syllables. In other cases, there may be pauses within a word, audible or silent blocking, or circumlocutions (substituting certain words to avoid problematic words). The severity of the stuttering usually varies from situation to situation and is more severe when there is special pressure to communicate.

Follow-Up

The speech therapist was correct. Over the next few months, the stuttering gradually resolved; Aaron, now age 4, is an articulate child without any trace of speech difficulty.

SNIPER

Leah, age 7, was referred by her teacher for evaluation because of her tearfulness, irritability, and difficulty concentrating in class. Two and a half months earlier Leah had been among a group of children pinned down by sniper fire on her school playground. Over a period of 15 minutes, the sniper killed one child and injured several others. After the gunfire ceased, no one moved until the police stormed the sniper's apartment and found that he had killed himself. Leah did not personally know the child who was killed or the sniper.

Before the shooting, according to her teacher, Leah was shy but vivacious, well-behaved, and a good student. Within a few days after the incident, there was a noticeable change in her behavior. She withdrew from her friends. She began to bicker with other children when they spoke to her. She seemed uninterested in her schoolwork and had to be prodded to persist in required tasks. The teacher noticed that Leah jumped whenever there was static noise in the public address system and when the class shouted answers to flashcards.

Leah's parents were relieved when the school made the referral, because they were uncertain about how to help her. Leah had been uncharacteristically quiet when her parents asked her about the sniping incident. At home she had become moody, irritable, argumentative, fearful, and clinging. She was apprehensive about new situations and fearful of being alone and insisted that someone accompany her to the bathroom. Leah regularly asked to sleep with her parents. She slept restlessly and occasionally cried out in her sleep. She always appeared to be tired, complained of minor physical problems, and seemed more susceptible to minor infections. Her parents were especially worried after Leah nearly walked in front of a moving car without being aware of it. Although she seemed less interested in many of her usual games, her parents noticed that she frequently engaged her siblings in nurse games, in which she was often bandaged.

When asked about the incident in the interview, Leah said that she had tried desperately to hide behind a trash can when she heard the repeated gunfire. She had been terrified of being killed and was "shaking all over," her heart pounding and her head hurting. She vividly told of watching an older child fall to the ground, bleeding and motionless. She ran to safety when there was a pause in the shooting.

Leah described a recurring image of the injured girl lying bleeding on the playground. She said that thoughts of the incident sometimes disrupted her attention, though she would try to think about something else. Lately, she could not always remember what was being said in class.

She no longer played in the area where the shooting had occurred. During recess or after school, she avoided crossing the playground on her way home from school each day and avoided the sniper's house and street. She was particularly afraid at school on Fridays, the day the shooting had occurred. Although her mother and father comforted her, she did not know how to tell them what she was feeling.

Leah continued to be afraid that someone would shoot at her again. She had nightmares about the shooting and dreams in which she or a family member was being shot at or pursued. She ran away from any "popping noises" at home or in the neighborhood. Although she said that she had less desire to play, when asked about new games, she reported frequently playing a game in which a nurse helped an injured person. She began to watch television news about violence and recounted news stories that demonstrated that the world was full of danger.

Discussion of "Sniper"

Leah experienced a traumatic event that involved actual or threatened death or serious injury to herself and to her classmates and evoked intense fear, helplessness, and horror. Within a few days of the trauma, she began to exhibit the characteristic symptoms of severe Posttraumatic Stress Disorder (DSM-IV-TR, p. 467). Because the duration of symptoms is less than 3 months, we further specify Acute.

Although adults sometimes have "flashbacks" in which they actually experience the situation as if it were currently happening, children rarely reexperience trauma in this way. As is typical for her age, Leah reexperienced the trauma in the form of recurrent, intrusive images and recollections of the event and recurrent, distressing dreams about it. She also incorporated themes from the event into repetitive themes in play.

Leah attempted to avoid thoughts and feelings associated with the trauma and places that reminded her of the event. This formerly vivacious little girl now exhibited numbing of general responsiveness. She became apathetic and uninterested in her schoolwork and detached from her former friends. She displayed persistent symptoms of increased arousal, including exaggerated startle reaction (to loud noises), irritability, difficulty concentrating, and sleep disturbance.

In making a multiaxial assessment, we check on Axis IV Problems Related to Interaction With Legal System/Crime and specify Victim of sniper attack. Because of the serious symptoms and impairment in her social relationships and schoolwork, we assign a current global assessment of functioning score of 45.

SHOELACES

George is a 16-year-old youth who was admitted to the hospital from a juvenile detention center following a serious suicide attempt. He had, in some way, wrapped shoelaces and tape around his neck, causing respiratory impairment. When found, he was cyanotic and semiconscious. He had been admitted to the detention center earlier that day; it had been noted there that he was quite withdrawn.

On admission, George was reluctant to speak, except to say that he would kill himself, and nobody could stop him. He did, however, admit to a 2-week history of depressed mood, difficulty sleeping, decreased appetite, decreased interest, guilt feelings, and suicidal ideation.

According to his parents, George had had no emotional difficulties until, at age 13, he became involved in drugs, primarily LSD, marijuana, and nonopioid sedatives. His grades dropped drastically, he ran away from home on several occasions after arguments with his parents, and he made a suicide gesture by overdosing on aspirin. A year later, following an argument with the principal, he was expelled from school. Unable to control his behavior, his parents had him evaluated in a mental health clinic, and a recommendation was made for placement in a group home. He apparently did well in the group home, and his relationship with his parents improved immensely with family counseling. He was quite responsible in holding a job and attending school and was involved in no illegal activities, including use of drugs.

Six months before admission to the hospital, however, George again began using drugs and, over a course of 2 weeks, engaged in 10 breaking-and-enterings, all of which he did alone. He remembers being depressed at this time, but cannot recall whether the mood change was before or after reinvolvement with drugs. He was then sent to the juvenile detention center, where he did so well that he had been discharged to his parents' care 3 weeks previously. One day after returning home, he impulsively left with his buddies in a stolen car for a trip to Texas, and he was picked up and readmitted to the detention center. George's depression began shortly thereafter, and, according to him, his guilt about what he had done to his parents led to his suicide attempt.

Discussion of "Shoelaces"

The serious suicide attempt that occasioned admission to the hospital is clearly a symptom of a Major Depressive Episode. There is a 2-week history of depressed mood with many of the characteristic symptoms of the depressive syndrome. Although there is mention of the patient's being depressed 6 months previously, it is not clear whether at that time he had the full depressive syndrome. There is also a reference to his having made a suicide gesture by overdosing on aspirin at age 13, but it is unclear whether that represented a Major Depressive Episode. Thus, the first-listed diagnosis would be Major Depressive Disorder, Single Episode, Severe Without Psychotic Features (DSM-IV-TR, p. 375).

Since age 13, the patient has displayed a repeated and persistent pattern of conduct in which the basic rights of others or major age-appropriate societal norms or rules have been violated. This has included behavior leading to expulsion from school, purchasing illegal drugs, and running away from home, culminating in the 10 breaking-and-enterings and the stealing of a car. This pattern of antisocial behavior justifies the diagnosis of a Conduct Disorder (DSM-IV-TR, p. 98). Since the onset of his conduct symptoms occurred after age 10, Adolescent-Onset Type (which has a better prognosis) is noted.

There have been many episodes of maladaptive use of substances, including LSD, marijuana, and sedatives. With the little information available, it is not possible to determine whether the criteria for Substance Dependence were ever met; therefore, a diagnosis of Substance Abuse would be indicated for each substance, that is, Cannabis Abuse (DSM-IV-TR, p. 236), LSD Abuse (DSM-IV-TR, p. 252), and Sedative Abuse (DSM-IV-TR, p. 286).

COMPULSIONS

Alan, a 10-year-old boy, is brought for a consultation by his mother because of "severe compulsions." The mother reports that the child at various times has to run and clear his throat, touch the doorknob twice before entering any door, tilt his head from side to side, rapidly blink his eyes, and suddenly touch the ground with his hands by flexing his whole body. These "compulsions" began 2 years ago. The first was the eye blinking, and then the others followed, with a waxing and waning course. The movements occur more frequently when he is anxious or under stress. The last symptom to appear was the repetitive touching of the doorknobs. The consultation was scheduled after the child began to make the middle finger sign while saying "fuck."

When examined, Alan reported that most of the time he did not know in advance when the movements were going to occur except for the touching of doorknobs. Upon questioning, he said that before he felt he had to touch a doorknob, he got the thought of doing it and tried to push it out of his head, but he couldn't because it kept coming back until he touched the doorknob several times; then he felt better. When asked what would happen if someone did not let him touch the doorknob, he said he would just get mad; once his father had tried to stop him and Alan had had a temper tantrum. Alan explained that the touching of the doorknobs didn't really bother him—what did was all the "other stuff" that he couldn't control.

During the interview the child grunted, cleared his throat, turned his head, and rapidly blinked his eyes several times. At times he tried to make it appear as if he had voluntarily been trying to perform these movements.

Personal history and physical and neurological examination were totally unremarkable except for the abnormal movements and sounds. The mother reported that her youngest uncle had had similar symptoms when he was an adolescent, but she could not elaborate any further. She stated that she and her husband had always been "very compulsive," by which she meant only that they were quite well organized and stuck to routines.

Discussion of "Compulsions"

The mother describes Alan's difficulties as "compulsions," and Alan's description of what goes on in his mind before he touches doorknobs seems to describe an obsession with an accompanying compulsion. He first gets the intrusive thought of touching the doorknob. He tries to resist the thought, but is unable to do so; in response to this obsession, he then touches the doorknob twice.

He acknowledges that if he resisted the compulsion to touch doorknobs, he would be extremely uncomfortable. However, because these obsessions and compulsions apparently do not cause marked distress, do not significantly interfere with his functioning, and are not particularly time consuming, the diagnosis of Obsessive-Compulsive Disorder is not given.

Alan is most disturbed by his motor tics (e.g., tilting his head from side to side, blinking his eyes, flexing his whole body) and verbal tics (e.g., clearing throat, saying "fuck"). Because the motor tics involve a series of coordinated movements, they are considered "complex motor tics." The combination of motor and verbal tics with a duration of over 1 year establishes the diagnosis of Tourette's Disorder (DSM-IV-TR, p. 114).

It is sometimes difficult to distinguish a complex motor tic from a compulsion because the observed behavior can be similar. A tic is an involuntary, sudden, rapid, recurrent, nonrhythmic, stereotyped motor movement or vocalization. In contrast, a compulsion is an intentional voluntary act that is either performed in response to an obsession or according to rules that must be applied rigidly. Alan, like many patients with Tourette's Disorder, also has obsessions and compulsions, even if not sufficiently impairing to warrant the additional diagnosis of Obsessive-Compulsive Disorder.

THE ENIGMA

A psychiatrist specializing in patients with mental retardation received a call from a pediatric colleague referring 17-year-old Libby. She was described as "cured from depression" and needing only follow-up medication.

Libby's arrival created a commotion in the waiting room. She was a small, slender person, markedly agitated and restless, who screamed unintelligibly in a high-pitched voice, while her anxious parents tried to calm her. She looked far from being cured.

The parents provided the following history. Before Libby reached age 1, she was diagnosed as having severe mental retardation. Extensive diagnostic evaluations failed to determine the etiology of the retardation. She has always been physically healthy. Libby is an only child, was reared at home, and attended special classes in public schools. She was cheerful, friendly, and affectionate. She was nonverbal, but managed to communicate through gestures and vocalizations. She learned some household tasks and liked to help her mother around the house.

Libby had never been separated from her parents until 6 months ago, when the parents went to Europe for a week and left Libby with a housekeeper. On their return, they found her agitated, unresponsive to their requests, and uninterested in her usual activities. She cried frequently, slept poorly, ate little, and spent most of the time roaming around the house aimlessly. The parents felt guilty about having gone away and tried to make amends by spending all their time with Libby and trying to do things with her that would make her happy.

Libby's parents wondered if she might be physically ill, but an examination and tests by her pediatrician were negative. The pediatrician gave her an antianxiety drug, but it had no effect. The school psychologist thought that Libby's behavior was an attention-getting device, reinforced by her parents' indulgence; the psychologist suggested setting firm limits and referred them to a child guidance clinic, where they were informed by the child psychiatrist that Libby was punishing them for abandoning her when they went on their vacation. He suggested giving Libby unlimited attention and affection.

When this regimen only made matters worse, another psychiatrist was consulted. He thought that Libby might be depressed and started her on an antidepressant. Libby did not improve. In desperation, the parents called every psychiatric hospital in the area, trying to have Libby admitted, but none was willing to take her. As one admitting social worker explained, psychiatric hospitals generally have no experience treating retarded, nonverbal patients. Libby was finally hospitalized on a pediatric ward, where an extensive medical evaluation failed to disclose the cause of her condition.

Libby's pediatrician decided to treat her in the hospital for a "psychotic depression." He therefore increased the dose of antidepressant and added an antipsychotic drug. Libby started to eat better, slept throughout the night, and was somewhat less agitated. She was discharged, but soon had a relapse. She again became irritable and agitated, slept poorly, and experienced a decrease in appetite.

During the diagnostic interview with the specialist, Libby was extremely agitated. She screamed often, in a high-pitched voice, would not sit in one place, and tugged at her mother's arm, indicating she wanted to go home.

Discussion of "The Enigma"

This case illustrates the difficulty in diagnosing people with Severe Mental Retardation (DSM-IV-TR, p. 49) who are unable to describe their subjective experiences. Libby seems depressed and agitated, but cannot tell us about a persistent depressed mood. It seems reasonable to make a provisional diagnosis of Major Depressive Disorder (DSM-IV-TR, p. 375), based on her crying, being uninterested, and having decreased appetite, insomnia, and psychomotor agitation, even though she has not consistently responded to antidepressant medication. Her pediatrician diagnosed a "psychotic depression," but we see no evidence of psychotic symptoms and assume that the antipsychotic medication was intended primarily to control her psychomotor agitation.

Follow-Up

The dosage of antidepressant was gradually decreased and eventually discontinued. For the next 3 months, Libby's mood and behavior varied. For several weeks she was calmer, and then she would again start to scream and become extremely agitated, aggressive, and very distractible.

Detailed family history disclosed that a maternal aunt experienced "depression" and responded well to maintenance treatment with lithium. Therefore, Libby was started on lithium, and the dosage was gradually increased until her serum level was between 0.5 and 0.7 mEq/L. She improved steadily and gradually and within a few months was her "old self" again. Her improvement continued even after the antipsychotic was gradually (over several months) discontinued.

The specialist who treated this patient noted the following, with which we concur:

> Patients like Libby are often dismissed as cases of nonspecific behavior disorders peculiar to retarded persons, or as exhibiting "attention-getting behaviors" stemming from parental overprotection as a compensation for their guilt feelings. In fact, Libby's case was seen by some as an example of such a mechanism.
>
> Libby's clinical presentation was in marked contrast to her usual condition. It was dominated by irritable mood, agitation, distrac-

tibility, and sleep disturbance, all of which are included in the diagnostic criteria for a Manic Episode [DSM-IV-TR, p. 362]. Her screaming could be seen as an equivalent of pressured speech. Symptoms such as grandiosity, flight of ideas, and excessive involvement in pleasurable activity could not, of course, be described by a severely retarded and nonverbal person. The clinical presentation was cyclic, and the periods of crying, decrease in activities, and loss of weight suggest a Major Depressive Episode [DSM-IV-TR, p. 356]. The family history was positive for a lithium-responding "depression." It is possible that Libby was in a Major Depressive Episode when she was put on the antidepressant, and she improved at first, but then developed manic symptoms apparently triggered by the medication. Her good response to lithium raises the question of whether these manic symptoms represent a Manic Episode of Bipolar I Disorder. However, there would have to be evidence of episodes of manic symptoms not precipitated by antidepressant medication for the diagnosis of Bipolar I Disorder to be made.

OMNIVOROUS GEORGE

George, a thin, pale 5-year-old boy, was admitted to the hospital for a nutritional anemia that seemed to result from his ingestion of paint, plaster, dirt, wood, and paste. He had had numerous hospitalizations under similar circumstances, beginning at age 19 months, when he had ingested lighter fluid.

George's parents subsisted on welfare and were described as immature. He was the product of an unplanned but normal pregnancy. His mother began eating dirt when she was pregnant, at age 16. His father periodically abused drugs and alcohol.

Discussion of "Omnivorous George"

Eating of nonnutritive substances may be developmentally appropriate for an infant, but its persistence up to age 5 warrants a diagnosis of Pica (DSM-IV-TR, p. 105). As in this case, it is commonly associated with a similar history in the mother and low socioeconomic status.

In some cultural settings, the eating of nonnutritive substances, such as clay, may be a sanctioned practice, in which case the diagnosis would not apply—but that certainly is not the case here. In other cases, the disturbance may be associated with other disorders, such as Autistic Disorder, Schizophrenia, or the neurological disorder Klein-Levin syndrome.

A PERFECT CHECKLIST

Billy, a 7-year-old African American child, was brought to a mental health clinic by his mother because "he is unhappy and always complaining about feeling sick." He lives with his parents, his younger brother, and his grandmother. His mother describes Billy as a child who has never been very happy and never wanted to play with other children. From the time he started nursery school, he has complained about stomachaches, headaches, and various other physical problems. They are most intense in the morning when he is getting ready to go to school. In the last few months, his somatic complaints have escalated, prompting a complete medical examination, including a neurological examination and electroencephalogram, results of all of which were normal.

Billy did well in first grade, but in second grade he is now having difficulty completing his work. He takes a lot of time to do his assignments and frequently feels he has to do them over again so that they will be "perfect." Because of Billy's frequent somatic complaints, it is hard to get him off to school in the morning. If he is allowed to stay home, he worries that he is falling behind in his schoolwork. When he does go to school, he often is unable to do the work, which makes him feel hopeless about his situation. In order to get through the day, he carries a note that he has instructed his mother to write for him: "You are not getting out of school early today. If you feel that you have to do your papers over and over again, please just do the best you can. Do not think about the time of day and it will go quickly."

His worries have expanded beyond school, and frequently he is clinging and demanding of his parents. He is fearful that if his parents come home late or leave and go somewhere without him that something may happen to them. For the past 2 weeks he has insisted that his little brother sleep with him because he is afraid to go to sleep at night alone.

Although Billy's mother acknowledges that he has never been really happy, in the last 6 months, she feels, he has become much more depressed. He frequently lies around the house, saying that he is too tired to do anything. He has no interest or enjoyment in playing. His appetite has diminished. He has trouble falling asleep at night and often wakes up in the middle of the night or early in the morning. Three weeks ago, he talked, for the first time, about wanting to die and said that maybe he would shoot himself.

Billy's mother became pregnant 2 months after she was married. She did not feel ready for a child. She was hypertensive during the pregnancy and was emotionally upset. Delivery was complicated because of increasing hypertension. At the time of delivery, Billy reportedly went into cardiac arrest. During the first week of his life, he developed projectile vomiting, which persisted for 2 weeks. He had nocturnal enuresis until a year ago.

During the assessment, Billy allowed his mother to go to another room to be interviewed; but after 20 minutes, he became very upset, began crying, and insisted on being taken to her. He then was willing to sit outside the room where his mother was, as long as the door was open and he could see her.

Billy was unable to finish a symptom checklist (designed for children his age) given at the time of the evaluation. He felt that he had to have a perfect checklist and requested that he be allowed to take the papers home so that he could finish them. He became very worried about not being able to complete the list; although he was told that it was not necessary for him to take the papers home, he insisted upon doing so.

Discussion of "A Perfect Checklist"

This case was submitted as an example of Dysthymic Disorder in a child with a recent superimposed Major Depressive Episode. There is little doubt about the latter, as Billy is clearly depressed, has lost interest and enjoyment in playing, and has trouble sleeping, poor appetite, low energy, and suicidal thoughts. In cases such as this, in which there has been a long history of depressed mood before the onset of a full depressive syndrome, the question is whether to regard the chronically depressed mood as a prodrome of the Major Depressive Disorder or to make another diagnosis of Dysthymic Disorder. The DSM-IV-TR rule is that in a child, a 1-year period of sustained depressed mood or irritable mood accompanied by at least three symptoms of the dysthymic syndrome justifies an additional diagnosis of Dysthymic Disorder. In Billy's case, however, we do not have enough information about specific symptoms before the recent episode of Major Depressive Disorder to justify the diagnosis of Dysthymic Disorder. Because this is the first episode and the symptoms cause marked impairment in functioning, the diagnosis would be Major Depressive Disorder, Single Episode, Severe Without Psychotic Features (DSM-IV-TR, p. 375).

Billy has many other symptoms, including perfectionism, worrying about his performance in school, somatic complaints, and anxiety about being separated from his mother. The perfectionism raises the question of Obsessive-Compulsive Personality Disorder or Obsessive-Compulsive Disorder. He is too young for us to consider a personality disorder diagnosis, and there is no evidence of frank obsessions or compulsions. His worrying about his work and school performance, accompanied by somatic complaints, suggests the additional diagnosis of Generalized Anxiety Disorder. However, because these symptoms apparently occur only during the presence of a mood disorder, the DSM-IV-TR rule is to regard these symptoms as associated features of the mood disorder rather than as an independent anxiety disorder.

The diagnosis of Separation Anxiety Disorder (DSM-IV-TR, p. 125) requires at least three of eight symptoms of excessive anxiety concerning separation from those to whom the child is attached. We count at least four: unrealistic worry about possible harm befalling major attachment figures, reluctance to go to school, avoidance of being alone (including clinging), and complaints of physical symptoms on school days.

The many somatic complaints suggest Undifferentiated Somatoform Disorder, but a more parsimonious approach is to regard these symptoms as a manifestation of either the Separation Anxiety Disorder or the Major Depressive Disorder.

ECHO

Richard, age 3½, a firstborn child, was referred at the request of his parents because of his uneven development and abnormal behavior. Delivery had been difficult, and he had needed oxygen at birth. His physical appearance, motor development, and self-help skills were all age appropriate, but his parents had been uneasy about him from the first few months of life because of his lack of response to social contact and the usual baby games. Comparison with their second child, who, unlike Richard, enjoyed social communication from early infancy, confirmed their fears.

Richard appeared to be self-sufficient and aloof from others. He did not greet his mother in the mornings, or his father when he returned from work, though, if left with a baby-sitter, he tended to scream much of the time. He had no interest in other children and ignored his younger brother. His babbling had no conversational intonation. At age 3 he could understand simple practical instructions. His speech consisted of echoing some words and phrases he had heard in the past, with the original speaker's accent and intonation; he could use one or two such phrases to indicate his simple needs. For example, if he said, "Do you want a drink?" he meant he was thirsty. He did not communicate by facial expression or use gesture or mime, except for pulling someone along and placing his or her hand on an object he wanted.

He was fascinated by bright lights and spinning objects and would stare at them while laughing, flapping his hands, and dancing on tiptoe. He also displayed the same movements while listening to music, which he had liked from infancy. He was intensely attached to a miniature car, which he held in his hand, day and night, but he never played imaginatively with this or any other toy. He could assemble jigsaw puzzles rapidly (with one hand because of the car held in the other), whether the picture side was exposed or hidden. From age 2 he had collected kitchen utensils and arranged them in repetitive patterns all over the floors of the house. These pursuits, together with occasional periods of aimless running around, constituted his whole repertoire of spontaneous activities.

The major management problem was Richard's intense resistance to any attempt to change or extend his interests. Removing his toy car, disturbing his puzzles or patterns, even retrieving, for example, an egg whisk or a spoon for its legitimate use in cooking, or trying to make him look at a picture book precipitated temper tantrums that could last an hour or more, with screaming, kicking, and the biting of himself or others. These tantrums could be cut short by restoring the status quo. Otherwise, playing his favorite music or a long car ride was sometimes effective.

His parents had wondered if Richard might be deaf, but his love of music, his accurate echoing, and his sensitivity to some very soft sounds, such as those made by unwrapping a chocolate in the next room, convinced them that this was not the cause of his abnormal behavior. Psychological testing gave him a mental age of 3 years in non-language-dependent skills (fitting and assembly tasks), but only 18 months in language comprehension.

Discussion of "Echo"

Richard demonstrates marked impairment in reciprocal social interaction and in verbal and nonverbal communication and a markedly restricted repertoire of activities, all beginning in the first few months of life. He doesn't seem interested in other children and never wants to play "baby games" with his parents. His speech is limited and peculiar (echoing words and phrases of others), and his play is abnormal in that he never engages in imaginative play. His interests are markedly restricted and stereotyped (doing puzzles and making patterns with kitchen utensils), and he has stereotyped motor mannerisms (flapping of his hands). These behaviors, beginning prior to age 3, are the characteristic signs of the Pervasive Developmental Disorder Autistic Disorder (DSM-IV-TR, p. 75).

ZOMBIE

An 11-year-old girl asked her mother to take her to a psychiatrist because she feared she might be "going crazy." Several times during the last 2 months she has awakened confused about where she is until she realizes she is on the living room couch or in her little sister's bed, even though she went to bed in her own room. When she recently woke up in her older brother's bedroom, she became very concerned and felt quite guilty about it. Her younger sister says that she has seen the patient walking during the night, looking like a "zombie," that she didn't answer when she called her, and that the patient has done that several times, but usually goes back to her bed. The patient fears she may have "amnesia" because she has no memory of anything happening during the night.

There is no history of seizures or of similar episodes during the day. An electroencephalogram and physical examination prove normal. The patient's mental status is unremarkable except for some anxiety about her symptom and the usual early adolescent concerns. School and family functioning are excellent.

Discussion of "Zombie"

This girl is not "going crazy," but rather is experiencing the characteristic features of Sleepwalking Disorder (DSM-IV-TR, p. 644): episodes of arising from bed during sleep and walking about, appearing unresponsive during the episodes, experiencing amnesia for the episode upon awakening, and exhibiting no evidence of impairment in consciousness several minutes after awakening. Psychomotor epileptic seizures are ruled out by the normal electroencephalogram and the absence of any seizurelike behavior during the waking state.

Although the process of dissociation is involved in Sleepwalking Disorder, because the disturbance begins during sleep, it is classified as a Sleep Disorder rather than as a Dissociative Disorder.

SLOW LEARNER

Janet, age 13, has a long history of school problems. She failed first grade, supposedly because her teacher was "mean," and was removed from a special classroom after she kept getting into fights with the other children. Currently in a normal sixth-grade classroom, she is failing reading and barely passing English, arithmetic, and spelling, but doing satisfactory work in art and sports. Her teacher describes Janet as a "slow learner with a poor memory" and states that she doesn't learn in a group setting and requires a great deal of individual attention.

Janet's medical history is unremarkable except for a tonsillectomy at age 5 and an early history of chronic otitis. She sat up at 6 months, walked at 12 months, and began talking at 18 months. Examination revealed an open and friendly girl who was very touchy about her academic problems. She stated that she was "bossed around" at school but had good friends in the neighborhood. Intelligence testing revealed a full-scale IQ of 97; wide-range achievement testing produced grade-level scores of 4.8 for reading, 5.3 for spelling, and 6.3 for arithmetic.

Discussion of "Slow Learner"

The differential diagnosis of academic problems includes consideration of poor schooling, Mental Retardation, Attention-Deficit/Hyperactivity Disorder, Oppositional Defiant Disorder, Conduct Disorder, and Learning Disorders. In this case, because other children in her class are apparently passing when she is not, it is reasonable to rule out inadequate schooling as an explanation for Janet's academic difficulties. Her average intelligence rules out a diagnosis of Mental Retardation. Although there is a mention of "fights with other children" and inability to "learn in a group setting," there is certainly no description of other behaviors that would justify a diagnosis of either Attention-Deficit/Hyperactivity Disorder, Oppositional Defiant Disorder, or Conduct Disorder.

There is positive evidence suggesting a Learning Disorder: she not only seems to have particular difficulty with reading in school but also performs significantly below her expected level on a reading achievement test. Her reading score of 4.8 is more than 1 year below her expected reading level. We thus gave Janet the diagnosis of Reading Disorder (DSM-IV-TR, p. 53). Given this diagnosis, it is reasonable to regard the fighting and difficulty learning in a group as associated features of the Learning Disorder.

There is now considerable research evidence suggesting that early, chronic otitis may be associated with later learning or language difficulties.

BRRR

Bruce is an attractive 6-year-old boy whose mother brought him to the emergency room because she was frightened that she could not prevent the child from setting fires, which he had done several times in the last year and a half. Although he had so far managed to put out all the fires he set himself, his mother was afraid that he would set the house afire while she and his sister were asleep. She complained that he was sneaky about setting the fires, making it impossible for her to control him or to know how many fires he had actually set.

Bruce says that he has set fires because a "man in my head tells me to." This "man" stays in his room when he is awake and "goes away" when he is asleep. The man makes a noise ("brrr"), which Bruce interprets as a command to "set fires." He is afraid to talk to anyone about the man or not to obey his commands, "because he might beat me up." His mother apparently does not take the voice seriously, stating that Bruce has offered a variety of different reasons for setting fires, depending on to whom he was talking. Both agree that he sets fires in retaliation against his mother when he is angry with her.

Bruce has been fascinated with setting fires for the past 2 years. His mother remembers that he and a friend set the first fire by burning holes in the plastic sheets on his and his sister's beds. His mother found out about the incident later and reacted by hitting him on his hands and telling him how dangerous fires were. During the next fire-setting incident, Bruce used a lighter to try to burn a door frame that his mother had just painted. This time he was not hit, but was forbidden to ride his bicycle for a week. His mother was sleeping during a third episode, in which he set the garbage on fire with a table lighter. He then took a broom and beat out the fire. His mother awoke to a funny smell and remembers that he was running all over the house in a peculiar manner. She related this incident with amusement at the child's antics.

The last two fires had taken place 3 weeks previously, when Bruce first tried to burn a dishtowel on a gas flame. After he burned the fringe, he rolled up the towel and threw it in the garbage. His mother, who was just outside the apartment at the time, sent him to bed and later explained to him again about the dangers of fire setting. During the last incident, he took a stretch monster toy that was kept in a styrofoam box and burned holes with a lighter on the sides of the box that corresponded to the monster's arms and feet.

Apart from these incidents, his mother remembers that Bruce would often find matches or go into the bathroom with a lighter and try to smoke. His mother has talked to him at length about fires and how they get bigger with alcohol and can be put out with water. He becomes excited during these discussions, but then promises never again to play with fire.

At the present time, his mother reports, Bruce is unhappy in school and misses his former friends from the neighborhood the family moved from 3 months before this evaluation. She says that he has made no new friends outside school and that he and his sister complain frequently of boredom.

Aside from the fire setting, there is no history of any other aggressive or antisocial behavior. His mother reports that Bruce has been difficult to discipline, but mainly because he ignores her. Bruce's schoolteacher was surprised to hear of his fire setting. She described him as a lovely, bright, obedient child who played and worked well with both the teacher and his peers. Upon further inquiry, she could say only that at times he became a "little wild" in play.

Bruce lives with his 10-year-old sister and 26-year-old mother, who herself was hospitalized as an adolescent after she had been truant from school for 7 months in retaliation for her mother's remarriage. In an initial discussion with the interviewer, she acknowledged that at times she becomes violently angry, to the point where she is unable to control herself.

The findings of Bruce's physical examination were within normal limits except for a second-degree burn on his hand, which his mother initially said came from her attempts to "teach him that fire hurts" by insisting that he put his hand in a gas flame. (She later denied this, but Bruce insisted that she had done it.)

When interviewed, Bruce was somewhat guarded and distrustful at first. This seemed to be a manifestation of shyness and fear of what his mother would say or do. Over the course of several evaluation sessions, Bruce's play revolved around themes of fires getting bigger and out of control. He knows that he can get burned and that a big fire could burn his house and "I would die." When talking about fires, his affect was either inappropriate (laughter) or blunted. When discussing the "man" and his command hallucinations, Bruce seemed to be genuinely frightened, as if he regarded the man as real and threatening. He denied suicidal ideation, although his mother reported that he had recently said that he wished to die.

Discussion of "Brrr"

Recurrent setting of fires may be a symptom of Conduct Disorder; Bruce, however, is described by his teacher as a "lovely, bright, obedient child who plays and works well with both the teacher and his peers," and he apparently engages in no antisocial activities other than fire setting. Political extremists may set fires to make a political statement. We doubt this is what Bruce is up to.

It does seem that Bruce has committed deliberate and purposeful fire setting on several occasions, that he derives pleasure from the fire setting, that he is very fascinated with fires, as evidenced by his excitement over his mother's discussions with him about the specifics of fires, and that there is no understandable goal, such as monetary gain from insurance. The diagnosis is therefore Pyromania (DSM-IV-TR, p. 671), within the group of Impulse-Control Disorders Not Elsewhere Classified.

Some readers may notice that the DSM-IV (and DSM-IV-TR) diagnostic criteria for this disorder require "tension or affective arousal before the act." This feature can only be inferred from the available information, as this subjective experience is often not easily documented in a very young person.

Other readers may be bothered by the "command hallucinations." It is hard to reconcile his mother's evaluation that the "man" in his head is one of a number of stories that he provides to explain his behavior with his behavior during the interview when he seemed genuinely frightened at thoughts of the "man." If the hallucinations were truly genuine, one would certainly expect other signs of disorganized or psychotic behavior, which have not been present. Therefore, we do not add a diagnosis of a psychotic disorder.

No Brakes

Jeremy, age 9, is brought by his mother to a mental health clinic because he has become increasingly disobedient and difficult to manage at school. Several events during the past month convinced his mother that she had to do something about his behavior. Several weeks ago he swore at his teacher and was suspended from school for 3 days. Last week he was reprimanded by the police for riding his bicycle in the street, something his mother had repeatedly cautioned him about. The next day he failed to use his pedal brakes and rode his bike into a store window, shattering it. He has not been caught in any more serious offenses, though once before he broke a window when he was riding his bike with a friend.

Jeremy has been difficult to manage since nursery school. The problems have slowly escalated. Whenever he is without close supervision, he gets into trouble. He has been reprimanded at school for teasing and kicking other children, tripping them, and calling them names. He is described as bad-tempered and irritable, even though at times he seems to enjoy school. Often he appears to be deliberately trying to annoy other children, though he always claims that others have started the arguments. He does not become involved in serious fights, but does occasionally exchange a few blows with another child.

Jeremy sometimes refuses to do what his two teachers tell him to do, and this year has been particularly difficult with the one who takes him in the afternoon for arithmetic, art, and science lessons. He gives many reasons why he should not have to do his work and argues when told to do it. Many of the same problems were experienced last year when he had only one teacher. Despite this, his grades are good and have been getting better over the course of the year, particularly in arithmetic and art, which are subjects taught by the teacher with whom he has the most difficulty.

At home Jeremy's behavior is quite variable. On some days he is defiant and rude to his mother, needing to be told to do everything several times before he will do it, though eventually he usually complies; on other days he is charming and volunteers to help; but his unhelpful days predominate. "The least little thing upsets him, and then he shouts and screams." Jeremy is described as spiteful and mean with his younger brother, Rickie; even when he is in a good mood, he is unkind to Rickie.

Jeremy's concentration is generally good, and he does not leave his work unfinished. His mother describes him as "on the go all the time," but not restless. His teachers are concerned about his attitude, not about his restlessness. His mother also comments that he tells many minor lies, though when pressed, he is truthful about important things.

Discussion of "No Brakes"

Jeremy's defiant and reckless behavior suggests the possibility of both Conduct Disorder and Attention-Deficit/Hyperactivity Disorder. Though he has annoyed other children and adults, he has not violated their basic rights or displayed any of the more serious forms of behavior, such as stealing, cruelty, truancy, running away from home, or destroying property, that would justify a diagnosis of Conduct Disorder. His encounter with the police was over a petty violation, and the damage he caused to a shop window was not done with any destructive intent. Although Jeremy does quite well academically, he has problems with teachers and peers. He has a high energy level but is not aimlessly hyperactive and does not appear to have the characteristics of Attention-Deficit/Hyperactivity Disorder.

The persistent argumentative, irritable, defiant, annoying, and resentful behaviors are characteristic symptoms of Oppositional Defiant Disorder (DSM-IV-TR, p. 102). We note the severity as Moderate.

Some clinicians consider Oppositional Defiant Disorder merely a mild form of Conduct Disorder, but many children with the disorder never develop any more serious behavioral problems.

LADY MACBETH

Interviewer: Tell me about when things were the hardest for you. When was that?

Patient: It was around Christmas time last year.

Interviewer: And you were how old then?

Patient: 13.

Interviewer: You're 14 now, right?

Patient: Yes.

Interviewer: When things were really at their worst, can you tell me what it was that was disturbing to you at that time?

Patient: Well, the major part about it was that, like all these things that I did, they were really stupid, and they didn't make any sense; but I'm still gonna have to do it and, it was sort of like being scared of what would happen if I didn't do it.

Interviewer: What were the things that you were doing?

Patient: In the morning when I got dressed, I was real afraid that there'd be germs all over my clothes and things, so I'd stand there and I'd shake them for half an hour. I'd wash before I did anything—like if I was gonna wash my face, I'd wash my hands first; and if I was gonna get dressed, I'd wash my hands first; and then it got even beyond that point. Washing my hands wasn't enough, and I started to use rubbing alcohol. It was winter time and cold weather, and this really made my hands bleed. Even if I just held them under water, they'd bleed all over the place, and they looked terrible, and everyone thought I had a disease or something.

Interviewer: And when you were doing that much washing, how much time every day did that take, if you added up all the different parts of it?

Patient: It took about 6 hours a day. In the morning I didn't have a whole lot of choice, because I had to get up at 6:00 A.M. and get ready for school. All I'd do was get dressed as best I could. I didn't even have time to brush my hair. At the time I never ate breakfast, so all these things . . . it was just so complex that I didn't have time to do anything.

Interviewer: You also told me about other things in addition to the washing and worrying about dirt: that you would have plans about how you would do other things.

Patient: Okay, well, they were like set plans in my mind that if I heard the word, like, something that had to do with germs or disease, it would be considered something bad and so I had things that would go through my mind that were sort of like "cross that out and it'll make it okay" to hear that word.

Interviewer: What sort of things?

Patient: Like numbers or words that seemed to be sort of like a protector.

Interviewer: What numbers and what words were they?

Patient: It started out to be the number 3 and multiples of 3 and then words like 'soap and water,' something like that; and then the multiples of 3 got really high, they'd end up to be 123 or something like that. It got real bad then.

Interviewer: At any time did you really believe that something bad would happen if you didn't do these things? Was it just a feeling, or were you really scared?

Patient: No! I was petrified that something would really happen. It was weird, because everyone would always say how sensible I was and intelligent. But it was weird because I tried to explain it in order to really make them understand what I was trying to say and they'd go, you know, like, 'Well, that's stupid,' and I knew it; but when I was alone, things would be a lot worse than when I was with this group, because if I was around friends, that would make me forget about most of this. But when I was alone it . . . like, my mind would wander to all sorts of things and I'd get new plans and new rituals and new ideas, and I'd start worrying more and more about people that could get hurt that I cared about and things that could really go bad if I didn't.

Interviewer: Who were the people you'd worry most would get hurt?

Patient: My family, basically my family.

Interviewer: Any particular people in your family?

Patient: Well, like my grandmother—she's 83 and you know, I was just worried that . . . I know that she's old and she's not gonna be around much longer, but I was worried that maybe something I did could cause her to get really, really sick or something.

Interviewer: Had anything like this ever been on your mind before you were 13, when this started?

Patient: Well, let's see . . . my mother, her family has always been mostly real neat people and extremely clean and so that could have affected it, because I was growing up in that sort of background. But I always like to be clean and neat, and I was never really allowed to walk around the house with muddy shoes or anything like that, so . . .

Interviewer: But your concerns about cleanliness, about how many times you did things—have they ever gotten in the way of your doing things that you wanted to do?

Patient: Uh-huh. Many times. Like, I was supposed to go somewhere with a friend, and we were gonna leave at 11:00 A.M. and I wanted to take a shower before I left. So I had to get up about 6:00 A.M. in the morning, and sometimes I just won't even make it with 5 hours to do it.

Interviewer: And that was since you were 13. But what about any time in your life before that—had anything like this ever happened? Or as far as you know was this the first?

Patient: It was the first time.

Interviewer: Have you at any time felt that you had some other special idea about forces beyond you . . . about your being able to control things magically or be in control?

Patient: I'm really scared of supernatural things. I don't like to say that I believe in superstitions and things, but I guess I really do because they frighten me. When I was little they weren't really bothering me or anything, but now I avoid it as much as I can. Like, the number 13 now, if it came up, you know, it wouldn't bother me, but I'd rather have the number 7 instead.

Interviewer: So you are superstitious, but you've never heard any special voice talking to you or . . .

Patient: Yeah, I have. It's like . . . if I tried to describe it, people would think that I saw little people dancing around or something, and that was wrong because all it was, it wasn't like a voice, it was just like a thought.

Interviewer: More like being able to hear yourself think?

Patient: Right.

Interviewer: Have you ever seen things that other people couldn't see?

Patient: No.

Interviewer: I know you are doing very well here in school and on the ward here at the hospital. Do you have any signs left of the problems that you used to have with your rituals and compulsions?

Patient: Well, everyone is compulsive to a point. I can see little things that I'll do. Like I will go over something twice, or three times, because that's a special number. Like, if I read something and I really don't understand it, maybe I would go over it one more time and then, say, one more time will make it three. But nothing really big. It's been really good, because I have gotten out and taken a shower, and gotten dressed, and washed my face and brushed my teeth, and all that stuff in like half an hour! That's really good for me because I wasn't able to do that before.

Interviewer: So, in general it's fair to say it's things that just you would notice now, and probably someone sharing the room with you wouldn't be able to tell the other things you are doing even though you know these little things are there. Good. . . . Well, thank you very much.

Discussion of "Lady Macbeth"

This adolescent girl articulately and vividly describes what it is like to have a severe form of Obsessive-Compulsive Disorder (DSM-IV-TR,

p. 462). She has both obsessions and compulsions, and both are a significant source of distress to her and interfere with her functioning.

The obsessions consist of ideas that (at least at some time during the course of the illness) intrude themselves into her consciousness and are experienced as inappropriate. For example, she gets the idea that maybe she did something that could cause her grandmother to get sick. Another example is the thought that there are germs on her clothes. The need to neutralize such distressing thoughts has led to various compulsions that are repetitive, and she feels driven to perform according to rules that must be applied rigidly. For example, if she heard a word that suggested germs or disease, she had to undo it ("cross that out") by saying the number 3 and multiples of 3, or words like "soap and water." Although these behaviors were designed to prevent discomfort or some dreaded event, the activity was not connected in a realistic way to what it was designed to prevent and was clearly excessive. For example, she washed her hands for hours to prevent becoming infected by the germs, to the point where her hands would actually bleed. Although emotionally she reacted as if the dangers were real ("I was petrified that something would really happen"), intellectually she always knew that her fears were irrational and were not about real-life problems (her friends would say that it was stupid, and she knew that it was). In rare cases, during a severe episode of the illness, the person may no longer recognize that the obsessions or compulsions are excessive or unreasonable; in such instances the diagnosis is specified as With Poor Insight.

Obsessional thoughts need to be distinguished from auditory hallucinations. This patient recognized that if she described some of her obsessional thoughts to people, they might think that she was hallucinating ("if I tried to describe it, people would think that I saw little people dancing around or something"). However, she is quite clear that it was just her own thoughts, not a voice.

Obsessive-Compulsive Disorder is sometimes associated with Obsessive-Compulsive Personality Disorder. Whereas Obsessive-Compulsive Disorder involves true obsessions and compulsions, Obsessive-Compulsive Personality Disorder involves such personality traits as perfectionism, interpersonal control, and excessive devotion to work or productivity. There is no evidence in this case of Obsessive-Compulsive Personality Disorder.

Major Depressive Disorder often occurs either before or during the course of Obsessive-Compulsive Disorder. In fact, on further questioning, this patient did describe an episode of Major Depressive Disorder that occurred early in the course of her Obsessive-Compulsive Disorder.

ROCKING AND READING

Twenty-two-year-old Betsy was referred for evaluation by the staff of her group home. She had been placed in the group home some 3 months previously, following court-ordered "deinstitutionalization" from a large residential facility for the retarded. The evaluation was requested because Betsy "didn't fit in" with other patients and had developed some problem behaviors, particularly aggression directed toward herself and, less commonly, toward others. Unlike other patients in the group home, she tended to "stay to herself" and had essentially no peer relations, although she did respond positively to some staff members. Her self-abusive and aggressive behaviors usually were triggered by changes made in her routine. Self-abusive behavior consisted of repeated pounding of her legs and biting of her hand.

Betsy had been placed in residential treatment when she was age 4 and had remained in some kind of residential setting ever since. Her parents had both died, and she had no contact with her only sibling. At the time of her transfer to the group home, she was reported to have had several abnormal electroencephalograms, but no seizures or other medical problems had been noted. When last given psychological tests, she achieved a full-scale IQ of 55, with comparable deficits in adaptive behaviors.

During the evaluation, Betsy spends much of her time reading a children's book she discovered in the waiting room. Her voice is flat and monotonic. She is unable to respond to any questions about the book she is reading and reacts to interruptions of her ongoing activity by pounding her legs with her fist. She rocks back and forth continually during the interview. She makes eye contact with the examiner initially, but otherwise seems oblivious of everyone around her. She neither initiates activities, imitates the play of the examiner, nor responds to attempts to interest her in alternative activities, such as playing with a doll. From time to time she repeats a single phrase in a monotonic voice, "Blum, blum." Physical examination reveals extensive bruises covering most of her lower extremities.

Betsy was the product of a normal pregnancy, labor, and delivery. She was noted to have been an unusually easy baby. Her parents had first become concerned when she failed to speak by age 2. Motor milestones were delayed. Her parents initially thought that she might be deaf, but this was obviously not the case, as she responded with panic to the sound of a vacuum cleaner. As a young child, Betsy had been observed to "live in her own world," had not formed attachments to her parents, had idiosyncratic responses to some sounds, and always became extremely upset when there were changes in her environment.

By age 4, Betsy was still not speaking, and placement in the state institution was recommended following a diagnosis of Childhood Schizophrenia. In the year after her placement, Betsy began speaking. However, she did not typically use speech for communication; instead, she merely repeated phrases over and over. She had an unusual ability to memorize and became fascinated with reading, even though she appeared not to comprehend anything she read. She exhibited a variety of stereotyped behaviors, including body rocking and head banging, requiring a great deal of attention from the staff.

Discussion of "Rocking and Reading"

Betsy has long-standing problems, including impairment in social interaction (lack of awareness of others and gross impairment in peer relations). Although she has some speech, it is markedly abnormal in its production (monotonic) and in its form and content (she repeats the same phrases over and over). She exhibits stereotyped behaviors (rocking) and a markedly restricted range of interests. All of these, beginning in early childhood, establish the diagnosis of Autistic Disorder (DSM-IV-TR, p. 75). Although the stereotypic and self-abusive behavior results in harm to herself, a separate diagnosis of Stereotypic Movement Disorder is not given because stereotypic behavior is a common characteristic feature of Autistic Disorder.

Although some cases of Autistic Disorder are associated with normal or, more rarely, high IQ, this case illustrates its frequent coexistence with Mild Mental Retardation (DSM-IV-TR, p. 49).

At the time of Betsy's placement in the state institution, she was diagnosed as having Childhood Schizophrenia. That diagnosis assumed a continuity between the childhood disorder and adult psychosis. However, there is considerable evidence from family and longitudinal studies that Autistic Disorder and the adult psychosis are not related; therefore, beginning with DSM-III, the childhood disorder has not been referred to as "Schizophrenia."

INTO EVERYTHING

Eddie, age 9, was referred to a child psychiatrist at the request of his school because of the difficulties he creates in class. He has been suspended for a day twice this school year. His teacher complains that he is so restless that his classmates are unable to concentrate. He is hardly ever in his seat, but roams around the class, talking to other children while they are working. When the teacher is able to get him to stay in his seat, he fidgets with his hands and feet and drops things on the floor. He never seems to know what he is going to do next and may suddenly do something quite outrageous. His most recent suspension was for swinging from the fluorescent light fixture over the blackboard. Because he was unable to climb down again, the class was in an uproar.

His mother says that Eddie's behavior has been difficult since he was a toddler and that as a 3-year-old he was unbearably restless and demanding. He has always required little sleep and been awake before anyone else. When he was small, "he got into everything," particularly in the early morning, when he would awaken at 4:30 A.M. or 5:00 A.M. and go downstairs by himself. His parents would awaken to find the living room or kitchen "demolished." When he was age 4, he managed to unlock the door of the apartment and wander off into a busy main street, but, fortunately, was rescued from oncoming traffic by a passerby. He was rejected by a preschool program because of his difficult behavior; eventually, after a very difficult year in kindergarten, he was placed in a special behavioral program for first- and second-graders. He is now in a regular class for most subjects, but spends a lot of time in a resource room with a special teacher. When with his own class, he is unable to participate in games because he cannot wait for his turn.

Psychological testing has shown Eddie to be of average ability, and his achievements are only slightly below expected level. His attention span is described by the psychologist as "virtually nonexistent." He has no interest in TV and dislikes games or toys that require any concentration or patience. He is not popular with other children, and at home he prefers to be outdoors, playing with his dog or riding his bike. If he does play with toys, his games are messy and destructive, and his mother cannot get him to keep his things in any order.

Eddie has been treated with a stimulant, methylphenidate, in small doses. While taking the drug, he was much easier to manage at school in that he was less restless and possibly more attentive.

Discussion of "Into Everything"

Eddie's behavior graphically demonstrates the characteristic inattention, impulsivity, and hyperactivity of Attention-Deficit/Hyperactivity Disorder (DSM-IV-TR, p. 92). He primarily shows symptoms of hyperactivity/impulsivity: he often has difficulty remaining seated, fidgets, runs about or climbs in situations where it is inappropriate, and has difficulty waiting his turn. He also displays some symptoms of inattention: he can't sustain attention, he doesn't seem to listen to what is being said to him, and he strongly dislikes activities that require patience and concentration.

The diagnosis of Attention-Deficit/Hyperactivity Disorder requires that some of the characteristic symptoms be present in two or more situations, such as at school and at home, in order to avoid giving the diagnosis to cases in which the disturbed behavior is apparently situation specific. In this case, it is clear that Eddie's disturbed behavior occurs both at home and at school. The diagnosis also requires that the onset of symptoms be before age 7. In Eddie's case, the symptoms apparently began when he was 3.

There are three types of this disorder: Predominantly Inattentive, Predominantly Hyperactive-Impulsive, and Combined. In this case, the appropriate type would be Predominantly Hyperactive-Impulsive.

TIM

Tim, age 6, was referred to the clinic by his general practitioner because of persistent soiling. A medical workup revealed no general medical condition that could account for these symptoms.

Tim had never gained control of his bowel habits. He was not constipated as an infant; but after a febrile illness at age 2, he had become constipated. Six months later he had impacted feces and was seen by a surgeon, who prescribed laxatives and suppositories. Following this, there was a pattern of alternating constipation, when he did not go to the toilet for several days, and runny diarrhea, when he soiled his pants many times a day. At age 4, Tim took laxatives regularly, and his stool became softer and more regular. At about the same time, his mother first attempted to toilet train him. He was made to sit on the toilet every evening until he "performed." Although he usually managed this, producing a tiny amount or, rarely, a normal stool, he continued to soil his pants frequently during the day. His mother said that within half an hour of changing his pants, he would be soiled again, and this pattern has continued until the present time.

Tim himself has been distressed about the soiling since starting school. He hates taking his clothes off for gym or on the beach. He worries that people will notice if, as occasionally happens, feces drop out of his pants. He is anxious when sitting on the toilet in the evenings and at first would do so only if bribed. Now he insists his mother stay in the bathroom with him.

Tim is also enuretic at night. He became dry by day at age 3½ but has continued to wet at night; because waking him at night has not prevented his wetting, his mother still puts him in diapers.

For the last month, since seeing a puppet show, Tim has awakened frequently with nightmares about witches. He often asks about witches, and his mother has tried to assure him that they do not exist. He has had a light on all night in his room for the past month. He never goes into his parents' bed, as they do not allow this because of his being wet.

His mother says that Tim has seemed rather preoccupied with death. He often asks why people have to die and if he or his parents will die first. He then works out how old he might be when his parents die. He has said that he doesn't want to be buried because then people would walk over him.

Apart from the problems of soiling and wetting, his mother feels he is a normal little boy who is happy and outgoing. He is very affectionate with his mother and likes to receive lots of kisses and hugs. His mother implied that this might be excessive for a boy. He is attached to his father, but not as much as to his mother. He likes to play and go out with his father, but with his mother he is clinging and likes to stay close to her.

Up until age 4, Tim had worried his parents because of seeming rather effeminate. He liked to dress in girls' clothes and talked of "when I grow up to be a girl." Now when playing he likes to take traditionally male roles, such as policemen or bus conductors.

There was initially some difficulty in Tim's adjustment at school. He used to scream when his mother left him, and he was reported to be very timid and afraid of other children. This lasted most of the first term; but he eventually began "to stand up for himself" and has been quite happy at school since then. He has several friends there, and the school is satisfied with his progress.

Tim's developmental milestones were all a little behind those of his two older sisters, but his mother could not recall them exactly. He sat at about 6 months, shuffled about on his bottom and did not crawl, and walked at 18 months. He spoke his first words at about that same time.

Tim's mother is a smartly dressed 35-year-old laboratory technician who seems timid and speaks quietly but at the same time is quite forceful and articulate in what she says. She seems to feel unsure of herself with Tim and thinks that bringing up a boy is much more difficult than bringing up her daughters. She is embarrassed, as a professional person, not to have sought help earlier. She recalls how she, too, had in childhood hated to use lavatories away from home.

Tim's father is an intelligent, distinguished-looking 40-year-old contractor. He was reticent during the interview. He readily admitted that he did not take an active part in the rearing of the children, but enjoyed them and was very fond of them. He explained that he was rather disgusted by the soiling and tried to keep out of the situation for fear of being too punitive.

Tim is small for his age and has a babyish, full face. In the interview he is at first very timid and shy and clings to his mother. However, he does allow his mother to leave the room after a short period and becomes much more assertive and outgoing once she leaves. He plays with family figures in the dollhouse and soon has the little boy figure on the toilet and all the other members of the family watching him. His speech is immature and difficult to understand, but his vocabulary is extensive.

Tim is also seen by a pediatrician. On physical examination, a fecal mass the size of a melon can be palpated in the lower abdomen, and soft feces can be felt in his rectum.

Discussion of "Tim"

Encopresis can sometimes be caused by general medical conditions, such as aganglionic megacolon and anal fissure. Because these have been ruled out in Tim's case, the diagnosis of Encopresis (Not Due to a General Medical Condition) is appropriate (DSM-IV-TR, p. 118). Because Tim's fecal incontinence is apparently associated with constipation and overflow incontinence, this would also be noted with the diagnosis. In addition, he continues to have nighttime wetting, warranting an additional diagnosis of Enuresis (Not Due to a General Medical Condition) (DSM-IV-TR, p. 121). Because the enuresis occurs only during sleep, Nocturnal Only is specified.

For the last month Tim has had nightmares about witches and has been scared of the dark and preoccupied with death. Because this is likely to be only a transient reaction, it does not warrant an additional diagnosis. If it persists or becomes more severe, however, then an additional diagnosis, such as Adjustment Disorder with Anxious Mood, should be considered.

Tim apparently went through a phase during which he showed some signs of possible disturbance in gender identity but now seems to have a clear sense of himself as a male. He also showed some signs of separation anxiety when he began school, but they were insufficient for a diagnosis of Separation Anxiety Disorder.

CARTOGRAPHER[*]

A psychiatric evaluation is requested by the teachers of C.B., a 13-year-old boy. He is of average intelligence, according to the Wechsler Intelligence Scale for Children (WISC; 1974), with better verbal than performance skills. He does well on tasks requiring rote learning, but his teachers are deeply puzzled and concerned about his poor comprehension of abstract ideas and his social naiveté. They find him appealing, but sadly vulnerable to the hazards of everyday life.

---

[*]From Wing L: "Asperger's Syndrome. A Clinical Account." *Psychological Medicine* 11:115–130, 1981.

His mother dates her son's problems from age 6 months, when his head was accidentally bruised. From that time on, he became socially aloof and isolated and spent most of his time gazing at his hands, which he moved in complicated patterns before his face. At age 1, he began to watch the passing traffic, but still ignored people. He continued to be remote, with poor eye contact, until age 5. He passed his motor milestones at the usual ages and, as soon as he was physically able, began to spend hours running in circles with an object in his hand, screaming if attempts were made to stop him. He performed many stereotyped movements as a young child, including jumping, flapping his arms, and moving his hands in circles.

At age 3, C.B. was able to recognize letters of the alphabet, and he rapidly acquired skill in drawing; he drew the salt and pepper shakers, correctly copying the names written on them, over and over again. For a time this was his sole activity. Following this, he became fascinated with pylons and tall buildings and would stare at them from all angles and draw them. C.B. did not speak until age 4, and then for a long time used only single words. Later, he repeated phrases and reversed pronouns.

After age 5, C.B.'s speech and social contact markedly improved. Until age 11, he attended a special school, where the staff tolerated a range of bizarre, repetitive routines. At one point, for example, he insisted that, before lessons could begin, all his class and the teacher should wear watches he made from plasticine. Despite all his problems, C.B. proved to have excellent rote memory, absorbed all he was taught, and could reproduce facts verbatim when asked. He was transferred to a regular public school at age 11.

C.B. uses good grammar and has a large vocabulary, but his speech is naive and immature and concerned mainly with his own special interests. He has learned not to make embarrassing remarks about other people's appearance, but tends to ask repetitive questions. He is not socially withdrawn, but prefers the company of adults to that of children his own age, finding it difficult to understand the unwritten rules of social interaction. He says of himself, "I am afraid I suffer from bad sportsmanship." He enjoys simple jokes, but cannot understand more subtle humor. He is often teased by his classmates.

C.B.'s main interest is in maps and road signs. He has a prodigious memory for routes and can draw them rapidly and accurately. He also makes large, complicated, abstract shapes out of any material that comes to hand and shows much ingenuity in ensuring that they hold together.

He has never engaged in pretend play, but is deeply attached to a toy panda, to which he talks as if it were an adult when he needs comfort.

C.B.'s finger dexterity is good, but he is clumsy and ill-coordinated in large movements and therefore is never chosen by the other children for sports and team games.

Discussion of "Cartographer"

C.B.'s many problems apparently began at an early age (6 months), with severe impairment in several developmental areas. He has shown grossly impaired social interaction, with a marked lack of awareness of the existence of others (totally ignoring the presence of others, watching only his hands or traffic) and no social play. Qualitative impairment in language development was indicated by his not speaking at all until age 4, and then speaking only single words, progressing to the use of repetitive phrases and reversed pronouns. Finally, he showed a markedly restricted repertoire of activities and interests, as manifested by stereotyped body movements (e.g., jumping, flapping his arms, moving his hands in circles), compulsive adherence to specific routines or rituals (e.g., insisting that his classmates wear plasticine watches), and preoccupation with a single narrow interest at a time (e.g., copying the names of the salt and pepper shakers). These characteristics indicate Autistic Disorder (DSM-IV-TR, p. 75), a Pervasive Developmental Disorder.

Since age 5, C.B.'s condition has improved considerably. He no longer exhibits bizarre behavior and gross distortions in language. Though he retains some signs of the illness (his speech is naive and immature; he has difficulty understanding the unwritten rules of social interaction), the full syndrome of Autistic Disorder is no longer present. Hence, the diagnosis is qualified as In Partial Remission.

This case was first published in 1981 as an example of Asperger's syndrome. However, the criteria for Asperger's Disorder in DSM-IV-TR require that there not be any significant general delay in language development, which is present in this case. This illustrates that in the past the term *Asperger's* has been used differently by different clinicians to indicate less severe cases of Pervasive Developmental Disorder.

Follow-Up

In the 7 years since his evaluation at age 13, C.B. has continued to make progress in practical and self-care skills and in the formal aspects of language (vocabulary and grammar). He still has an odd vocal intonation; a stilted, pedantic style of speech; and difficulty in initiating or taking turns in conversation. He retains his tendency to deliver monologues on the subjects that interest him. He has been unable to find work and most of the time stays within his own home, where he lives with his parents. He has no friends with whom he associates, but he has become adept at using citizens' band radio and regularly contacts a wide network of other radio enthusiasts. His circumscribed interests are now his radio, the progress of football teams, and maps. He remains somewhat clumsy and ill-coordinated in gross motor skills.

C.B.'s behavior is quiet and amenable, and he presents no problems for his parents or his sister, all of whom are very fond of him. The main concern is what will happen to him when his parents can no longer provide him with a home. They know that he is socially odd and naive and, despite the radio network, isolated, and that he lacks the ability to plan for himself and to cope with the demands of everyday life. Despite his skills, C.B. remains as innocent and vulnerable as a young child.

Reference

Wechsler D: Manual for the Wechsler Intelligence Scale for Children—Revised. New York, The Psychological Corporation, 1974

I'm Not Right Up Here[*]

Phillip, age 12, was suspended from a small-town Iowa school and referred for psychiatric treatment by his principal. The following note came with him:

---

[*] From Jenkins RL: *Behavior Disorders of Childhood and Adolescence.* Springfield, IL, Charles C. Thomas, 1973, pp. 60–64.

This child has been a continual problem since coming to our school. He does not get along on the playground because he is mean to other children. He disobeys school rules, teases the patrol children, steals from the other children, and defies all authority. Phillip keeps getting into fights with other children on the bus.

He has been suspended from cafeteria privileges several times for fighting, pushing, and shoving. After he misbehaved one day at the cafeteria, the teacher told him to come up to my office to see me. He flatly refused, lay on the floor, and threw a temper tantrum, kicking and screaming.

The truth is not in Phillip. When caught in actual misdeeds, he denies everything, and takes upon himself an air of injured innocence. He believes we are picking on him. His attitude is sullen when he is refused anything. He pouts and when asked why he does these things, he points to his head and says, "Because I'm not right up here."

This boy needs help badly. He does not seem to have friends. His aggressive behavior prevents the children from liking him. Our school psychologist tested Phillip, and the results indicated average intelligence, but his school achievement is only at the third- and low fourth-grade level.

The psychiatrist learned from Phillip's grandmother that he was born when his mother was a senior in high school. Her parents insisted that she keep the baby and help rear him; most of his upbringing has been by his grandparents, however.

Phillip was "3 months premature" and a "blue baby," requiring oxygen for 24 hours. Shortly after his birth, Phillip's mother ran off with a man, married him, and had a second child. The marriage broke up, and she left this child with its father. Phillip has had no contact with his mother since she left him.

Phillip's toilet training was not successful, and he remained a bedwetter for some years. At age 5, his maternal grandparents adopted him because they were afraid that his mother might some day claim him. He showed anxiety at separation from his grandmother when he began school.

He was then in a serious car accident, in which his grandmother was injured and one person in the other car killed. Phillip did not appear to be injured, but seemed to have some transient memory loss, probably a direct, immediate result of the impact. Subsequently, he had nightmares, fear of the dark, and an exacerbation of his fear of separation from his grandmother.

Phillip's school progress was not good. He repeated third grade and then was in a special class for underachievers. His grandmother recalls that Phillip's teacher complained that he "could never stay in his seat."

A few months before the consultation, Phillip was seen in a mental health clinic and placed on some mild tranquilizers. A 3-month return appointment was arranged, but the school suspended him before that date.

Discussion of "I'm Not Right Up Here"

Phillip's antisocial behavior began when he was in grade school, and a pattern of fighting, lying, and stealing has persisted for many years. This disturbance of conduct, lasting more than 6 months, justifies the diagnosis of Conduct Disorder (DSM-IV-TR, p. 98). Because the disturbance began before age 10, it is noted as Childhood-Onset Type.

Because his behavior problems did not cause more than minor harm to others and he does not have many of the other symptoms of Conduct Disorder, such as cruelty to animals or people, using a weapon, setting fires, or running away from home, the severity is noted as Moderate.

Follow-Up

Phillip was admitted to the children's unit of a state mental hospital. After 8 months he was discharged as having received "maximal hospital benefit," with a statement that "the prognosis is not favorable." He returned to school in his small community. Over the next 2 years, Phillip's behavior gradually deteriorated, with much involvement in name calling, fights, and refusals to obey school personnel. He was suspended following the discovery in his locker of a tape recorder that was missing from a school office.

At this time his grandparents recognized that they could no longer cope with him and accepted his commitment for long-term treatment in the state mental hospital. Phillip's course in the hospital was stormy. He made himself unpopular with his peers by repeatedly stealing from them. When caught, he would lie or refuse to answer. He had a foul mouth and used derogatory, insulting language. As a result of his behavior, he spent much time in seclusion. While in seclusion he destroyed his mattress by cutting it with a piece of glass. He was generally hostile and uncooperative and, when crossed, would become combative. Hospital personnel controlled him only with difficulty and frequently had bruised shins to show for it. When Phillip lost control, he seemed to do so completely, and communication became impossible until he had been overpowered and had time to cool down.

His relations with staff began to improve as they persisted in showing interest and goodwill in spite of his assaultiveness. His relations with his peer group improved much more slowly. Real progress began when he was assigned to work with some of the maintenance staff. He enjoyed this work and often did a good job.

When Phillip was age 16, he was transferred from the adolescent ward to a closed adult men's ward. Here his combativeness rapidly diminished and his adjustment accordingly improved. Phillip ascribed this improvement to the fact that he was no longer in contact with other poorly controlled adolescents, who tended to stir him up and provoke him. After about 3 months, he was returned to the home of his grandparents and, when last seen (6 weeks later), was making a satisfactory adjustment. He attended school in the morning and worked in a gas station in the afternoon in a school–work program. (Note: The improvement in Phillip's behavior provides some hope that he will not be one of the many children with Conduct Disorder who go on to develop Antisocial Personality Disorder.)

HE BREAKS HIS TOYS

Johnny, age 8, was brought to a clinic for evaluation by his mother, who said, "There is something wrong with his brain." When asked to be more specific, she replied with a vague litany of complaints that were frequently self-contradictory.

> He was always slow to learn things, slower than any of my other children. But I know he's really very smart. Sometimes he just amazes me with what he remembers or can figure out. He doesn't do much, for example, at school or with activities outside school. Sometimes I think it's because he's lazy, and other times I think he's depressed, and other times I think maybe it's because he is sick a lot. He gets a lot of stomachaches. He's re-

ally such a sweet boy, I mean he's so nice with his four sisters and our pets. But sometimes he's so nasty I get afraid. For example, he gets frustrated with some of his toys, and then he gets destructive. He's broken more toys than all of my other three children put together. He seems to like people, but he only has one friend at school. He refuses to try out for soccer or anything like that where he could play with the other boys. Sometimes I think he just doesn't care about anything. He's always dropping dishes and things around the house.

A more detailed history revealed that the pregnancy, birth, and early medical history had been unremarkable, but minor problems had appeared in the first year of life. These included being slow to sit up, crawl, and walk. Because Johnny was the fourth child in the family, the mother had not "had time" to record the actual ages when these milestones were reached. She could only pinpoint that "he was much older than any of the other children when he did finally manage to do those things," adding that the pediatrician had nonetheless assured her that Johnny was not retarded. "A good thing he did," she laughed, "because later when Johnny had so much trouble learning to use the knife and fork, and to tie his shoelaces, and to button his shirts, I did worry about that."

Asked if there were any remaining concerns along these lines, the mother replied "none at all." Apparently, Johnny excelled in reading and did well in all his other school subjects, except for handwriting and physical education.

His medical history was also unremarkable. During the preschool years there had been only "the normal childhood illnesses" (chicken pox, earaches, and flu) and "an awful lot of bruises and scraped knees." The stomachaches had started "some time around age 7," but again, the pediatrician had assured the mother that they were not cause for concern.

Examination revealed a pleasant, but rather quiet, boy with appropriate affect, good concentration, and apparently normal cognitive skills. Although quiet and reserved, Johnny did not appear apathetic; indeed, he became quite enthusiastic when describing a book he had just read. During the interview, Johnny denied any problems in school or with peers. When specifically asked, he did admit to occasional stomachaches and to nonparticipation in group activities, which he attributed to simply "not liking that stuff."

Psychological testing performed in the school setting revealed above-average intelligence and academic performance. However, Johnny scored well below the norm on a test of motor development requiring tasks involving running, balancing, coordination, and motor speed. The psychologist noted that he showed good concentration and attention during the testing.

Discussion of "He Breaks His Toys"

Many features of this case are typical of Developmental Coordination Disorder (DSM-IV-TR, p. 58). These include late gross motor milestones (standing, sitting, walking), early history of bruises (from bumping into things) and falls, reported "destructiveness" (dropping things or breaking toys when trying to manipulate them), and difficulty with tasks requiring fine motor coordination (buttoning clothes, tying shoelaces, and handwriting) and with sports, such as ball games.

The stomachaches, "laziness," "depression," and "apathy" probably represent Johnny's efforts to avoid physical education class, tests in which handwriting is necessary, and the embarrassment of repeated failures in team sport situations. Similarly, Johnny's "bad temper" and "frustration" are probably not evidence of disturbance in attention or conduct, but rather a manifestation of his motor difficulties. As often happens, it is these secondary problems that have brought him to professional attention.

One may wonder why a disorder of physical coordination appears in a classification of mental disorders. It is true that the defining features of the disorder are more physical than behavioral or psychological, and therefore one could argue that the disorder should more properly be considered a general medical condition, rather than a mental disorder. However, it seems reasonable to classify it with the other developmental disorders of childhood because of the absence of a specific known etiology and because the behavioral consequences of the disorder (e.g., irritability and avoidance behavior) are treated by mental health professionals.

DOLLS

Rocky is an 8-year-old boy for whom his parents seek treatment because "he wants to be a girl." The patient's major playmate is his younger sister;

although his parents are trying to foster friendships with other boys, Rocky prefers to play with girls or to be with his mother or a female baby-sitter. He refuses to participate in rough play with boys and physical fighting, although he is well built, above average in height for his age, and well co-ordinated. At home he engages in much make-believe play, invariably assuming female roles. When playing house with his younger sister, he plays the "mother" or "big sister" role and leaves the male role to her. He likes to imitate female TV figures, such as Brenda from *Beverly Hills 90210* or Bart Simpson's sister, Lisa. Similarly, he likes to playact female characters from various children's books.

Rocky has never been interested in toy cars, trucks, or trains, but is an avid player with dolls (baby, Barbie, and family dolls) and enjoys playing with kitchen toys. He also likes to play wedding, pregnancy, a female teacher, or a lady doctor. He is good at drawing and is very interested in drawing female figures. Although his parents try to restrict the activity, he engages in a lot of cross-dressing. Sometimes he uses a quilt or a towel around his middle for skirts, or a T-shirt or nightgown for a dress. He does not use any female underwear or bathing suits. He likes bows in his hair and may use an underskirt or a veil on his head to imitate long hair. He loves dancing, preferably in dresses. He is very interested in jewelry, has plastic necklaces, and pretends at times to wear earrings. Also, he pretends to apply lipstick (with Chapstick) and would use real lipstick and perfume if his mother would let him. He states, "I want to be a girl," often when he is unhappy (e.g., when he started kindergarten, when he felt in competition with his younger sister).

On physical examination, the boy was found to have normal male genitalia. His intellectual development is apparently normal. Although somewhat reluctant, he is able to describe much of what his parents have related about his toy and game preferences. He says that he does not want to be a boy because he is afraid he will have to play with soldiers or play army with other boys when he grows bigger. He wishes a fairy could change him into a girl. What he likes about being a girl is wearing dresses, long hair, and jewelry. His drawings are all of female figures.

Family history, pregnancy, birth, and early development are all normal. The parents do not show any overt psychopathology. The patient's problems seem to have started with the birth of his younger sister, when he was 2. For the first 4 months of her life, his sister had digestive problems and required a great deal of parental attention and care. Rocky then began to display definite signs of regression—he played the baby role again, wanting to drink from a bottle and be held and carried. His mother gave in to some extent. Both parents and baby-sitters think that cross-dressing and wanting to be a girl date back to that time, although, before the birth of his sister, there were already some instances of the patient's imitating long hair by wearing a towel on his head. When the patient was 4, his sister got a baby doll, which he took from her. Around this same time he spent a vacation with his sister at their grandparents and complained that his sister got more attention than he, ending with the familiar "Why can't I be a girl? Why didn't God make me a girl? Girls get to dress up, get to wear pretty things."

From age 3 on, Rocky was enrolled in nursery school, and he initially displayed much separation anxiety. He appeared more sensitive than the other children, always seemed to feel threatened by them, and did not stand up for himself. His teacher noted from the beginning that he dressed up very frequently, said that he wanted to be a mother when he grew up, and refused to engage in rough-and-tumble activities. In the third grade his classroom teacher closed off the doll corner because of his preoccupation with doll play.

Discussion of "Dolls"

There should be little question about the diagnosis in this case. This boy has a strong and persistent identification of himself as a female. He frequently states his desire to be a girl—not just play a female role. He is preoccupied with female stereotypical activity, preferring to play with girls and pretending that he is a girl, and frequently cross-dresses. He plays exclusively with stereotypically female toys such as dolls. When imitating characters from books and TV, he always chooses female characters. There is also evidence of a persistent discomfort with being a boy. He rejects stereotypical male toys and activities and shows an aversion toward rough-and-tumble play.

These are the characteristic features of Gender Identity Disorder as seen in a male (DSM-IV-TR, p. 581). When this disorder is diagnosed in a female, the desire to be male because of a profound discontent in being a female needs to be distinguished from the desire merely to have the perceived cultural advantages associated with being a male.

DOWN'S SYNDROME

A 15-year-old boy was brought to the emergency room by his mother, who, clutching the on-call resident's arm, pleaded, "You've got to admit him; I just can't take it anymore." The patient had been taken home from a special school by his mother 6 months previously. The mother showed the resident papers from the school that indicated that the patient's IQ was 45. He had had several placements, beginning at age 8. On visiting days, the boy always pleaded with his mother, "Mommy, take me home." After a year or so away, the patient would be brought home by his mother, who had always been racked with guilt because of his retardation and her inability to manage him in the home. The patient was an only child whose parents had been divorced for the past 4 years. The father had moved to another city.

During the last 6 months at home, the patient had increasingly become a behavior problem. He was about 5 feet, 9 inches tall and weighed close to 200 pounds. He had become destructive of property at home— breaking dishes and a chair during angry tantrums—and, more recently, physically assaultive. He had hit his mother on the arm and shoulder during a recent scuffle that began when she tried to get him to stop banging a broom on the apartment floor. The mother showed her bruises to the resident and threatened to call the mayor's office if the hospital refused to admit her son.

On examination, the boy was observed to have the typical signs of Down's syndrome, including thick facial features, slightly protruding tongue, epicanthic fold of the eyelids, and Simian crease of the palms of the hands. With indistinct and slurred speech, the boy insisted that he "didn't mean to hurt anybody."

Discussion of "Down's Syndrome"

This boy's IQ of 45 indicates significantly subaverage general intellectual functioning. The need for placement in special schools since age 8 suggests that there have been severe concurrent deficits or impairments in adaptive behavior. These two features, with onset before age 18, indicate the Axis II diagnosis of Mental Retardation (DSM-IV-TR, p. 49). Because the IQ level is between 35 and 55, the severity level is Moderate.

The diagnosis of Mental Retardation should be made when the criteria are met, regardless of the presence of another diagnosis. In the presence of significant Mental Retardation, the issue of a Learning Disorder is moot, as the specific deficit would have to be out of proportion to the deficits in other areas of development. A Pervasive Developmental Disorder can coexist with Mental Retardation; but unlike in this case, only when there is no interest or pleasure in social contact. Therefore, no diagnosis is warranted on Axis I.

This child, as is often the case, presents for admission because of destructive and aggressive behavior, not because of impairment in intellectual functioning. This aggressive behavior is presumably a persistent pattern; nevertheless, the additional diagnosis of Conduct Disorder is not justified because there are none of the other characteristic features of this disorder, such as stealing, lying, and running away from home.

In this case, Mental Retardation is apparently a result of Down's syndrome, which would be noted on Axis III.

The presence of any clinically relevant psychosocial or environmental problems is unclear from the available information. Therefore, one would not check any items from the Axis IV Psychosocial and Environmental Problems Checklist.

The patient's highest level of functioning in the past year is very poor, owing to marked impairment in all areas of functioning; therefore, an appropriate highest global assessment of functioning (GAF) rating is only about 20. Because of the increase in dangerous behavior recently, necessitating the visit to the emergency room, the current GAF is rated 10.

THIN TIM

Eight-year-old Tim was referred by a pediatrician who asked for an emergency evaluation because of a serious weight loss during the past year for which the pediatrician could find no medical cause. Tim is extremely concerned about his weight and weighs himself daily. He complains that he is too fat, and if he does not lose weight, he cuts back on food. He has lost 10 pounds in the past year and still feels that he is too fat, though it is clear that he is underweight. In desperation, his parents have removed the scales from the house; as a result, Tim is keeping a record of the calories that he eats daily. He spends a lot of time on this, checking and rechecking that he has done it just right.

In addition, Tim is described as being obsessed with cleanliness and neatness. Currently he has no friends because he refuses to visit them, feeling that their houses are "dirty"; he gets upset when another child touches him. He is always checking whether he is doing things the way they "should" be done. He becomes very agitated and anxious about this. He has to get up at least two hours before leaving for school each day in order to give himself time to get ready. Recently, he woke up at 1:30 A.M. to prepare for school.

Discussion of "Thin Tim"

The emergency evaluation is because of Tim's recent weight loss. He has lost 10 pounds in the last year, during which time a boy of his age might have been expected to gain about that amount. This means he is actually 20 pounds below his expected weight for his age. Although Anorexia Nervosa is unusual in a male and in one so young, his refusal to maintain a normal weight suggests this diagnosis (DSM-IV-TR, p. 589). Tim also has the other characteristic features of the disorder: fear of becoming fat, feeling fat even when obviously underweight.

Although not the focus of attention, Tim's preoccupation with various recurrent thoughts concerning dirtiness causes him considerable distress. Moreover, he has to check whether he is doing things the way they "should" be done, and such activities apparently interfere with his normal functioning (he has to get up several hours before school in order to get ready). Although he does not seem to experience these recurrent thoughts and repetitive acts as inappropriate, it is reasonable to assume that the thoughts do intrude into his consciousness and are beyond his control and that his lengthy "getting ready" routines are performed in response to these thoughts. Thus, they represent true obsessions and compulsions. Because the content of these obsessions and compulsions is unrelated to Tim's Eating Disorder, an additional diagnosis of

Obsessive-Compulsive Disorder (DSM-IV-TR, p. 462) is made and is listed second, as the initial focus of attention is the eating problem.

There is phobic avoidance (he won't visit friends' houses because they might be dirty), but the additional diagnosis of a Specific Phobia is not made because phobic avoidance is a commonly associated feature of Obsessive-Compulsive Disorder.

NIGHTTIME VISITOR

Nina was age 8 when her guidance counselor at school referred her to the Family Treatment Center in Cleveland because of disruptive, aggressive behavior. Her 11-year-old brother, Don, and her 9-year-old sister, Sara, were also evaluated, together with her mother.

Several months earlier Nina had been admitted to the hospital with vaginal bleeding and a discharge. A diagnosis of vaginal warts (*condyloma acuminatum*) was made, and the vaginal culture proved to be positive for gonorrhea. When questioned by a social worker whom the pediatrician asked to see the children, Nina revealed that she and Sara had been sexually molested by their father for the past 2 years. According to her, he would come into their bedroom regularly at night and have vaginal intercourse with her and, more rarely, with Sara. The girls noticed that if they were awake, their father often would not bother them. Nevertheless, Nina was so frightened that she would close her eyes and feign sleep during the molestation. Their father threatened them with beatings if they divulged the secret, so they had never told anyone.

Their brother, Don, after witnessing one of the molestations, told their mother. She did not believe him and told her husband, who then proceeded to beat Don. In fact, Don had often been beaten by his father. After Don's disclosure, Nina and Sara told their mother what had been happening, but she scolded them for "making up stories."

When the social worker talked with the mother about these events, she admitted that she had suspected that her children were telling the truth, but was afraid of confronting her husband about his sexual abuse because she feared his murderous rage. During their 12-year marriage, he had frequently beaten her, but she never thought of leaving him because her religion forbade divorce.

After the medical confirmation of the sexual abuse, the children were temporarily placed in foster care, the father was jailed, and the family court cited the mother for neglect because she had failed to intervene to protect the children from the father's sexual abuse. The children were subsequently placed with their maternal grandmother and then returned to their mother after she agreed to a psychiatric evaluation and treatment for herself and her children.

When interviewed at the Family Treatment Center, Nina is a sad, unusually quiet child who rarely smiles. She describes that, since the abuse started 2 years ago, she spends most of her time in her room alone doing little more than watching television. She often has difficulty falling asleep and reports nightmares about her father coming into her room. Nina has talked with the children in school about being molested and now believes that they all dislike her because of it. When she testified in court, she was certain that she would be sent to jail because she had done something wrong. She also fears that her father will return and attack her. At home, she is generally irritable and often fights with Sara and Don, and feels "picked on" by her mother, whom she feels has always favored her siblings.

Discussion of "Nighttime Visitor"

Nina's difficulties are almost certainly related to the trauma of having been repeatedly sexually abused by her father. Does this kind of trauma qualify as the type of extreme stressor that is required for the diagnosis of Posttraumatic Stress Disorder? The stressor criterion for this disorder requires that the person has experienced, witnessed, or been confronted with an event that involves actual or threatened death or injury, or threat to one's physical integrity. In addition, the diagnosis requires that the person's response involve intense fear, helplessness, or horror. It is a reasonable inference that sexual intercourse with a child is experienced as a "threat to one's physical integrity," and Nina clearly reacted with intense fear.

The reexperiencing of the trauma (nightmares of her father) is also characteristic of Posttraumatic Stress Disorder. This diagnosis also requires at least three symptoms indicating persistent avoidance of stimuli associated with the trauma or numbing of general responsiveness. We find evidence of a feeling of estrangement from others (her classmates), restricted range of affect (she is unusually quiet and rarely smiles), and diminished participation in significant activities (doing little other than watching television). In addition, the diagnosis requires persistent symptoms of increased arousal. Nina has difficulty falling asleep and is generally irritable at home.

Thus, Nina would meet the criteria for the diagnosis Posttraumatic Stress Disorder (DSM-IV-TR, p. 467). Because her symptoms had persisted for more than 3 months, the diagnosis would be specified as Chronic.

Nina's reaction to having been sexually abused by her father and not protected (or even believed) by her mother has included depressed mood, nightmares about the trauma, anger, inappropriate self-reproach and guilt, and the feeling that schoolmates dislike her. This suggests the possible additional diagnosis of a Mood Disorder, but there is no evidence that the depressed mood is accompanied by the characteristic symptoms of a Major Depressive Episode, other than self-reproach and guilt. Although the sexual abuse had been going on for 2 years, there is no description of a persistent depressed mood that would justify a diagnosis of Dysthymic Disorder. In fact, during this time Nina seems to have been more frightened than depressed.

Follow-Up

After the evaluation of the family, individual psychotherapy was recommended for Nina, Sara, and their mother. In addition, family treatment was instituted in order to improve the relationship between the children and their mother and to help establish structure and discipline in the home. Nina's mother was encouraged to allow the children to express their feelings of having been betrayed by her. At home Nina began to overeat and steal money from her mother's purse, as a way of expressing anger toward her mother and of getting more attention.

In the treatment setting, Nina acted frightened and needy, and she clung to her female therapist. She expressed her yearnings for nurturance and safety by caring for doll babies and stuffed animals. She was frequently involved in "traumatic play," in which she acted out various elements of the trauma. These dramas often involved a witch who poisoned children and devils and monsters who attacked them when they tried to run away.

No One Hits the Baby

Four-year-old Carol was referred for an evaluation when her teacher made a complaint to the state Central Registry for Child Abuse Reports. A family evaluation by a social worker revealed the following.

Carol is the older of two children, both of whom live with their parents in a two-bedroom apartment. Her problems began with the birth of her sister 3 months ago. Her teachers noticed a change in her behavior at school. She began pushing other children and hit a classmate with a wooden block, causing a laceration of the classmate's lip. When Carol's teacher took her aside to talk about her behavior, she noticed what seemed to be belt marks on Carol's abdomen and forehead.

Carol's sister was "colicky" and slept for only short periods throughout the day and night. She stopped crying only when her mother held her. Her mother therefore had little time for Carol, and Carol's father took over her care on evenings and weekends. He began to drink more than usual, half a bottle of wine each evening, and became increasingly irritable. He and his wife argued over her attention to the infant and the requirement that he take care of Carol. Carol, who was a bright, curious, talkative 4-year-old, asked constant questions and often wanted to hold the baby. When refused, she would lie on the floor and have a tantrum. Since her sister's birth, she had begun to have difficulty falling asleep and awoke repeatedly during the night.

Carol's father was unable to cope with her demands for attention and often told her to shut up and slapped her when she did not obey. On many occasions he responded to her tantrums or repeated questions by hitting her with his belt.

Carol is a lively and attractive little blue-eyed blond, dressed in jeans, T-shirt, and sneakers. She relates appropriately and warmly to the interviewer and easily separates from her parents in the waiting room. Her intelligence appears above average, as indicated by her fund of knowledge, vocabulary, and drawings of a person and of geometric forms. About her sister, Carol says, "She's a bad girl. She cries all the time. I get hit when I cry, but no one hits the baby." When asked about fights at the day-care center, she replies, "I hit Robert (her playmate) because he pulls my hair." She says she is afraid to go to sleep because she has bad dreams of an old man killing her.

Discussion of "No One Hits the Baby"

We shall focus on the diagnosis of Carol's difficulties as she is the "identified patient," but we should note that her problems are actually the consequence of her father's psychopathology. We assume that Carol's reaction to having a baby sister would not have been remarkable were it not for her father's physical abuse of her.

Researchers have only recently begun to study the psychological consequences of physical and sexual abuse of children. It would seem that children who are physically or sexually abused are at risk for developing several disorders. Major Depressive Disorder, Separation Anxiety Disorder, Oppositional Defiant Disorder, and Conduct Disorder are frequent initial reactions to sexual or physical abuse. In adolescents, suicidal behavior and psychoactive substance abuse are also frequent. It is unclear how often Posttraumatic Stress Disorder is an initial reaction. Major Depressive Disorder, various personality disturbances, and (more rarely) Dissociative Identity Disorder are long-term consequences that are seen in adults. It is certainly clear that children who themselves have been physically or sexually abused are likely to abuse their own children. The cases in which this kind of multigenerational abuse has been identified have generally involved more serious and long-term abuse than Carol has experienced.

Carol's changed behavior includes temper tantrums at home, fighting with other children at school, and having trouble falling asleep. These few symptoms are not indicative of a syndrome that would justify the diagnosis of any of the above disorders. Therefore, we are left with the residual diagnosis of Adjustment Disorder With Mixed Disturbance of Emotions and Conduct (DSM-IV-TR, p. 683).

Follow-Up

Carol, along with her mother and father, began a family therapy program that included parenting training and behavioral therapy for Carol, coordinated with the day-care center. Her father was persuaded to join Alcoholics Anonymous, has stopped drinking, and has been able to control his anger at his daughter. Six months later, Carol's aggressive behavior had ceased. She was doing well with peers and in her academic work, was sleeping throughout the night, and had stopped having temper tantrums.

BABY SUSAN

Susan was admitted to the hospital at age 6 months by an aunt for evaluation of failure to gain weight. She had been born into an impoverished family after an unplanned, uncomplicated pregnancy. During the first 4 months of her life, she gained weight steadily. Regurgitation was noted during the fifth month and increased in severity to the point where she was regurgitating after every feeding. After each feeding, Susan would engage in one of two behaviors: 1) she would open her mouth, elevate her tongue, and rapidly thrust it back and forward, after which milk would appear at the back of her mouth and slowly trickle out; or 2) she would vigorously suck her thumb and place fingers in her mouth, following which milk would slowly flow out of the corner of her mouth.

In the past 2 months Susan had been cared for by a number of people, including her aunt and paternal grandmother. Her parents were making a marginal marital adjustment. Nevertheless, Susan often smiled and was responsive to all of her caregivers

Discussion of "Baby Susan"

Failure to gain weight or weight loss in an infant, once general medical conditions, such as congenital anomalies, have been ruled out, suggests either Rumination Disorder of Infancy, Feeding Disorder of Infancy or Childhood, or Reactive Attachment Disorder of Infancy or Early Childhood. It is clear that in this case the child is not gaining weight because of the regurgitation of food after each feeding, indicating the presence of Rumination Disorder of Infancy (DSM-IV-TR, p. 106). Typically, the child strains and arches the back and makes sucking movements with his or her tongue. The food is ejected from the mouth or chewed and reswallowed. Often the child gives the impression of gaining considerable satisfaction from the activity. As in this case, the disorder usually appears between 3 months and 12 months.

There is a suggestion in this case that the quality of parental care may have been inadequate. However, the absence of any evidence of inappropriate social relatedness rules out the diagnosis of Reactive Attachment Disorder of Infancy or Early Childhood. Because the cause of the weight loss is the regurgitation, the residual diagnosis of Feeding Disorder of Infancy or Early Childhood is not given.

SHE WANTS TO BE A BOY

Kelly, a 16-year-old Canadian girl from British Columbia, is referred to a gender identity clinic at the suggestion of her family physician and with her parents' agreement and participation. According to her mother, "Kelly wants a sex change. She wants to be a boy very desperately." Kelly echoes this, saying that she has wanted to be a boy "since I was 2." The current referral was precipitated by Kelly's relationship with another girl, Anna, who has been living with the family for the past few months. Kelly's mother became agitated about the girls' relationship, feeling that it was sexual: "They always have their legs crossed, arms around each other, and once were lying naked with their breasts exposed reading dirty books."

Since reaching puberty, Kelly has continued to show a number of signs suggesting that she is very uncomfortable with being a female. She found her menstrual periods "horrible" and disliked having to wear a bra. Kelly has continued to say that she wants to be a boy, including having a penis. Last year, she learned of the possibility of sex-reassignment surgery. She knows that it would include a mastectomy, removal of her internal reproductive organs, and hormone injections. She is not sure whether she could have a penis surgically constructed.

During the interview, Kelly is asked why the idea of being a boy is so important to her, and why she cannot pursue her life goals and remain a girl. She then states that at the present time her sole reason for wanting to be a boy is that she wants to play in the National Hockey League. Kelly claims that a few months ago she had been asked to try out for a minor league team owned by the Los Angeles Kings. She feels that if she had a penis, she would have a better chance of getting on the team.

Kelly's physical appearance is ambiguous with regard to her biological sex. Her hair is short, she is dressed casually in blue jeans, and she wears no makeup. She does, however, wear one earring. Kelly says that she does not care if others perceive her as a male or as a female, preferring to be seen as a "human being." As she speaks, it becomes clear that she prefers that people not ask her if she is a male or a female, though she does not actually say that she wants others to perceive her as a male.

Kelly quit school after the seventh grade. She claims that she is now in a youth group, training to be in the military. She very much enjoys this because even though she is known to be a female, "They treat you like a buddy—the same as the other guys." She takes great delight in ordering around her cadet peers, relishing "being mean; they all hate me" when she demands that they do 500 pushups. Kelly spoke in great detail about using a submachine gun and said she had been practicing weapon use for several years. She is attracted by "gory things, blood, and living dangerously." Kelly says that the thought of war appeals to her because "they push you so hard and you are down on your knees, begging them to stop."

Kelly's mother tried to find out about her sexuality by having her read a "pornographic" book and underline those passages that excited her or, as Kelly put it, gave her a "twingy" feeling, during which she felt "weird inside." The passages that elicited such a feeling involved love-making between women. Kelly says that she is not sure if boys or girls turn her on. She jogs whenever she begins to have "twingy feelings" and denies that she has ever masturbated. "I think it's sick."

She denies ever experiencing sexual images either in dreams or fantasy. She says she has never had any sexual experiences with another person and has no desire to marry. When asked about lesbianism, she claims not to want to know very much about the gay subculture: "It's their life."

When she appeared for the physical examination, she apologized for not having shaved her legs. An endocrine evaluation was performed and indicated that the sex chromosomes were XX, there were no abnormally elevated levels of testosterone, and there were no signs of physical hermaphroditism.

Discussion of "She Wants to Be a Boy"

Kelly has a strong and persistent identification with being male (cross-gender identification) that goes far beyond just a desire for the perceived cultural advantages of being male. She has a stated desire to become a male, including the consideration of having a sex change operation. She has a stated desire to live and be treated as a male. In addition, she indicates a persistent discomfort with being female. All of these features are characteristic of Gender Identity Disorder (DSM-IV-TR, p. 581). The disorder is further specified by indicating sexual attraction. Although she seems to be most sexually excited by passages in a book depicting lesbian relationships, her lack of any sexual fantasies or experiences and her denial of either a heterosexual or homosexual orientation suggest Sexually Attracted to Neither Male nor Female Type.

Follow-Up

At a 4-year follow-up, Kelly remained preoccupied with changing her sex, yet she continued to live in an ambivalent gender role; for example, she was employed in a typically "masculine" occupation, but claimed that no one asked, or cared, if she was male or female. In the past year, Kelly made an application to an adult gender identity clinic with the hope that she would eventually be able to have a sex change operation. She failed to keep her appointment.

TINY TINA

Tina, a small, sweet-faced, freckled 10-year-old child, has been referred by a pediatrician who was unsuccessful in treating her for refusing to go to school. Her difficulties began on the first day of school one year ago when she cried and hid in the basement. She agreed to go to school only when her mother promised to go with her and stay to have lunch with her at school. For the next 3 months, on school days, Tina had a variety of somatic complaints, such as headaches and "tummy aches," and each day would go to school only reluctantly, after much cajoling by her parents. Soon thereafter she could be gotten to school only if her parents lifted her out of bed, dressed and fed her, and drove her to school. Finally, in the spring, the school social worker consulted Tina's pediatrician, who instituted a behavior-modification program with the help of her parents. Because this program was of only limited help, the pediatrician had now, at the beginning of the school year, referred Tina to a psychiatrist.

According to her mother, despite Tina's many absences from school last year, she performed well. During this time she also happily participated in all other activities, including Girl Scout meetings, sleepovers at friends' houses (usually with her sister), and family outings. Her mother wonders if taking a part-time bookkeeping job 2 years ago, plus the sudden death of a maternal grandmother to whom Tina was particularly close, might have been responsible for the child's difficulties.

When Tina was interviewed, she at first minimized any problems about school, insisting that everything was "okay" and that she got good grades and liked all the teachers. When this subject was pursued, she became angry and gave a lot of "I don't know" responses as to why, then, she often refused to go to school. Eventually she said that kids teased her about her size, calling her "Shrimp" and "Shorty"; but she gave the impression, as well as actually stating, that she liked school and her teachers. She finally admitted that what bothered her was leaving home. She could not specify why, but hinted that she was afraid something would happen, though to whom or to what she did not say; but she confessed that she felt uncomfortable when all of her family members were out of sight.

On the Rorschach (1921) there was evidence of obsessive rumination about catastrophic events involving injury to members of her family and themes concerning family disruption.

Discussion of "Tiny Tina"

All of Tina's problems involve a fear of going to school. The question is: Is it school that she is really afraid of, or is it separating herself from her parents? The evidence that she is really afraid of school is her claim that the other children tease her and her willing participation in other activities away from home, such as sleepovers and Girl Scout meetings. But Tina herself concludes that it is really her fear that something bad will happen when her family is out of her sight that is behind her refusal to go to school. We are inclined to accept this explanation. An enforced 6 hours away from her family every day is apparently more troubling to her than an occasional hour at a Girl Scout meeting or, surprisingly, a sleepover, usually with her sister.

In the absence of any more pervasive disorder, the excessive distress about separation from the family and unrealistic worry about harm befalling them, reluctance to go to school, and complaints of physical symptoms on school days, over a period of more than 4 weeks, all indicate Separation Anxiety Disorder (DSM-IV-TR, p. 125). We should not quarrel with a clinician who wished to make this diagnosis provisional pending further clarification of Tina's distress about being teased. If she is excessively fearful of the possibility of being humiliated or embarrassed in public, then the diagnosis of Social Phobia should be considered as an alternative or as an additional diagnosis.

Reference

Rorschach H: Psychodiagnostics: A Diagnostic Test Based on Perception. Bern, Switzerland, Hans Huber, 1921

SEIZURE

A 16-year-old female junior-high-school student was hospitalized on the psychiatric service for behavior problems. She had been in trouble with school authorities since age 12 for truancy and petty thefts. More recently, she was expelled from junior high school when she and two friends were caught smoking marijuana in the locker room. Finally, a series of thefts from neighborhood stores and an incident in which she and a companion set a fire in a vacant lot brought her into court and prompted a judge to remand her to a psychiatric ward for evaluation. Her parents said they were unable to control her, that she was a "born liar," and that when she became angry with them, she frequently had stayed out all night, without telling them where she had been.

On the ward, the girl befriended other adolescents. The staff found her to be demanding and affectively volatile. She frequently stormed out of community meetings when decisions were made that did not go her way. She tried to have the ward recreational activities revolve around her and was very enthusiastic about them at first, but later appeared angry and pouting when she was not permitted to monopolize the activity. Beneath her superficial bravado, however, the nursing staff found her to be insecure and dependent.

One evening about a week into her hospitalization, after being refused a pass to go out of the hospital, the patient stormed down the hall to her room. Minutes later, a scream was heard; and when the first nurse reached her, the patient was writhing on the floor on her back, making jerking movements of her pelvis, arms, and legs and rolling her eyes upward. When the staff and patients had congregated near her room, her violent shaking stopped. She lay nearly still, eyes closed, with a slight trembling visible over her body. She had not bitten her tongue or voided urine or feces. When her arm was raised above her face and dropped, it fell to the side of her head each time, rather than striking her face. Finally, the nurse, noting her to be fully alert, asked her some questions, which she answered appropriately, although she stated that she could not yet move. Fifteen minutes later, she walked to the examining room to be evaluated by the doctor on call.

Discussion of "Seizure"

The doctor on call would have no difficulty in making a diagnosis of the behavioral problems that led to this girl's hospitalization. For at least 4 years, she has been getting into trouble. She has repeatedly been truant, stolen from stores, and recently set a fire. She lies to her parents and stays out all night. This repetitive and pervasive pattern of violating the basic rights of others and major age-appropriate societal norms or rules indicates Conduct Disorder (DSM-IV-TR, p. 98). Because the onset of the conduct problems was after age 10, we would indicate Adolescent-Onset Type, which generally has a better prognosis than Childhood-Onset Type. Because the number of conduct problems that this girl has is more than enough to make the diagnosis, but their effect on others is not extremely harmful, we would rate the severity of the Conduct Disorder as Moderate.

The immediate diagnostic problem for the doctor on call is how to characterize her "fit." There are several features that suggest it was not a genuine epileptic seizure. During a genuine grand mal seizure, one would expect urinary, and possibly fecal, incontinence. One would also expect a period of postictal (postseizure) confusion during which the patient would not be fully alert and able to protect herself from hitting herself in the face when her hand was dropped.

Because there is a close temporal relationship between her being upset and the "fit," it is reasonable to assume that the fit is related to a psychological conflict or need. There are three diagnostic possibilities: Conversion Disorder, Factitious Disorder With Predominantly Physical Signs and Symptoms, and the V code Malingering. Both Malingering and Factitious Disorder assume that the symptom is consciously faked. In this case, we do not see any evidence to support the notion that the patient was conscious of intentionally producing the symptom. Without additional evidence of her conscious production of the "seizure," we would prefer to give her the benefit of the doubt, assume that the symptom was not under her control, and diagnose it as Conversion Disorder (DSM-IV-TR, p. 498). We would indicate our lack of certainty by qualifying the diagnosis as Provisional. If the patient were later to acknowledge that, angry with the staff, she decided to give them a hard time by faking the fit, we would change the diagnosis to Malingering. In the unlikely event that she developed a pattern of exhibiting fake fits for no purpose other than to be a patient, we should change the diagnosis to Factitious Disorder.

NO FRIENDS

Emily is a 7-year-old girl who was brought to an outpatient mental health clinic for children by her mother because of difficulties with peer relationships. A recent telephone call from Emily's second-grade teacher convinced her mother that it was necessary to seek professional help for Emily. The teacher was becoming increasingly concerned about Emily's reluctance to interact with the other children in the class. During recess,

Emily stands off to the side of the playground with her head down, looking extremely uncomfortable. In the classroom she never initiates conversation with the other children and has great difficulty responding even when approached by another child. It is now 6 months into the school year, and Emily's extreme discomfort around her peers has not improved at all. Indeed, she does not have a single friend in the classroom.

Emily's discomfort in interacting with peers dates back to kindergarten. Her teachers in kindergarten and first grade had commented on her report card that she was very withdrawn and nervous with the other children. However, her second-grade teacher was the first to take an active role in trying to get Emily the help she needed.

Emily's mother had tried repeatedly to get Emily involved with other children in the neighborhood. In fact, she would take Emily by the hand and lead her to neighbors' homes where there were children of the same age to try and make friends for her child. Unfortunately, when she did this, Emily would start to shake or cry and would not be able to say a word to the neighbor's child. Emily has never been asked to attend a birthday party for another child.

Her behavior at home is quite different. Emily is warm and outgoing with her family, in marked contrast to the withdrawn and anxious child observed by her teachers and peers.

Discussion of "No Friends"

Many children are socially reticent—that is, they are slow to warm up in an unfamiliar social situation. However, such children overcome their initial shyness and do not demonstrate the extreme and persistent social isolation that we see in Emily's case. In an adult, Emily's behavior would suggest the possibility of Avoidant Personality Disorder. However, because Emily is so young, the diagnosis of a personality disorder is not appropriate. Emily is clearly afraid of situations in which she is exposed to unfamiliar people, and we suspect that she is afraid of acting in a way that will be humiliating or embarrassing. These features, plus her capacity for social relationships with familiar people (her family), warrant the diagnosis of Social Phobia (DSM-IV-TR, p. 456). Generalized Type is noted because the anxiety is present in virtually all social interactions with her peers.

STAR WARS

Susan, a 15-year-old, was seen at the request of her school district authorities for advice on placement. She had recently moved into the area with her family and, after a brief period in a regular class, was placed in a class for the emotionally disturbed. She proved very difficult to control, with a very poor understanding of schoolwork at about the fifth-grade level, despite an apparently good vocabulary. She disturbed the class by making animal noises and telling fantastic stories, which made other children laugh at her.

At home Susan is aggressive, biting or hitting her parents or brother if frustrated. She is often bored, has no friends, and finds it difficult to occupy herself. She spends a lot of time drawing pictures of robots, spaceships, and fantastic or futuristic inventions. Sometimes she has said she would like to die, but she has never made any attempt at suicide and apparently has not thought of killing herself. Her mother says that from birth she has been different and that the onset of her current behavior has been so gradual that no definite date can be assigned to it.

Susan's prenatal and perinatal history are unremarkable. Her milestones were delayed, and she did not use single words until age 4 or 5. Ever since she entered school, there has been concern about her abilities. Repeated evaluations have suggested an IQ in the low 70s, with achievement somewhat behind even that expected at this level of ability. Because her father was in the service, there have been many moves; results of her earlier evaluations are not available.

The parents report that Susan has always been difficult and restless and that several doctors have said she is not just mentally retarded but has a serious mental disorder. The results of an evaluation done at age 12 because of difficulties in school showed "evidence of bizarre thought processes and fragmented ego structure." At this time she was sleeping well at night and was not getting up with nightmares or bizarre requests, though this apparently had been a feature of her earlier behavior. Currently she is reported to sleep very poorly and tends to disturb the household by getting up and wandering around at night. Her mother emphasizes Susan's unpredictability, the funny stories that she tells, and the way in which she talks to herself in "funny voices." Her mother regards the stories Susan tells as childish make-believe and preoccupation and pays little attention to them. She says that since Susan went to see the movie *Star Wars* she has been obsessed with ideas about space, spaceships, and the future.

Her parents are in their early 40s. Her father, having retired from military service, now works as an engineer. Susan's mother has many unusual beliefs about herself. She claims to have grown up in India and to have had a very bizarre early childhood, full of dramatic and violent episodes. Many of these episodes sound highly improbable. Her husband refuses to let her talk about her past in his presence and tries to play down this material and Susan's problems. The parents appear to have a rather restricted relationship, in which the father plays the role of a taciturn, masterful head of household and the mother bears the brunt of everyday family duties. The mother, in contrast, is loquacious and very circumstantial in giving her history. She dwells a great deal on her strange childhood experiences. Susan's brother is now age 12 and is an apparently normal child with an average school career. He does not spend much time in the house or with the family, but prefers to play with his friends. He is ashamed of Susan's behavior and tries to avoid going out with her.

In the interview Susan presents as a tall, overweight, pasty-looking teenager, dressed untidily and with a somewhat disheveled appearance. She complains vociferously of her insomnia, though it is very difficult to elicit details of the sleep disturbance. She talks at length about her interests and occupations. She says she made a robot in the basement that ran amok and was about to cause a great deal of damage, but she was able to stop it by remote control. She claims to have built the robot from spare computer parts, which she acquired from the local museum.

When pressed on details of how the robot worked, Susan became increasingly vague; when asked to draw a picture of one of her inventions, she drew a picture of an overhead railway and went into what appeared to be complex mathematical calculations to substantiate the structural details, which in fact consisted of meaningless repetitions of symbols (e.g., plus, minus, divide, multiply). When the interviewer expressed some gentle incredulity, she blandly replied that many people did not believe that she was a supergenius. She also talked about her unusual ability to hear things other people cannot hear and said she was in communication with some sort of creature. She thought she might be haunted, or perhaps the creature was a being from another planet. She could hear his voice talking to her and asking her questions; he did not attempt to tell her what to do. The voice was outside her own head and was inaudible to others. She did not regard the questions being asked her as upsetting; they did not make her angry or frightened.

Her teacher comments that although Susan's reading is apparently at the fifth-grade level, her comprehension is much lower. She tends to read what is not there and sometimes changes the meaning of the paragraph. Her spelling is at about the third-grade level, and her mathematics, a little bit below that. She works hard at school, though very slowly. If pressure is placed on her, she becomes upset, and her work deteriorates.

Discussion of "Star Wars"

At the present time Susan exhibits several psychotic symptoms. She apparently is delusional in that she believes she has made a complicated invention and that she is in communication with "some sort of creature." She has auditory hallucinations of a voice talking to her and asking her questions. The presence of delusions and hallucinations, in the absence of a full mood syndrome or a general medical condition or use of a substance that could account for the disturbance, raises the question of Schizophrenia.

The DSM-IV-TR criteria for Schizophrenia require that for a significant portion of time since the onset of the disturbance, one or more major areas of functioning, such as work, interpersonal relations, or self-care is markedly below the level achieved prior to the onset of the disturbance (or when the onset is in childhood or adolescence, failure to achieve expected level of interpersonal, academic, or occupational achievement). Certainly the onset of Susan's illness was in childhood, and she has failed to achieve the expected level of social development for someone her age. Therefore, our diagnosis of Susan's condition is Schizophrenia (DSM-IV-TR, p. 312), further classified as Continuous because she is apparently delusional all of the time. Because her behavior is somewhat disorganized and she does not have catatonic symptoms or disorganized speech, the type would be noted as Undifferentiated.

Susan's IQ level above 70 mercifully spares her from the additional diagnosis of Mild Mental Retardation. One could argue for the V code Borderline Intellectual Functioning. However, it is not Susan's limited intellectual capacity, but rather her bizarre behavior, that is creating difficulties at school.

The early onset of her illness raises questions about a Pervasive Developmental Disorder, such as Autistic Disorder. However, it is unlikely that, if she had such a disorder, she would have been able to function in a regular elementary school.

Chapter 3

Cases Illustrating Multiaxial Assessment

$\mathbf{D}$SM-IV encourages the use of a multiaxial system for evaluation (DSM-IV-TR, p. 27), as did DSM-III and DSM-III-R. A multiaxial system involves an assessment on several axes, each of which refers to a different domain of information that may help the clinician plan treatment and predict outcome. There are five axes in the DSM-IV-TR multiaxial classification:

Axis I	Clinical Disorders
	Other Conditions That May Be a Focus of Clinical Attention
Axis II	Personality Disorders
	Mental Retardation
Axis III	General Medical Conditions
Axis IV	Psychosocial and Environmental Problems
Axis V	Global Assessment of Functioning

The discussion of each case in this chapter provides an assessment on each of the five axes and concludes with a summary of the multiaxial evaluation for that case.

INFECTED

$\mathbf{J}$erry Johnson is a short, stocky man whose long red hair is worn in a ponytail. He was 19 when he was transferred to an inpatient research unit. He had spent the previous 2 months in a local community hospital after swallowing an unknown number of aspirin in a suicide attempt. He lives with his family—an alcoholic father, a hard-working, martyred mother, and an older sister—in a working-class neighborhood of Boston. As he tells it, his troubles began about 6 months ago during his sophomore year at college,

387

when his friends decided he was too old to be a virgin and chipped in to buy him a few hours with a prostitute. He had intercourse with her twice, and the second time his condom came off. After she left, he says, "I beat my chest with male pride"; but a week later he noticed a discharge from his penis, went scurrying to his doctor, and received a diagnosis of chlamydia. He then began to worry that he was infected with the human immunodeficiency virus (HIV) and since that time has had two HIV tests (both negative). He has repeatedly called an HIV hot line to ask questions about acquired immunodeficiency syndrome (AIDS). Because a doctor told him that one could not be absolutely sure about being HIV negative until 2 years had elapsed, he became convinced that he, in fact, was infected, and worried about spreading the infection to his family. He noticed changes in the surface of his penis that he was convinced were evidence of AIDS. The medication he was given for chlamydia caused thrush, which just confirmed his conviction. He became very depressed, thought about ways to kill himself, began stuffing himself with junk food (gaining 10 pounds), and was preoccupied with guilt about what he had done.

After the suicide attempt, he was treated with antidepressants at the community hospital. Because he continued to make veiled suggestions that he was still suicidal, even though his mood had improved, he was transferred to the psychiatric hospital, where he was placed on constant observation and given a new antidepressant.

As further history was collected, it became clear that he had been troubled long before the "tryst." The last of three siblings, he was the one who did best in school, and was thus chosen to redeem the family. In junior high school he was preoccupied with thoughts of being contaminated, feared he could contaminate others with his germs, and felt that he shouldn't associate with immigrants who might give him a disease. At the same time, he began to question the strict religion in which he had been reared. He became a born-again Christian, then joined a Satanic cult, but finally returned to his family's church at age 16. At the same time he began to focus more seriously on his studies in high school, receiving A's in his humanities courses and doing respectably well in science and math. Because there was no money to send him to the college of his choice, he began his freshman year at a community college. He then started to worry about his own sexual orientation after several homosexual students made overtures to him; and this concern persists.

Discussion of "Infected"

The history indicates that even before onset of the presenting problem, the patient had a long history of emotional problems that included childhood fear of contamination and adolescent concerns about sexual orientation and religious identity. The childhood worry about contamination suggests the possibility of Obsessive-Compulsive Disorder, but there is insufficient information about its clinical significance to make a retrospective diagnosis. However, the concern with contamination apparently has provided a fertile ground for what now has become the most prominent disturbance—the patient's conviction that he has been infected with HIV.

This episode began with sex with a prostitute, which apparently did result in his developing a venereal disease, chlamydia. Given that he had sex with a prostitute, it is certainly understandable that Jerry might become worried about the possibility of HIV infection. However, despite having two negative HIV tests, he remained convinced that he was infected, and cited the physical changes on his penis from chlamydia and the thrush that resulted from the antibiotic treatment as evidence.

Jerry's preoccupation with the idea that he has a serious disease, despite appropriate medical evaluation and reassurance, suggests the diagnosis of Hypochondriasis. In Hypochondriasis, the intensity with which the person holds the unrealistic belief is on a continuum. At one end of the continuum are patients who fully recognize that their concerns are unrealistic, but yet are preoccupied with the possibility of having the disease. At the other end of the continuum are patients who are only able to acknowledge the remote possibility that they do not have the illness. When a patient is firmly convinced that he or she has an illness, the belief is of delusional intensity and the diagnosis of a psychotic disorder should be considered.

In this case, we would conclude that Jerry's belief for a considerable period of time has crossed over the line of intact reality testing and is of delusional proportions, thus ruling out the diagnosis of Hypochondriasis. It should be noted that the judgment that his belief is delusional is made even while recognizing that there is a remote possibility that the HIV tests were negative because he had not yet developed antibodies to HIV infection. In a similar fashion, a husband could have a delusion of jealousy, a conviction that his wife is unfaithful based on illogical reasoning, even if it turns out that his wife has been having an affair.

The delusion of being infected with HIV resulting from sex with a prostitute is not bizarre, as such a situation could certainly occur. Therefore, the appropriate Axis I diagnosis is Delusional Disorder, Somatic Type (DSM-IV-TR, p. 329).

Because the depressive symptoms that led to the suicide attempt and subsequent hospitalization are certainly clinically significant, an additional Axis I diagnosis of Depressive Disorder Not Otherwise Specified (DSM-IV-TR, p. 381) is made. Note that even if the criteria for a Major Depressive Episode were met, the diagnosis of Major Depressive Disorder would not be made because it is superimposed on Delusional Disorder.

There is no evidence of an Axis II personality disorder. On Axis III we would note the history of chlamydia and thrush, since these infections triggered his delusion of having AIDS. Since the case does not describe psychosocial or environmental problems relevant to the diagnosis, treatment, or prognosis, we note Deferred on Axis IV. His current GAF score on Axis V would be 35, since he has impaired reality testing (his delusion of having AIDS).

Multiaxial Evaluation

Axis I   Delusional Disorder, Somatic Type
            Depressive Disorder Not Otherwise Specified
Axis II   None
Axis III   History of chlamydia and thrush
Axis IV   Deferred
Axis V   GAF = 35 (current)

Follow-Up

Jerry remained in the hospital for 5 months. Although he did not appear depressed and refused all antidepressant medication because of the side effects, the staff were reluctant to release him because they were afraid he was minimizing his symptoms and still harbored the belief that he had AIDS. They feared that perhaps he had a suicide plan. In psychotherapy, Jerry began to focus on becoming independent from his family. By the time he was discharged, his concern about illness had diminished to the point that he spoke only of an "unknown virus" that had changed the look of his penis.

One year later Jerry completed his sophomore year at school, where he did well—mostly A's and B's. In addition, he obtained a half-time job for the summer. At that time he no longer felt that he was a "basket case." He was mildly depressed much of the time, mostly about his lack of romantic success, and he sometimes had trouble concentrating because of "obsessing about girls and how to get them." He no longer believed he had AIDS, was "much better" at making friends than he used to be, and now had a real social life. He wanted to continue in therapy, but couldn't afford it.

MISERY

An orthopedic surgeon in Seattle requested a psychiatric consultation on Peggy Sandler, a single 28-year-old graduate student who was recovering from a recent spinal fusion, because he thought she was not complying with physical therapy.

The psychiatrist noted that Ms. Sandler was an attractive young woman with a below-the-knee amputation of her left leg. She was oddly ingratiating and cheerful and didn't seem to be appropriately troubled by her deteriorating medical condition. She reported that 5 years previously she had been thrown to the ground by a boyfriend, injuring her back. Over the next 2 years she had multiple surgical procedures on her back. Finally, a fusion left her pain free until 6 months ago, when she was diagnosed with spinal degenerative changes and was referred for physical therapy.

Amazed that she didn't volunteer any information about her amputation, the psychiatrist asked how it happened and learned that shortly after the original surgery to her back, she had been in a motorcycle accident, sustaining burns to her left ankle. This became a chronic injury and ultimately lead to amputation of her leg a year and a half ago. She reported this calmly and denied any distress over the disfigurement or disability. She also calmly reported that fluctuating swelling of her stump and recurrent ulcers had interfered with her being successfully fitted with a prosthesis. Thus, she had remained in a wheelchair. She had also been hospitalized several times many years earlier for colitis and kidney stones.

The psychiatrist called the surgeon who had performed her amputation. He reported that the original burn had quickly progressed to a chronic injury, with chronic pain and swelling of the left leg. When the leg proved unresponsive to medical management, the patient received a series of skin grafts, all of which failed because of infection and edema. She was instructed to keep her leg elevated, but did not comply, and her leg continued to deteriorate. She saw many doctors and was followed in a pain clinic but continued to experience pain, massive edema, and recurrent infections. Ms. Sandler repeatedly urged her surgeon to amputate her leg, claiming that it was painful and of no use to her. Ultimately he complied.

The surgeon who performed the amputation also reported that Ms. Sandler had recently had several admissions for left-sided weakness and numbness. Physical findings were inconsistent, the workup was negative, and she was discharged with a diagnosis of conversion disorder. It was shortly thereafter that her back pain recurred. The surgeon also commented that various physicians involved in the management of her leg injury had raised the possibility that her symptoms might be self-induced.

Ms. Sandler is an only child, born to a middle-class family. By her own account, after graduating from college, she moved from job to job for a number of years, generally leaving because of medical problems and repeated hospitalizations. At the time of admission, she was a part-time graduate student being supported by social security. No one had accompanied her to the hospital, and she had no visitors during her hospitalization. She asked that her doctors not contact her family.

Ms. Sandler was transferred to an inpatient rehabilitation unit, where she quickly developed a string of largely unexplained medical problems, including a urinary tract infection, gastroenteritis with diarrhea and fever, painful swelling of the right hand and wrist, a rash on her back and torso, and atypical mental status changes, including difficulty doing rudimentary calculations and inconsistent memory deficits. Meanwhile, she repeatedly refused to comply with safety procedures on the unit, leaving her wheelchair unlocked and her bed rail down, despite constant reminders by the staff. Over time she generated a good deal of anger and frustration among most staff members, although a few found her a particularly sad and pathetic case.

After her previous surgeon had been contacted, the staff became suspicious about the role that she might be playing in the development of her symptoms. Ms. Sandler's room was searched and furosemide (a diuretic), cathartics, and an exercise band that could serve as a tourniquet were found. These were believed possibly to explain many of her symptoms as well as the unexplained metabolic abnormalities that had been noted in her chart. Careful review of her chart revealed that her urinary tract infection had been diagnosed on the basis of positive cultures in the absence of cells in the urine, most consistent with a fecal contaminant. It remained unclear if or how she might have factitiously elevated her temperature, even while observed, or how she might have induced the bitelike lesions on her back and torso.

Discussion of "Misery"

When a clinician attempts to obtain a history from a patient, there is a basic assumption that the patient is doing the best that he or she can do to provide accurate information. In this case, the referral was triggered by noncompliance with the surgeon's therapeutic recommendation. The first suggestion that things might not be as they appeared was the patient's striking nonchalance about her disability (the leg amputation)—referred to as *la belle indifférence*. Suspicions were further raised when additional history became available from her previous surgeon. Finally, compelling evidence was obtained that indicated that she had deliberately produced many of her puzzling physical symptoms and metabolic abnormalities, suggesting a diagnosis of either Factitious Disorder or Malingering.

The distinction between these two conditions depends on the underlying motivation. In Malingering, there are clear external incentives—for example, the man who, in order to avoid military service, puts sugar in his urine to simulate diabetes. In contrast, in Factitious Disorder the motivation is presumed to be a psychological need to assume the sick role. In this case there do not appear to be any clear external incentives, and one can only presume that, for unknown reasons, Ms. Sandler has a pathological need to perpetuate being a medical patient. Because her symptoms are primarily physical, the Axis I diagnosis would be Factitious Disorder With Predominantly Physical Signs and Symptoms (DSM-IV-TR, p. 517), a disorder that was first called Munchausen syndrome, after an eighteenth-century baron who wrote many fantastic tales.

We assume that people with Factitious Disorder also have severe personality disturbance. However, in the absence of any specific information about this patient's long-term personality functioning, we would note Diagnosis Deferred on Axis II. On Axis III we list the left leg amputation and her recent spinal fusion. Undoubtedly, Ms. Sandler has multiple psychosocial problems, but because of lack of any specific information, at this point we note Deferred on Axis IV. Her Axis V GAF rating of 33 reflects her major impairment in her thinking and judgment.

Multiaxial Evaluation

Axis I   Factitious Disorder With Physical Signs and Symptoms
Axis II   Diagnosis Deferred
Axis III   Left leg amputation, recent spinal fusion
Axis IV   Deferred
Axis V   GAF = 33 (current)

Follow-Up

A team meeting was convened, and Ms. Sandler was told that it was suspected that she had factitious symptoms, implying that she was actively involved in inducing at least some of her symptoms. She was informed that this is a serious and potentially life-threatening mental illness and that inpatient psychiatric hospitalization was recommended for further evaluation and management. She did not comment on the diagnosis, appeared unconcerned, and agreed to transfer to a psychiatric ward.

Ms. Sandler was in an acute psychiatric unit for 4 months. During that time she developed no new medical problems and made no complaints of pain or physical discomfort. Instead, she developed a series of psychiatric symptoms. She initially presented with rapid alternations of mood, appearing first hypomanic, racing around the unit in her wheelchair and claiming to be up all night, then depressed, curling up on her bed with the lights out and refusing to eat or interact with others. Her presentation was thought by some staff members to result from factitious Bipolar Disorder, whereas others attributed her symptoms to genuine affective instability or true dissociative phenomena.

Ms. Sandler's behavior on the unit was provocative and impulsive. She was labile and suspicious. She split staff, threw tantrums, said she was suicidal, and barricaded herself in her room. She improved on an anticonvulsive medication and an antipsychotic, but nevertheless spent the second half of her hospitalization refusing to participate in activities and with restricted privileges because of her threats of self-destructive behavior if she was allowed to leave the unit.

In psychotherapy, she gradually revealed a history of daily physical abuse at the hands of her parents throughout childhood and early adolescence. Her therapist believed that this history was genuine and diagnosed a Dissociative Disorder on the basis of the symptoms she described. Other staff members remained unconvinced of the veracity of her story of childhood abuse, but were impressed with the array of features characteristic of Borderline Personality Disorder.

Ms. Sandler agreed to a voluntary transfer to long-term hospitalization. One day before the planned transfer, she changed her mind, saying she wanted to "get on with my life," and submitted a sign-out letter. She went to court, where she was granted discharge by the judge. She signed out against medical advice and was lost to follow-up.

EATING AND BUYING

Ellen Farber, a single 35-year-old insurance company executive, came to a psychiatric emergency room of a university hospital with complaints of depression and the thought of driving her car off a cliff. An articulate, moderately overweight, sophisticated woman, Ms. Farber appeared to be in considerable distress. She reported a 6-month period of increasingly persistent dysphoria and lack of energy and pleasure. Feeling as if she were "made of lead," Ms. Farber had recently been spending 15–20 hours a day in her bed. She also reported daily episodes of binge eating, when she would consume "anything I can find," including entire chocolate cakes or boxes of cookies. She reported problems with intermittent binge eating since adolescence, but these episodes had recently increased in frequency, resulting in a 20-pound weight gain over the past few months. In the past her weight had often varied greatly as she had gone on and off a variety of diets. She denied preoccupation with thinness or a history of episodes of vomiting or other weight-reduction procedures to compensate for the binge eating.

She attributed her increasing symptoms to financial difficulties. Ms. Farber had been fired from her job 2 weeks before coming to the emergency room. She claimed it was because she "owed a small amount of money." When asked to be more specific, she reported owing $150,000 to her former employers and another $100,000 to various local banks. Further questions revealed that she had always had difficulty managing her money and had been forced to declare bankruptcy at age 27. From age 30 to age 33, she had used her employer's credit cards to finance weekly "buying binges," accumulating the $150,000 debt. She denied past or present symptoms of mania, obsessive thoughts, or a compulsion to buy, but rather reported that spending money alleviated her chronic feelings of loneliness, isolation, and sadness. Experiencing only temporary relief, every few days she would impulsively buy expensive jewelry, watches, or multiple pairs of the same shoes.

Two years ago, when her employers noticed the massive credit card bills, Ms. Farber had nothing she could sell to reduce the debt. Her employers allowed her to pay off the debts by continuing to work for them and giving them part of her salary. However, she could not stop her spending. She financed further purchases by a process she called "check kiting." She would open a checking account at one bank, overdraw from that account to open a second account at another bank, and then overdraw from the second account to open an account at a third bank. Over 2 years this escalating process led to her additional $100,000 debt. When the banks discovered the fraudulent practice 2 weeks ago, they contacted Ms. Farber's employers, who promptly fired her, which led to her current desperate state.

In addition to lifelong feelings of emptiness, Ms. Farber described chronic uncertainty about what she wanted to do in life and with whom she wanted to be friends. She had many brief, intense relationships with both men and women, but her quick temper led to frequent arguments and even physical fights. Although she had always thought of her childhood as happy and carefree, when she became depressed, she began to recall episodes of abuse by her mother. Initially, she said she had dreamt that her mother had pushed her down the stairs when she was only 6, but she then began to report previously unrecognized memories of beatings or verbal assaults by her mother.

Ms. Farber was admitted to the hospital for inpatient management of her depression.

Discussion of "Eating and Buying"

Ms. Farber enters the hospital when she can see no way out of her escalating personal difficulties. She apparently has a Major Depressive Episode, with symptoms of depressed mood, overeating, oversleeping, and loss of energy and interest. In the absence of a history of a prior episode, on Axis I we would diagnose Major Depressive Disorder, Single Episode (DSM-IV-TR, p. 375). However, in this case her depression is only the tip of the iceberg.

She has long-standing problems with eating and spending. The recurrent binge eating, without the compensatory behaviors associated with Bulimia Nervosa, indicate Binge-Eating Disorder, an Axis I diagnosis that is included in a DSM-IV-TR appendix for diagnoses requiring further study (DSM-IV-TR, p. 787), and listed as an example of Eating Disorder Not Otherwise Specified. Like most people with Binge-Eating Disorder, she is overweight and has a history of marked weight changes.

Her financial problems are the result of an inability to resist what she calls "buying binges," which somehow alleviate her feelings of emptiness and sadness. Although there is an antisocial quality to much of her behavior, she has no history of childhood antisocial behavior or other evidence of Antisocial Personality Disorder. Our official classification does not recognize a pathological spending disorder (perhaps analogous to Pathological Gambling), although there is a self-help group, Debtors Anonymous, for people with this problem. For such individuals, the diagnosis of Impulse-Control Disorder Not Otherwise Specified (DSM-IV-TR, p. 677) can be given. Like many people who have trouble controlling impulses, Ms. Farber now has serious legal problems resulting from the consequences of her behavior.

It is likely that an underlying personality disorder fuels her binge eating and binge buying. She has the characteristic features of the Axis II diagnosis of Borderline Personality Disorder (DSM-IV-TR, p. 710): uncertainty about who she is and with whom she wants to be, chronic feelings of emptiness, intense and unstable interpersonal relationships, inappropriate and intense anger, and impulsivity (eating and buying). As is often the case with people with Borderline Personality Disorder, there are memories of childhood physical abuse.

We would note Ms. Farber's being overweight on Axis III and her employment and financial problems on Axis IV. Since she has suicidal ideation and has been too depressed to work, we would give an Axis V GAF rating of 35.

Multiaxial Evaluation

Axis I	Major Depressive Disorder, Single Episode
	Eating Disorder Not Otherwise Specified (Binge-Eating Disorder)
	Impulse-Control Disorder Not Otherwise Specified
Axis II	Borderline Personality Disorder
Axis III	Overweight
Axis IV	Unemployed, financial problems
Axis V	GAF = 35 (current)

NOTHING MATTERS

Lois Pitman was admitted to a psychiatric unit in a university hospital because she was depressed and suicidal. She is a divorced 41-year-old African American mother of three adolescents. She says she has been using an increasing amount of cocaine in the preceding weeks, because cocaine makes her "feel numb so that nothing matters." This escalation in drug use and thoughts of suicide coincided with an investigation of the family by child protective services, initiated after Ms. Pitman's older daughter made charges of sexual molestation against her mother's live-in boyfriend. The boyfriend denied the charges. Ms. Pitman was devastated by the accusation and unsure about whom to believe. She did not understand how her boyfriend could have done such a thing.

Although she is a registered nurse, Ms. Pitman's license was suspended 5 years ago because of drug use, and she has been unemployed since then. She has completed a number of drug treatment programs, but has been unable to stay sober. She has had a series of stormy relationships with boyfriends. The family lives in a neighborhood characterized by frequent violence and heavy drug trafficking. Ms. Pitman has been mugged several times and nearly raped on several other occasions. Her son was once grazed by a bullet as a result of a "drive-by" shooting.

In addition to two previous hospitalizations precipitated by suicide threats, Ms. Pitman has had an extensive history of outpatient treatment with a variety of therapists. She has often been noncompliant with treatment recommendations, frequently "acted out" strong feelings toward her therapists with suicide gestures and sexual promiscuity, and repeatedly abused substances. Various therapists have described her as "untrusting, bordering on paranoid," "hostile," and "dependent."

Over the course of several years, Ms. Pitman has reported myriad symptoms and has been given a variety of diagnoses by different therapists. She has described frequent episodes characterized by sad and irritable mood, sleep disturbance (difficulty falling asleep, awakening frequently during the night), weight loss, loss of interest and pleasure, decreased energy, restlessness, free-floating anxiety, low self-esteem and a sense of futility, guilty ruminations, a number of somatic complaints, and frequent suicide attempts, usually with the expectation of rescue.

On some occasions she has reported feeling "paranoid" and having the sensation that her vaginal area was emitting a foul odor. Throughout this time Ms. Pitman has abused a variety of drugs. Until a year ago she had used benzodiazepines, alcohol, and cocaine indiscriminately. For the past year, she has used only cocaine.

A wide range of medications has been prescribed, including antidepressants, anxiolytics, and, occasionally, neuroleptics, without any significant benefits. During her last hospitalization, Ms. Pitman was described as particularly difficult. She hurled racial epithets at the staff and precipitated an explosion of racial tensions on the ward. She would speak only to African American personnel and would dismiss suggestions made by white clinicians. At the end of that hospitalization, the discharging physician concluded that the diagnostic entity that most succinctly captured her array of behaviors and symptoms was Borderline Personality Disorder.

Several weeks into the current hospitalization, Ms. Pitman began having intense flashbacks of being sexually abused by her father. She admitted having had flashbacks of sexual abuse in the past, but had not told anyone about them because she felt "no one would believe" her. She eventually reported that this abuse began when she was age 7 and ended shortly after she began to menstruate, when she was age 12.

Discussion of "Nothing Matters"

We agree that the diagnosis that best describes Ms. Pitman's lifetime difficulties is the Axis II diagnosis of Borderline Personality Disorder (DSM-IV-TR, p. 710). Although there is no information about identity problems, she certainly has a pervasive pattern of instability of interpersonal relationships (stormy relationships with boyfriends and therapists), affects (often sad or irritable), and control over impulses (sex and drugs). She also has transient stress-related episodes of paranoid ideation, a common feature of the disorder.

In addition, she has had recurrent episodes of Major Depressive Disorder (DSM-IV-TR, p. 376), and her inability to control her use of mood-altering substances suggests Cocaine Dependence (DSM-IV-TR, p. 242) and a history of Alcohol Dependence (DSM-IV-TR, p. 213) and Benzodiazepine Dependence (DSM-IV-TR, p. 285), all noted on Axis I.

Ms. Pitman's concern about her daughter being sexually molested has led her to have flashbacks of her own sexual abuse as a child. Mental health professionals who treated her did not aggressively inquire about a history of sexual or physical abuse. Such an inquiry is particularly important in patients like Ms. Pitman who have Borderline Personality Disorder, as there has been considerable evidence showing that childhood physical or sexual abuse is common in people who develop this disorder.

The stigma associated with having been sexually victimized and the anticipation of further abuse by the criminal justice system should they report having been molested lead many women to suffer in silence. The perceived sense of social stigmatization may be magnified for African American women. Ms. Pitman, like many sexually abused women, told no one about having been abused as a child.

Many people with Borderline Personality Disorder, although they may have flashbacks of childhood traumas, do not experience continuous trauma as adults. In contrast, Ms. Pitman was continuously victimized by the dangerous conditions of her life and threats to her personal safety and her children's safety. The flashbacks are dissociative symptoms indicating Ms. Pitman's inability to successfully master her childhood trauma. Perhaps if she lived in a less threatening environment, she would not have had the recurrent flashbacks of the abuse. The reexperiencing of the trauma in flashbacks suggests the additional diagnosis of Posttraumatic Stress Disorder. However, we do not have sufficient information about the other characteristic symptoms of the disorder, such as avoidance behavior and numbing of general responsiveness, to make this diagnosis.

Ms. Pitman does not seem to have any general medical condition to list on Axis III. On Axis IV, however, we would note several of her psychosocial and environmental problems. We would assign an Axis V GAF rating of 30 to reflect her suicidality, heavy drug use, and depression.

Multiaxial Evaluation

Axis I   Major Depressive Disorder, Recurrent
           Cocaine Dependence
           Alcohol Dependence
           Benzodiazepine Dependence
Axis II   Borderline Personality Disorder
Axis III   None
Axis IV   Child protective services investigation, unemployed, dangerous neighborhood
Axis V   GAF = 30 (current)

THE JOURNALIST WITH UNCERTAIN NEWS

Marvin, a 35-year-old journalist, went to his internist because of fatigue, sore throat, and headaches. These symptoms had developed 3 months earlier, a few weeks after he learned that he was positive for the human immunodeficiency virus (i.e., his blood test indicated the presence of antibodies to HIV). He was given a complete physical examination and was told that he was in otherwise good health, except for mild allergies that accounted for his sore throat, and that the results of the the routine laboratory examinations of blood and urine were all negative. Nevertheless, he worried that his symptoms of fatigue, sore throat, and headaches might be the prodrome of acquired immunodeficiency syndrome (AIDS). He began to have frequent and intrusive thoughts about dying and had recurrent fantasies of cancerous disfigurement, protracted illness, and complete dependence on others. Having followed the news coverage about AIDS, he understood that a positive test did not indicate that he would necessarily get AIDS, but this did not prevent him from ruminating about a painful and prolonged death. His internist suggested that he see a psychiatrist.

Marvin describes his physical symptoms to the psychiatrist and relates them to his constant and increasing anxiety. He says that he is now having trouble concentrating at work. He has begun to question the value of his career compared with the pursuit of other interests. He has become increasingly concerned about the possible debilitating effects of job-related stress and worries that such stress may itself compromise his immune system. He contemplates quitting his job and retiring to his country home, where life would be simpler.

Last week his anxiety escalated when he heard that two acquaintances had recently been diagnosed as having AIDS. He now finds that he avoids reading anything in the newspaper about AIDS and being in any social situation in which this topic is likely to be discussed.

When he is in a situation that takes his mind off his problems, such as an engrossing movie or concert, Marvin can experience pleasure. His appetite and sleep have remained unchanged except for the recurrence of a nightmare in which he has a mysterious illness and is left alone to die in a hospital.

Marvin has never sought psychiatric help before and says that until now he always regarded himself as a happy person, proud of his professional achievements and fulfilled in his long-term relationship with his male lover. He hopes that therapy will help reduce "stress," which will "help my immune system fight off AIDS."

Discussion of "The Journalist With Uncertain News"

Like most people who are told that they are HIV positive, Marvin has become increasingly anxious and preoccupied with thoughts of his illness and death. In his case the anxiety is severe enough to interfere with his occupational functioning.

Marvin's nightmares and intrusive thoughts about illness and death suggest Posttraumatic Stress Disorder, in which a traumatic event is reexperienced in a number of ways. What is the event in this case? His nightmares and intrusive thoughts are of what he fears will happen (becoming ill and dying) and are not about being told or knowing that he is HIV positive. Therefore, he is not reexperiencing a traumatic event.

Marvin is depressed and anxious, but the full clinical picture of Major Depressive Disorder or an Anxiety Disorder (such as Generalized Anxiety Disorder) is not present. Thus we are left with the Axis I residual category of Adjustment Disorder With Mixed Anxiety and Depressed Mood (DSM-IV-TR, p. 683). The type would be noted as Acute to indicate that the symptoms have been present for less than 6 months. If the symptoms of the ongoing stress of knowing that he is HIV positive persist beyond 6 months, the type would be changed to Chronic.

In a person with evidence of HIV infection, it is important to exclude a general medical condition, such as central nervous system infections or tumor, as the cause of psychiatric symptoms. This distinction is often difficult because HIV-related illnesses may present with psychiatric symptoms. In addition, mental disorders may coexist with, and be exacerbated by, HIV-related physical illness. In this case there is no evidence of active HIV-related physical illness, although Marvin's symptoms of fatigue and headache will need periodic medical reevaluation.

On Axis II we would note None, since there is no suggestion of a personality disturbance. On Axis III, the HIV infection should be listed. On Axis IV, his knowledge that he is HIV positive would be noted. The Axis V GAF rating is 55 because of the moderate symptoms (e.g., difficulty concentrating at work).

Multiaxial Evaluation

Axis I   Adjustment Disorder With Mixed Emotional Features
Axis II   None
Axis III   HIV infection

Axis IV   Knowledge of being HIV positive
Axis V   GAF = 55 (current)

SICKLY

A 38-year-old married woman came to a mental health clinic with the chief complaint of depression. In the past month she had been feeling depressed, had experienced insomnia, had frequently wept, and had been aware of poor concentration, fatigue, and diminished interest in activities.

The patient relates that she was sickly as a child and has been depressed since her father deserted the family when she was 10. Apparently, she was taken to a doctor for this, and the doctor recommended that her mother give the patient a little wine before each meal. Her adolescence was unremarkable, although she describes herself as having been shy. She graduated from high school at 17 and began working as a clerk and bookkeeper at a local department store. She married at about the same age, but the marriage was not a success; she had frequent arguments with her husband, in part related to her sexual indifference and pain during intercourse.

At 19 she began to drink heavily, with binges and morning shakes, which she would relieve by having a drink as soon as she got up in the morning. She felt guilty that she was not caring adequately for her children because of her drinking. At 21 she was admitted to a mental hospital, where she was diagnosed with alcoholism and depression. She was treated with antidepressants. After discharge she kept drinking almost continually; when she was 29, she was again hospitalized, this time on the alcohol treatment unit. Since then she has remained abstinent. She has subsequently been admitted to psychiatric hospitals for a mixture of physical and depressive symptoms and once was treated with a course of electroconvulsive therapy, which produced little relief.

The patient describes nervousness since childhood; she also spontaneously admits being sickly since her youth with a succession of physical problems doctors often indicated resulted from her nerves or depression. She, however, believes that she has a physical problem that has not yet been discovered by the doctors. Besides nervousness, she has chest pains and has been told by a variety of medical consultants that she has a "nervous heart." She often goes to doctors for abdominal pain and has been diagnosed as having a "spastic colon." She has seen chiropractors and osteopaths for backaches, for pains in the extremities, and for anesthesia of her fingertips. Three months ago, she experienced vomiting, chest pain, and abdominal pain and was admitted to a hospital for a hysterectomy. Since the hysterectomy she has had repeated anxiety attacks, fainting spells that she claims are associated with unconsciousness that lasts more than 30 minutes, vomiting, food intolerance, weakness, and fatigue. She has had surgery for an abscess of the throat.

The patient is one of five children. She was reared by her mother after her father left. Her father was said to have been an alcoholic who died at 53 of liver cancer. Despite a difficult childhood financially, the patient graduated from high school and worked 2 years. She was forced to quit because of her sickliness.

She married her present husband at age 17 and has remained married. Her husband is said to be an alcoholic who has had some periods of work instability. They have argued about sex and finances. They have 5 children, ranging in age from 2 to 20 years old.

The patient currently admits to feeling depressed, but thinks that it is all because her "hormones were not straightened out." She is still looking for a medical explanation for her physical and psychological problems.

Discussion of "Sickly"

It is first necessary to separate the immediate problem that prompted the patient's current consultation (depression) from her long-standing problems (physical symptoms and excessive use of alcohol). She is apparently now having a recurrence of a Major Depressive Episode (1 month of depressed mood, accompanied by diminished interest, insomnia, poor concentration, and fatigue.) The mood disturbance is diagnosed on Axis I as Major Depressive Disorder, Recurrent, Mild (DSM-IV-TR, p. 376).

Nearly all of the patient's many physical symptoms that have plagued her for so many years are apparently not adequately explained by a known general medical condition. She has received "physical" diagnoses from doctors in the past, such as "nervous heart" and "spastic colon," but these do not represent disorders with known pathophysiology. Therefore, the physical symptoms suggest a Somatoform Disorder. In her case, the large number of symptoms involving multiple organ systems suggests the Axis I category Somatization Disorder (DSM-IV-TR, p. 490). The cardinal feature of Somatization Disorder is a history of many physical complaints beginning before age 30 and occurring over a period of several years, which result in treatment-seeking or functional impairment. In addition, the diagnosis requires four pain, two gastrointestinal, one sexual, and one pseudoneurological symptom. This patient reports pain during intercourse, chest pain, abdominal pain, backaches, and extremity pain; vomiting, food intolerance, and diarrhea (colitis); sexual indifference; and periods of "unconsciousness" and weakness (pseudoneurological symptoms).

The patient has also had periods of heavy alcohol consumption, with binge drinking, accompanied by morning shakes, which she treated by drinking more alcohol, and difficulty functioning as a mother. These problems all indicate the Axis I diagnosis of Alcohol Dependence (DSM-IV-TR, p. 213). Because the patient has not had any difficulties attributable to alcohol use for more than a year, the course is noted as In Sustained Full Remission. (We prefer In Sustained Full Remission to not noting the history of Alcohol Dependence because of the need for continued evaluation and the possibility of relapse in this case.) The order in which these diagnoses have been discussed indicates their order as listed on Axis I and reflects their relative importance as factors determining the current evaluation.

On Axis II we are tempted to note Personality Disorder Not Otherwise Specified (Provisional) to indicate our suspicion that the patient's pattern of relating to herself and others (apart from the Axis I diagnoses) is maladaptive. However, the chronic and pervasive psychopathology described in this case can be entirely accounted for by her Axis I diagnoses. Therefore, we note Diagnosis Deferred on Axis II.

Since her physical symptoms in the past have apparently not been due to a general medical condition and there is no indication of a current general medical condition, we would note None on Axis III.

This woman's life situation is probably fraught with psychosocial and environmental problems. Arguments with her husband

and his alcoholism and work instability are mentioned. Since these problems may affect the treatment and prognosis of her Somatization Disorder, they would be noted on Axis IV.

Owing to her inability to work because of her "sickliness" and the interpersonal problems with her husband, a GAF rating of 50 is given on Axis V for both current and the highest level of functioning in the past year, to indicate serious impairment. Note that her depressive symptoms would put her in the 51–60 range; but her poor occupational functioning, because of her Somatization Disorder, warrants a score in the next lower range.

Multiaxial Evaluation

Axis I   Somatization Disorder
          Major Depressive Disorder, Recurrent, Mild
          Alcohol Dependence, In Sustained Full Remission
Axis II   Diagnosis Deferred
Axis III None
Axis IV   Multiple problems with husband
Axis V   GAF = 50 (current and highest level past year)

PARANOID AND DANGEROUS

Tracy Shaw, age 32, overweight and wild looking, was brought to the psychiatric emergency room by the police after she had furiously shattered a full-length mirror in the principal's office of her child's school. The psychiatrist who examined her described her as "paranoid and dangerous to others" and recommended immediate hospitalization by two-physician certification if she refused to admit herself voluntarily.

Ms. Shaw refused voluntary admission. She stated that her suspicions concerning her child's unfair treatment in school were well founded and that she would harm no one. She acknowledged that she was particularly irritable and angry because she was premenstrual. Her husband supported her decision and assumed responsibility for her and for bringing her back to see the psychiatrist the next day. That evening her menses began.

When Ms. Shaw saw the psychiatrist the next day, she appeared to be a "different" person. She was relaxed, her anger and irritability had dissipated, and she displayed a sense of humor. However, she retained her conviction that the school principal owed her an explanation of his unfair treatment of her child.

Ms. Shaw gave a history of monthly premenstrual symptoms beginning at menarche but worsening since her 20s. The symptoms were not the same every month. Some months she would become depressed, with thoughts of suicide; other months she would crave chocolate and gain 5–10 pounds in 1 week; some months she would break out in hives; and there were months when she was free of symptoms. The symptoms were always predictable in their timing, occurring the week before her menses and remitting with its onset.

Ms. Shaw was the oldest daughter of a chronically depressed and fearful mother and an alcoholic businessman father. Before marriage, she was the caretaker of her family. Her mother recovered significantly during Ms. Shaw's adolescence, only to fail rapidly and die when her daughter left home and married after high school.

Currently, Ms. Shaw is the mother of four grade-school children; in addition, she has primary responsibility for a sibling with alcoholism who is dying of cancer, as well as for her handicapped husband, who has been severely depressed and vocationally incapacitated since surgery 1½ years ago. She lives with her in-laws. Both her husband and his parents have significant alcohol problems.

Ms. Shaw is still the family caretaker. "I can't live with myself unless I do it all. I feel guilty if I do something for myself." She can cope with the demands of her life and is not usually depressed, except during her premenstruum, when "the whole world closes in" and she feels "pulled down."

Discussion of "Paranoid and Dangerous"

The uncontrolled behavior that led to Ms. Shaw's psychiatric evaluation suggested to the psychiatrist that she was psychotic and potentially dangerous to others and therefore in need of involuntary hospitalization. Fortunately, Ms. Shaw was able to convince the psychiatrist that she was not psychotic, but that she experienced episodic difficulties that always occurred in the few days before her menses and remitted when her menses began. Her symptoms vary from cycle to cycle and include depression, anger, irritability, and overeating. Between episodes she is apparently completely free of such symptoms.

This pattern of recurrent dysphoric episodes beginning in the premenstrual phase and remitting with the onset of menses suggests the Axis I diagnosis of Premenstrual Dysphoric Disorder (DSM-IV-TR, p. 774), a diagnosis that is not in the official classification but is included in an appendix to DSM-IV-TR and is given as an example of Depressive Disorder Not Otherwise Specified in the DSM-IV-TR text. In order to confirm this diagnosis, it would be necessary to have Ms. Shaw make daily ratings of her mood and behavior for at least two cycles to document her impression that the changes are always associated with the menstrual cycle. In addition, it would be necessary to establish that at least five associated symptoms (e.g., decreased interest in usual activities, marked lack of energy, sleep disturbance, and other physical symptoms) have been present for most of the time during each symptomatic premenstrual phase.

Since we are unsure about the presence of a personality disturbance, on Axis II we would note Diagnosis Deferred. On Axis III we note that when seen in the emergency room she was premenstrual. On Axis IV we would note the severe family stresses. Her Axis V GAF rating of 52 reflects her impulsive violent behavior in the principal's office and the difficulties she was undoubtedly having during the few days prior to that incident.

Multiaxial Evaluation

Axis I   Depressive Disorder Not Otherwise Specified (Premenstrual Dysphoric Disorder)
Axis II   Diagnosis Deferred
Axis III Premenstrual (in emergency room)
Axis IV   Handicapped husband, dying sibling
Axis V   GAF = 52 (current)

The Socialite

Dorothea Cabot, a 42-year-old socialite, has never had any mental problems before. A new performance hall is to be formally opened with the world premiere of a new ballet; Dorothea, because of her position on the cultural council, has assumed the responsibility for coordinating that event. However, construction problems, including strikes, have made it uncertain whether finishing details will meet the deadline. The set designer has been volatile, threatening to walk out on the project unless the materials meet his meticulous specifications. Dorothea has had to calm this volatile man while attempting to coax disputing groups to negotiate. She has also had increased responsibilities at home as her nanny has had to leave to visit a sick relative.

In the midst of these difficulties, her best friend has been decapitated in a tragic auto crash. Dorothea herself is an only child, and her best friend had been very close to her since grade school. People have often commented that the two women were like sisters.

Immediately following the funeral, Dorothea becomes increasingly tense and jittery and able to sleep only 2–3 hours a night. Two days later she happens to see a woman driving a car just like the one her friend had driven. She is puzzled, and after a few hours she becomes convinced that her friend is alive and that the accident had been staged, along with the funeral, as part of a plot. Somehow the plot is directed toward deceiving her, and she senses that she is in great danger and must solve the mystery to escape alive. She begins to distrust everyone except her husband and to believe that the phone is tapped and that the rooms are "bugged." She pleads with her husband to help save her life. She begins to hear a high-pitched, undulating sound, which she fears is an ultrasound beam aimed at her. She is in a state of sheer panic, gripping her husband's arm in terror, as he brings her to the emergency room the next morning.

Discussion of "The Socialite"

A severe psychosocial stressor (the death and funeral of her friend, noted on Axis IV) preceded the development of Dorothea's psychotic symptoms (persecutory delusions and, later, auditory hallucinations) in a thus far short-lived illness. Thus, this is a rather straightforward example of the Axis I diagnosis of Brief Psychotic Disorder

With Marked Stressors (DSM-IV-TR, p. 332). We make the diagnosis Provisional pending follow-up to make sure that she has returned fully to her premorbid level of functioning, which is likely to be the case because of the clear relationship between the stressor and the development of the psychotic symptoms.

Because the predominant symptoms are persecutory delusions involving themes that some clinicians would consider bizarre ("ultrasound beams aimed at her"), both Delusional Disorder and Schizophreniform Disorder need to be considered. However, these diagnoses require a duration of illness of at least 1 month. If the patient does not fully recover, we would favor the diagnosis of Delusional Disorder, Persecutory Type (DSM-IV-TR, p. 329), because we do not regard the delusion involving "ultrasound beams" to be bizarre as ultrasound waves do exist.

Because of her good premorbid functioning, we can feel confident in noting No Diagnosis on Axis II. Likewise, she has no general medical condition that would warrant listing on Axis III. Axis IV would list her friend's death, work difficulty, and the absence of her nanny. Finally, on Axis V we would rate 30 for her current functioning, since her behavior is considerably influenced by her paranoid ideas.

Multiaxial Evaluation

Axis I   Brief Psychotic Disorder With Marked Stressors
Axis II   No Diagnosis
Axis III None
Axis IV   Death of a friend, work difficulty, absence of nanny
Axis V   GAF = 30 (current)

WORTHLESS WIFE

Connie, a 33-year-old homemaker and mother of a 4-year-old son, Robert, is referred by her general practitioner to a psychiatric outpatient program because of her complaint that she has been depressed and unable to concentrate ever since she separated from her husband 3 months previously.

Connie left her husband, Donald, after a 5-year marriage. Violent arguments between them, during which Connie was beaten by her husband, had occurred for the last 4 years of their marriage, beginning when she became pregnant with Robert. There were daily arguments during which Donald hit her hard enough to leave bruises on her face and arms. During their final argument, about Connie's buying an expensive tricycle for Robert, her husband had held a loaded gun to Robert's head and threatened to shoot him if she didn't agree to return the tricycle to the store. Connie obtained a court order of protection that prevented Donald from having any contact with her or their son. She took Robert to her parents' apartment, where they are still living.

Connie is an only child and a high-school and secretarial-school graduate. She worked as an executive secretary for 6 years before her marriage and for the first 2 years thereafter, until Robert's birth. Before her marriage Connie had her own apartment. She was close to her parents, visiting them weekly and speaking to them a couple of times a week. Connie had many friends whom she also saw regularly. She still had several friends from her high-school years. In high school she had been a popular cheerleader and a good student. In the office where she had worked as a secretary, she was in charge of organizing office holiday parties and money collections for employee gifts. She had no personal history of depression, and there was no family history of violence, mental illness, or substance abuse. Her parents had been happily married for 25 years.

Connie met Donald at work, where he was an accountant. They married after a 3-month courtship, during which time Connie observed Donald using cocaine twice at parties. When she expressed concern, he reassured her that he was only "trying it to be sociable" and denied any regular use.

Donald, a college graduate, is the oldest of three siblings. His father drank a pint of bourbon each night and often beat Donald's mother. Donald's two younger brothers both have histories of substance abuse.

During their first year of marriage, Donald became increasingly irritable and critical of Connie. He began to request that Connie stop calling and seeing her friends after work, and refused to allow them or his in-laws to visit their apartment. Connie convinced Donald to try marital therapy, but he refused to continue after the initial two sessions.

Despite her misgiving about Donald's behavior toward her, Connie decided to become pregnant. During the seventh month of the pregnancy, she developed thrombophlebitis and had to stay home in bed.

Donald began complaining that their apartment was not clean enough and that Connie was not able to shop for groceries. He never helped Connie with the housework. He refused to allow his mother-in-law to come to the apartment to help. One morning when he couldn't find a clean shirt, he became angry and yelled at Connie. When she suggested that he pick some up from the laundry, he began hitting her with his fists. She left him and went to live with her parents for a week. He expressed remorse for hitting her and agreed to resume marital therapy.

At her parents' and Donald's urging, Connie returned to her apartment. No further violence occurred until after Robert's birth. At that time, Donald began using cocaine every weekend and often became violent when he was high.

In the 3 months since she left Donald, Connie has become increasingly depressed. Her appetite has been poor and she has lost 10 pounds. She cries a lot and often wakes up at 5:00 A.M. and is unable to get back to sleep. Ever since she left Donald, he has been calling her at her parents' home and begging her to return to him. One week before her psychiatric evaluation, Connie's parents took her to their general practitioner. Her physical examination was normal, and he referred her for psychiatric treatment.

When seen by a psychiatrist in the outpatient clinic, Connie is pale and thin, dressed in worn-out jeans and dark blue sweater. Her haircut is unstylish, and she appears older than she is. She speaks slowly, describing her depressed mood and lack of energy. She says that her only pleasure is in being with her son. She is able to take care of him physically, but feels guilty because her preoccupation with her own bad feelings prevents her from being able to play with him. She now has no social contacts other than with her parents and her son. She feels worthless and blames herself for her marital problems, saying that if she had been a better wife, maybe Donald would have been able to give up the cocaine. When asked why she stayed with him so long, she explains that her family disapproved of divorce and kept telling her that she should try harder to make her marriage a success. She also thought about what her life would be like trying to take care of her son while working full time and didn't think she could make it.

Discussion of "Worthless Wife"

When Connie comes to treatment, she has all of the characteristic symptoms of a Major Depressive Disorder, Single Episode (DSM-IV-TR, p. 375), noted on Axis I. Her mood is persistently depressed and she feels worthless, has trouble concentrating, has lost weight, and has difficulty sleeping.

The question that many readers may ask is whether Connie has a personality disturbance that has kept her in a relationship with a man who has been mentally and physically abusive. As is typically the case, there is no evidence that Connie has chosen someone because he is abusive or because she gets any particular gratification from being victimized. Instead, what has kept her in the marriage is a combination of her low self-esteem and social pressures against leaving her husband. In more extreme cases of physical abuse, the wife may actually fear for her life or the lives of her children if she leaves her abusive husband.

Therfore, on Axis II, we would note None. Because of her current depressive symptoms, we would assign a GAF rating of 52.

Multiaxial Evaluation

Axis I   Major Depressive Disorder, Single Episode
Axis II   None
Axis III   None
Axis IV   Marital separation
Axis V   GAF = 52 (current)

Follow-Up

Connie received medication and individual psychotherapy for her depression. She also participated in group therapy with other women who had been abused by their spouses.

After 6 months of therapy, Connie was no longer depressed. She bought new clothes and had her hair cut in a more flattering and youthful style. She found employment as an executive secretary and placed Robert in a day-care center, where she participated in parent programs. She reported that she and Robert had fun together in the evening and on weekends. She again began seeing her friends. With financial assistance from her parents, she began divorce proceedings against Donald and requested sole custody of Robert.

A Child Is Crying

Fifteen-year-old Cindy was brought to a mental health clinic by her father after he received a call from the counselor at school, who was concerned that Cindy was depressed and possibly suicidal. Her father had also been concerned about her because she had seemed sad and withdrawn for the past month.

The household consists of Cindy, her father, her mother, and two younger siblings. According to Cindy, she has been depressed ever since she had a fight with her mother 2 years ago. During the fight her mother threw a pot of hot water and burned Cindy on the shoulder. She was taken to a medical emergency room and treated for the burn. Since then, she stays out of her mother's way.

Cindy's mother has a long history of mental problems, with multiple hospitalizations and long-term outpatient treatment. She is reported by the father to be chronically "psychotic" and to have marked mood swings. There have been many conflicts in the marriage over the years, and the couple is now in the process of getting a divorce and selling their home. For the past 2 years, since the incident with the boiling water, Cindy's mother has occupied the third floor of their house and has had little contact with the family.

Before the incident with her mother, Cindy was very socially involved, taking dancing and music lessons and participating in both church and school activities. She was a straight-A student.

Cindy says that her mood has been much worse in the past 6 months. She feels depressed almost every day, all day long. She worries about her mother and feels that the fight was probably her fault. She has lost interest in school and social activities and has not really paid attention to her schoolwork for the past 6 months. Her grades have dropped from A's to B's and C's. She is tired all the time and takes a nap when she comes home from school. At night she has trouble falling asleep and in the morning often has trouble getting up.

In the past 3 weeks, Cindy has become anxious and has had two ex-periences in which she felt "spacey and unreal." She often hears the voice of a young child crying for help; but when she looks to see if there is someone outside the door, there is never anyone there. At times, re-cently, especially when she feels guilty about the fight with her mother, she is convinced she doesn't deserve to live and has considered killing herself. Three weeks ago, while she was washing dishes, she thought about cutting her wrists with a knife; but the thought of how upset her father would be kept her from doing anything.

The psychiatrist who evaluated Cindy recommended an elective ad-mission to the hospital. However, both she and her father felt that she would be able to follow through with outpatient treatment. She was given the telephone number of the emergency room and the following day called to say that the voices were getting worse, and she was afraid she might hurt herself. She was directed to go immediately to the emer-gency room and was subsequently admitted to the hospital.

Discussion of "A Child Is Crying"

Cindy has been depressed for 2 years, but in the past 6 months has had the characteristic symptoms of a Major Depressive Episode: un-remitting depressed mood, loss of interest in most activities, de-creased energy, insomnia, excessive guilt, and thoughts of suicide. More recently, she has had auditory hallucinations of a child crying, which is congruent with her depressed mood, and has experienced depersonalization (felt "spacey and unreal").

In the absence of a history of either a Manic Episode or a Hypomanic Episode or of a substance or a general medical condi-tion that directly caused the disturbance, the diagnosis is Major De-pressive Disorder (DSM-IV-TR, p. 375), noted on Axis I. It is further qualified as Single Episode (because there was no prior episode), and Severe With Mood-Congruent Psychotic Features (because of the hallucinations). This case illustrates that the characteristic symp-toms of Major Depressive Disorder do occur in children.

We do not know whether, before the onset of the Major Depres-sive Episode 6 months ago, Cindy had 1 or more years of persistent symptoms of Dysthymic Disorder, such as feelings of inadequacy or pessimism, or social withdrawal. Thus, we would note the need to rule out this additional diagnosis.

There is no indication of an Axis II personality disorder or of an Axis III general medical condition. On Axis IV, we would note parental separation. Because of her suicidal ideation and auditory hallucinations her Axis V GAF rating would be 35.

Multiaxial Evaluation

Axis I   Major Depressive Episode, Single Episode, Severe With Mood-Congruent Psychotic Features

Axis II   None

Axis III   None

Axis IV   Parental separation

Axis V   GAF = 35 (current)

Chapter 4

International Cases

Spirit-Possession: Two Cases From West Africa

Individual or mass dissociative phenomena often occur in Africa. From 1984 on, a mass spirit-possession movement flourished in an ethnic group in Guinea-Bissau, West Africa. The movement first took hold in a socially marginal group of barren women. Later, more than a thousand young women and young men were "called by their highest being."

This calling is best understood as a dissociative phenomenon that occurs in two phases. During the first, a somnambulistic trance phase, the members of the movement run around and do "crazy" things until they establish contact with one of the leaders of the movement. They then talk about their personal problems, confess their sins, and start digging for medicinal roots while in a trance state. During the second phase, they hear voices inside their heads transmitting messages and orders from God. These messages have been interpreted as a form of rebellion on the part of the younger generation against their position of dependence within the male gerontocracy, as a rebellion of their ethnic group against the state, and as an economic and psychological revitalization.

The ideology of the movement is an amalgamation of traditional, Islamic, and Christian influences and new, political, Western influences to which their culture has been exposed in recent decades. The following two cases are of individuals who were engaged in this movement.

THE LEADER OF THE MOVEMENT

The 35-year-old woman who is a leader of the spirit-possession movement lives in a small village in the southern part of Guinea-Bissau. She tells her story to a psychiatrist who is interested in the movement.

During the rice-planting season I became ill. I went to my father's house; but in spite of visits to several diviners, I was unable to discover the cause of my illness. A year later I lost my only child, and within 1 month, it happened: I felt pain all over my body. One afternoon I suddenly jumped up from my stool, ran around, and did not know what was happening to me. My head was shaking, and my body was thrown to all sides. While I was running around, our God opened my mouth and made me announce that he was calling me. Before that time I had had dreams that I can't remember anymore. But one dream I can still remember. A white man with white long hair, dressed in a white robe, visited me in my dream. He handed me a book like your writing pad, and a pen, and taught me how to write.

Then it also became clear to me that my strange sickness came from our highest being. It soon became clear to me that I should follow God. He guided me and gave me orders. He taught me and forced me to speak through my mouth. He told me that our people should get rid of their ancestor spirits and ancestor shrines. The people were not to hold big mourning feasts and slaughter their whole herd of cattle anymore. They were to stop beating the great slit drum during mourning feasts to mock praise or mock the cattle-stealing achievements of the guests. I was also to tell people that they were to refrain from witchcraft, not to eat pork and not to drink alcohol, and that they were to stop stealing and should work hard instead.

About once or twice a day, God forced me to rush around until I knelt down in a clearing He pointed out to me. Then He guided my hand, in which I was holding a digging knife, and made me dig a hole. There I found a root, the healing properties of which were explained to me by God. God gives me His orders by means of voices, which I hear in my head. Usually it is the voice of my father's dead younger brother, whom I took care of before his death. I loved that brother, but whether that sort of thing is mutual is difficult to tell. Once I heard the voice of one of my aunts. Sometimes God enters my body, which gets hot when I have visions. Mostly it happens when I lie in bed before I fall asleep, and sometimes during the day or in a dream. It is like a cinema. I see colored moving pictures, which come and go and which show God's way. These orders are more important than the voices; and if I don't accept them, my body hurts, and I feel like somebody who is very ill and who may die. If I accept, my body feels fine. But I can't see God's face. Sometimes when I see the pictures, He sits down in a long white garment, which covers His face. He can also give me an order just like that. For instance, as we sit here, He may tell me to stand up and clean the whole place.

The people here around me all hear things. But with some of them who say they hear things, it is not true. Then God's voice tells me that this or that person is not clairvoyant or that he or she is a witch. Apart from what my voices tell me, I can also see those things in a sort of dream, both during the day and before I fall asleep. Besides that I can smell a witch. That is our most important weapon against witchcraft.

Discussion of "The Leader of the Movement"

This woman has symptoms that would be considered psychotic if they were experienced by someone from a society that did not share the beliefs of her culture. She believes she has special powers, and she has auditory, visual, tactile, and olfactory hallucinations. In her local society, however, these phenomena are quite common. Her culture ascribes to her the role of healer and accepts her unusual experiences as normal for someone in that role. Indeed, she is a successful healer. She listed the names of 40 women who had tried unsuccessfully to conceive, but had become pregnant and given birth after she treated them.

In the Guinean lingua franca, Crioulo, this woman's behavior would be called *abri cabessa* (i.e., "open head"), an expression used to describe a variety of conditions, ranging from psychotic to culturally accepted religious experiences. Examples include when a clairvoyant or someone with intuitive gifts enters a state in which he or she can foresee the future, or when people enter into a trance during important ceremonies, meaning that the head "opens," and the soul of a deceased ancestor enters.

Local culture would assign her a role as a healer, and her behavior would not be seen as something to be treated. When an initiation as a healer does not end the complaints or the deviant behavior (e.g., the "healer" exhibits bizarre psychotic behavior not in keeping with the role of healer), the culture could ascribe it to witchcraft or to a spell that has more power than can be neutralized by healers or doctors.

DSM-IV-TR lists trance states as an example of Dissociative Disorder Not Otherwise Specified (DSM-IV-TR, p. 532). This is as close as we can come to a diagnosis of this puzzling case.

INTERNATIONAL SPIRIT

In a region of Africa called Guinea-Bissau, where the "movement" is active, a 20-year-old man, N'Daffa, is admitted to the hospital. He left his village the day before, swam across a turbulent bay, and then walked naked into the center of the city. When stopped by a policeman, he took a bite out of the policeman's hand and then ran to the house of a doctor whom he knew. With the help of seven strong men, he was subdued so that a nurse could inject him with a tranquilizer. He was then carried off to the hospital. His family was called and arrived at the hospital, where they observed him from a safe distance.

The patient is dressed by a nurse in the hospital and is interviewed by a doctor while lying on the bed tied in sheets. He tells the Dutch doctor that hundreds of people are going to die and that he can kill people by pointing at them with his forefinger. The doctor now has to give him water and food, because he is the only one the young man trusts; he attacks anyone else approaching him.

The family says they want to take him to the woman leader of the "movement," but the police refuse and insist that he be taken to the mental health center in the capital. During the night the man develops a bronchopneumonia with high fever, for which he is given an antibiotic in addition to the antipsychotic already administered to him. The next morning N'Daffa is carried onto an airplane in a comatose state, accompanied by his brother. His brother stays with him during his hospitalization in the mental health center.

The brother gives the following history. N'Daffa was reared as the third child of a peasant family consisting of his father and his father's two wives, four sons, and three daughters. His father died when he was 10 years old. N'Daffa took part in the funeral ritual without difficulties, as he did in other ceremonies, such as those celebrating passage from one age group to another. His calm and cheerful character always made him popular. He looked down somewhat on others and did not care what they thought of him. He was not very interested in decorating his body with painting or beads, as is the custom, nor did he show much interest in competitive games with his peers.

N'Daffa's troubles apparently began suddenly 2 days before he was admitted to the hospital. He awoke during the night to urinate and felt a slight earthquake (which all the people in the south had felt, but which is extremely rare for that area). He then started seeing strange things. He went to bed again, and when he woke up, he went out to fetch wood. During the course of the day he felt better. The next evening he felt worse, and he swam across the bay—normally nobody would dare to undertake such a thing—to find a healer. He was unable to find a healer and arrived in the city naked, where he eventually was taken to the hospital.

At the mental health center N'Daffa is again examined. He gives answers to questions that make no sense. He says he saw a spirit that looked like a white woman with long hair. He talks to himself and utters unintelligible phrases, calls the names of people he knows, and tells the other patient in his room that they are both "international spirits." He claims that he can still kill other people by pointing his finger at them and that he is going to be a "scientist."

After 3 days in the mental health center, N'Daffa is back to his usual self. A normal conversation is possible; the "spirit has gone." He no longer has strange ideas. His temperature has dropped, and on auscultation his lungs are clear. The psychiatrist is skeptical about his total recovery from the effects of his experiences with the "movement." He nevertheless tries reducing his dosage of antipsychotic medication, which produces an immediate return of N'Daffa's symptoms. The dosage is then increased, and by the end of the fifth day, N'Daffa is again his old self. Both his brother and the visiting relatives urgently ask for his release because they still want to participate with him in a ceremony with one of the women in the "movement" in the south.

After 1 week N'Daffa leaves the mental health center and takes the plane back to the south. On his way home he participates in a "movement" ceremony. The woman leader of the "movement" concludes that his disease is an appeal by God for him to become a healer in the new movement.

Although N'Daffa takes a supply of medication with him sufficient for 4 weeks, he stops taking the medicine after 2 weeks. He does not show up for follow-up in the local hospital, which is 1 day's trip from his village. Three months later he says that he is immortal, that he speaks all languages, and that he can still kill people with his index finger. Three months after that, he is again back to normal, working in the fields, talking and behaving as he always has. He will soon be initiated as a healer.

Discussion of "International Spirit"

Although the psychiatrist has his doubts, the patient's deviant behavior, not seen in other members of the movement, makes him inclined to diagnose a psychotic disorder. Unlike the healer in the previous case, N'Daffa's behavior is deviant even for those involved in the movement: he is incoherent, his behavior is bizarre (nudism, indiscriminate aggression), and his beliefs (e.g., that he can kill people by pointing his finger at them and that he is going to be a "scientist") are not in keeping with the ideology of the movement.

It is not surprising that his symptoms are controlled with antipsychotic drugs but return as soon as the drugs are withdrawn. Although N'Daffa describes his psychotic experiences in terms of the spirit-possession movement, his behavior is disorganized, and he is unable to function. His initial episode lasts only about 10 days, with apparent full return to his premorbid level of functioning, so the DSM-IV-TR diagnosis Brief Psychotic Disorder (DSM-IV-TR, p. 332) would be made. His subsequent episode lasts more than 1 month, but less than 6 months, so we, along with the local psychiatrist, change the diagnosis to Schizophreniform Disorder (DSM-IV-TR, p. 319). Since the onset of the episode of illness was within 4 weeks of the first noticeable change in his usual behavior or functioning and his social and occupational functioning before the episode were good, we specify With Good Prognostic Features.

Other Cases From Africa

THE ELEVENTH PREGNANCY

Nkechi M. is a 38-year-old housewife from the middle belt area of Nigeria. She is admitted to the inpatient unit following referral by her half-brother, who is a surgeon.

The patient complains of heat, heaviness, and pain in the precordial and sternal areas of her chest. She also describes epigastric pain and a sensation of "something moving" in the suprapubic region. Other symptoms include intermittent crawling sensations in the head and legs and dizziness. These symptoms are of 3 months' duration. Her half-brother has examined her for duodenal ulcer by gastroscopy, but no ulcer was found. Symptomatic treatment of a possible duodenal ulcer, with antacids and cimetidine, a drug that inhibits gastric-acid secretion, was not helpful. Later, when an antianxiety agent, lorazepam, was given, she experienced short-lived relief. Gynecologic evaluation was normal.

Nkechi looked depressed on the ward but denied any depressed feelings. When confronted with her depressed appearance, she listed all her symptoms and inquired from the examiner whether they were not enough to make anyone unhappy. When giving her history, she was irritable and demanded that she be given "pills" to eliminate her uncomfortable feelings, instead of being asked "all these questions."

Nkechi is one of 15 children from a polygamous family in which there are 3 wives. Her father died 2 years ago at a ripe old age. Her mother is the youngest wife, about 60 years old, and is now looking after Nkechi's children. She has five full siblings, three brothers and two sisters. She is the youngest and has enjoyed a close relationship with her parents, especially her father. Her eldest sister, who lives in Lagos, has had a great influence on her.

Nkechi had the equivalent of a junior-high-school education, after which she went to typing school. She was employed as a government typist when she married a government driver, who was a Muslim. She gave up her job to rear her family, but refused to renounce her Christian upbringing. She regretted giving up her job, which she thought had more prospects than that of her husband. She had 10 children, 6 girls and 4 boys, who were given Muslim names by their father but were taken regularly to a Christian church by Nkechi.

She thought she had too many children, but did not discuss limiting the size of her family with her husband. She thought he would be outraged and blame it on their religious differences. When she "took in" (became pregnant) again earlier in the year of the consultation, she made clandestine and rather clumsy attempts at terminating the pregnancy, such as using abortifacients and presenting to several hospitals with symptoms suggestive of inevitable abortion. Eventually, she aborted.

When her husband and sister realized that she had had an abortion, they were very angry. Her sister demanded to know why "you have done this kind of thing . . . I didn't know you were that kind of person." Nkechi now regretted terminating the pregnancy, recalling that her eldest sister had 13 children. "Maybe," she said, "this eleventh child would have been a special gift from God. I believe that all this movement I am having inside my belly is a punishment from God for what I did." At times she thought that God wanted her life as well, especially when she found herself exhausted after very little exertion, or having palpitations for no apparent reason. She found it particularly terrifying to lie awake at night, unable to sleep or having "useless and bad dreams."

The lorazepam was gradually discontinued, and the patient was given diazepam when needed for sleep. The physician wanted Nkechi to give up the idea that pills for her stomach symptoms were a solution to her problems. Nkechi did not take to this approach easily. When she was upset—for example, when the physician was late for an appointment or an expected visitor did not turn up—she demanded a reinstatement of the lorazepam prescription. When she was reminded of the disappointment that had preceded the exacerbation of symptoms, she charged that she was being accused of telling lies about sensations in her body. On one occasion she actually informed the doctor that she had been using a private stock of lorazepam. (The nurses disputed this and found no such tablets during a locker search.) On another occasion, when she was demanding discharge from the hospital on the grounds of desiring to go home to look after her children, confrontation with her weepy and miserable mood was more successful. She pointed out how long she had been in the hospital (4 weeks) and how nobody was prescribing drugs that her brother promised her would be used in relieving her internal heat, palpitations, and other symptoms. Sympathetic comments changed her tirade into an account of how difficult it had been to bring up 10 children, the oldest of whom was only 22 years old and still dependent on her.

She achieved much symptom relief and was discharged with a prescription for night diazepam. She never kept any outpatient appointments, since she had traveled a long way to seek help. However, the half-brother confirmed that she never needed any more treatment for "ulcers" or similar complaints.

Discussion of "The Eleventh Pregnancy"

The Nigerian psychiatrist who contributed this case noted that complaints emphasizing somatic symptoms rather than upsetting emotions are common in African patients. Adjustment, Anxiety, and

Depressive disorders and various disorders involving cognitive impairment often present with somatic symptoms as the chief complaint. Even cases of Schizophrenia can be missed if attention is focused only on the chief complaint of somatic symptoms.

The most common somatic symptoms seen in African patients with mental disorders are internal heat (not fever), crawling sensations in parts of or all over the body (e.g., worms, ants), peppery sensations on the skin, breathlessness, and dizziness. The sensations often are localized in parts of the body of current or dominant concern. Hence, students often complain of head or visual disturbances (sometimes referred to as "Brain Fag Syndrome"); infertile and menopausal women often present with suprapubic and back complaints.

The most common treatment approaches are the use of benzodiazepines or, more frequently, a combination of benzodiazepines and tricyclic antidepressants. Psychotherapy is not emphasized, as in the case presented. This case illustrates the kind of resistance that often discourages physicians from trying psychotherapeutic approaches. The patients are often given a prescription, to be renewed in 2 or 3 weeks; and patients then use their own support systems, which include religious organizations and traditional healers. This patient was admitted to the hospital because her significant relatives turned against her, and also because she had a physician half-brother who could arrange for modern psychiatric treatment.

We suspect that Nkechi has a Depressive Disorder, but she denies depressed mood, and there is no evidence of anhedonia or of the other symptoms that characterize the full depressive syndrome. Since her primary complaints are of physical symptoms that cannot be adequately explained by a known general medical condition, and since the duration is less than 6 months, the diagnosis is Somatoform Disorder Not Otherwise Specified (DSM-IV-TR, p. 511).

POSTPARTUM PIETY

Zela is a 30-year-old high-school teacher living in Lagos, Nigeria. She is married and has five children. The birth of her last child was complicated by hemorrhage and sepsis, and she was still hospitalized in the gynecology ward 3 weeks after delivery when her gynecologist requested a psychiatric consultation. Zela was agitated and seemed to be in a daze. She said to the psychiatrist, "I am a sinner. I have to die. My time is past. I cannot be a good Christian again. I need to be reborn. Jesus Christ should help me. He is not helping me." A diagnosis of Postpartum Psychosis was made. An antipsychotic drug, chlorpromazine, was prescribed, and Zela was soon well enough to go home.

Three weeks later, she was readmitted, this time to the psychiatric ward, claiming that she had had a "vision of the spirits" and was "wrestling with the spirits." Her relatives reported that at home she had been fasting and "keeping vigil" through the nights and was not sleeping. She had complained to the neighbors that there was a witch in her house. The "witch" turned out to be her mother. Zela's husband, Peter, who was studying engineering in Europe, hurriedly returned and took over the running of the household, sending his mother-in-law away and supervising Zela's treatment himself. She improved rapidly on an antidepressant medication and was discharged in 2 weeks. Her improvement, however, was short-lived. She threw away her medications and began to attend mass whenever one was given, pursuing the priests to ask questions about scriptures. Within a week she was readmitted.

On the ward she accused the psychiatrist of shining powerful torch-lights on her and taking pictures of her, opening her chest, using her as a guinea pig, poisoning her food, and planning to bury her alive. She claimed to receive messages from Mars and Jupiter and announced that there was a riot in town. She clutched her Bible to her breast and accused all the doctors of being "idol worshipers," calling down the wrath of her God on all of them.

After considerable resistance, Zela was finally convinced to accept electroconvulsive treatment, and she became symptom free after six treatments. At this point, she attributed her illness to a difficult childbirth, the absence of her husband, and her unreasonable mother. She saw no further role for the doctors, called for her priest, and began to speak of her illness as a religious experience that was similar to the experiences of religious leaders throughout history. However, her symptoms did not return, and she was discharged after 6 weeks of hospitalization.

Discussion of "Postpartum Piety"

The African psychiatrist who submitted this case says that the usual diagnosis for cases of this kind is Postpartum (Puerperal) Psychosis, Depressed Type. However, if the disturbance persisted well beyond the postpartum period, as it did in this case, the diagnosis would be changed to some other psychotic disorder. Most patients with Puerperal Psychosis seek treatment by traditional healers or spiritual church healers. Zela's case demonstrates the way in which even highly educated Nigerians, such as this patient and her family, understand illness in terms of witchcraft or demonology.

This woman had recurrent, brief, psychotic episodes beginning shortly after the birth of her child. Her psychotic symptoms included delusions of guilt and visual and auditory hallucinations with religious content. Although the diagnosis and successful treatment given by her African psychiatrist assumed the presence of depression, the case report actually does not describe depressed mood or anhedonia.

In discussing the diagnosis from the perspective of DSM-IV-TR, let us first consider the initial evaluation. At that time Zela was delusional, agitated, and in a daze. Psychotic symptoms with a duration of at least 1 day and no more than 1 month that occur in the absence of a full mood syndrome and are not due to the direct effects of a substance or a general medical condition are diagnosed as Brief Psychotic Disorder (DSM-IV-TR, p. 332). Since the onset was within 4 weeks postpartum, With Postpartum Onset can be specified. This diagnosis is noted as Provisional, pending the expected recovery within a month.

Many clinicians believe that the biological effects of parturition are responsible for postpartum psychoses. However, because of the difficulty of separating the psychological and physiologic stresses associated with pregnancy and delivery, DSM-IV-TR would not consider such cases to be Psychotic Disorder Due to a General Medical Condition.

What about the diagnosis of the two later psychotic episodes? The second episode also seemed to last less than 1 month. The DSM-IV-TR classification does not adequately deal with recurrent and apparently brief psychotic experiences separated by periods of full remission. Therefore, the only option would be to repeat the diagnosis of Brief Psychotic Disorder for the second episode. The duration of the third episode is more ambiguous. The observation that she became symptom free after six electroconvulsive treatments suggests that remission may have occurred within a month, which would justify, once again, the same diagnosis. If there were significant residual symptoms that necessitated the 6-week hospital stay, then the diagnosis would be changed to Schizophreniform Disorder (DSM-IV-TR, p. 319) because of the bizarre delusions, prominent hallucinations, and duration of disturbance greater than 1 month. We would specify With Good Prognostic Features because of the onset of psychotic symptoms within 4 weeks of the first noticeable change in usual behavior or functioning, her good premorbid functioning, and the absence of blunted affect.

Follow-Up

During the following year, Zela had several brief relapses, with vivid and frightening dreams, which she described as a "loss of definition between reality and dream." Her priest believed that she was going through a difficult religious experience. Her mother thought that witchcraft might be the source of her problems and proposed a traditional religious solution. However, it was her husband who prevailed, and each relapse was treated with medication.

Zela returned to the psychiatry department 2 years later to visit the staff and to offer condolences on the death of one of the professors who had treated her. She reported that she was well and living a full life. This was in spite of her having occasional experiences of "presences" and "spirits." She recalled that the first time she reported these experiences to her husband, Peter, his response was, "Oh my God! Where are those tablets?" She herself, however, had a religious explanation of her experiences.

Although she is thought by some to be excessively religious, Zela has been able to function quite satisfactorily at her job and at home without any further psychiatric support.

PSEUDOCYESIS

A single 24-year-old Xhosa man from a small farming community in South Africa was referred for evaluation of his mental condition after murdering a male witch doctor.

According to the patient, he initially consulted the witch doctor for a cough and was treated with "herbs." However, the witch doctor then had anal intercourse with the patient as the passive partner on 3 successive days. Over the next few days, the patient came to realize that he was pregnant by the witch doctor. He consulted the witch doctor again, and herbs were prescribed, apparently "to take away the baby." The patient fully complied with the prescription, but discovered that his "pregnancy" continued. He returned to the witch doctor a few weeks later—on the day of the murder. By this time, he believed he had developed a *linea nigra* (a line extending from the naval to the pubis that often becomes pigmented during pregnancy) and that his lower abdomen was slightly distended. This time, however, the witch doctor said he could not help him, and that he should see "the white man's doctor." The patient apparently then became incensed and fatally stabbed the witch doctor.

On psychiatric examination, the patient was found to have a fixed, unshakeable belief that he was pregnant. He "proved" this to the examiner by pointing to his stomach, to indicate that something was moving inside. Other than the delusion that he was pregnant and its ramifications, he exhibited no other features of major psychopathology. He was well nourished and appropriately dressed. His speech was coherent and logical, and his affect and behavior were normal. He appeared to be intelligent and related well. He expressed remorse for his actions and guilt about the homosexual affair. The psychiatrist was surprised to find that on physical examination, the patient did have a *linea nigra,* and his lower abdomen was slightly distended. Findings of the remainder of the physical examination were normal.

The patient had no previous history of mental illness and had been functioning well as a machine operator. He had always held witch doctors in high regard, as he believed they could effect cures others could not, but had never before consulted one. He had had several female sexual partners, but had never before had a male partner. There was no history of substance abuse and no family history of mental illness.

Discussion of "Pseudocyesis"

A man's persistent belief that he is pregnant would be considered a bizarre delusion in most cultures and would therefore suggest the diagnosis of Schizophrenia or Schizophreniform Disorder. However, this man lives in a society in which the power of the witch doctor to perform miraculous acts is taken for granted. We therefore are reluctant to classify his belief that the witch doctor has impregnated him as a bizarre delusion. Furthermore, the diagnosis of Schizophrenia or Schizophreniform Disorder almost invariably involves other psychotic symptoms, such as hallucinations and marked impairment in general functioning, which are entirely absent in this case.

The presence of a nonbizarre somatic delusion, in the absence of hallucinations, bizarre behavior, or a mood syndrome, indicates a diagnosis of Delusional Disorder, Somatic Type (DSM-IV-TR, p. 329). This presentation of Delusional Disorder is apparently rare in Africa, as it is in this country.

Follow-Up

The patient was judged to be not responsible for the murder because he was mentally ill. He remained in the hospital and was treated with antipsychotic medication. At first, he steadfastly insisted that he was pregnant, although he did not know how far along in his pregnancy he was or whether the baby would ever come out. "Men don't generally get pregnant, but I am. This is so because God has willed it." When 9 months went by and he had not delivered a child he began to wonder if he in fact was still pregnant. Shortly thereafter he concluded that a large bowel movement he passed was in fact the baby. He then no longer believed that he was pregnant, but it was unclear whether he still believed that he once was. The stigmata of pregnancy (*linea nigra,* abdominal distension) disappeared. The last follow-up was about 1½ years after the murder, at which time the patient exhibited no disturbance in ideation, mood, or behavior.

CENTRAL AND SOUTH AMERICA

BONI KINWI SEEQUIT

Psychiatric consultation was requested by a thoracic surgeon for a 21-year-old Indian man from the Cuna tribe that inhabits the San Blas Islands on the Atlantic side of the Isthmus of Panama. The man had attempted to kill himself by shooting a bullet into his chest. When he was seen, he was already recovering from his wounds and was about to be discharged from the surgical ward.

The patient was cooperative and reported that on the day of the attempt, he felt well and had no particular preoccupations or concerns. He had performed his usual activities until noon, when he had lunch and then took a siesta in a hammock. He expected to visit a *nele* (a native healer) that afternoon for a medicinal bath. About half an hour later, he suddenly stood up, took the gun, and shot himself. At the time of this impulsive act, the patient was completely aware of his actions but could do nothing to resist the urge. He said that he felt the shotgun was alive and overpowered him. He was taken to the nearest rural hospital, where the initial emergency treatment was provided before he was sent to a major general hospital in Panama City.

When examined, the patient was alert, well oriented to time and place, and intellectually unimpaired. There was no evidence of thought disorder or hallucinations, and his mood was well modulated, without any symptoms of depression. Neurologic examination and EEG revealed no abnormality. There was no history of alcohol or drug abuse.

When asked about the reason for shooting himself, the patient answered that he did not want to kill himself and that he was suffering the "illness of suicide" *(boni kinwi seequit)*. The same explanation was given by his father and his *nele,* who explained that this illness affects only males and is usually apparent in childhood. The diagnosis is made when there is a history of the child's being aggressive and disrespectful toward his parents and having dreams of being killed. A diagnostic ritual is performed by the *nele,* and a series of medicinal baths are prescribed. It is believed that the illness is caused by possession by a spirit.

The patient's family had migrated to the jungle in an area west of the Panama Canal near the site of a hydroelectric plant. He lived in this area until age 10, when he was sent to Panama City to work as a servant. He also went to school and 7 years later finished junior high school, at which time his father insisted on taking him back to the village because he did not want his son to be influenced by the alien culture of the city and lose his traditions and beliefs.

The patient returned to his village reluctantly and 2 years later was forced to marry a girl he hardly knew but who had been chosen for him according to tribal traditions. He remembered being angry, but compliant. Three months before the suicide attempt, his first child was born. The patient did not relate any of these events to the attempt, which was the first he had ever made; he insisted on the version of the "suicide illness" diagnosed shortly after his return from the city to his village.

Discussion of "Boni Kinwi Seequit"

There is no DSM-IV-TR category that adequately describes the puzzling situation in which a young man who is apparently living a normal, routine life suddenly picks up a gun and shoots himself. There is no suggestion of any of the disorders that are frequently associated with suicidal behavior, such as Major Depressive Disorder, Alcoholism, a severe personality disorder, or a psychotic disorder.

What significance is there in the fact that while he was shooting himself, the patient felt that he could not resist the urge and that the shotgun was alive and overpowered him? The inability to resist the urge suggests an Impulse-Control Disorder Not Elsewhere Classified. However, patients with such disorders (e.g., Pathological Gambling, Kleptomania) are well aware that the impulses they have difficulty controlling are their own.

A Latin American psychiatrist who commented on this case noted that "suicide illness" appears to be common among members of the Cuna tribe. Treatment varies; depending on the decisions made by the *nele,* patients may be ostracized, killed, or forced to take potions that occasionally kill them. The treatment also includes medicinal baths, a custom based on the theory that diseases enter the body through the skin and are also cured through the skin.

There are two DSM-IV-TR categories that could capture this patient's "suicide illness," both examples of Dissociative Disorder Not

Otherwise Specified (DSM-IV-TR, p. 532). In both categories there is a narrowing of awareness of immediate surroundings or stereotyped behaviors or movements that are experienced as being beyond one's control; the disturbance is indigenous to particular locations and cultures and is not a normal part of accepted cultural or religious practice. In the first, Possession Trance, customary sense of personal identity is replaced by a new identity attributed to the influence of a spirit. Although "suicide illness" is believed by the subculture to be caused by possession of a spirit, there is no mention that the patient had the experience of a new identity when engaging in the suicidal behavior. In the other category, Dissociative Trance Disorder, the dissociation occurs in the absence of a new sense of identity.

EL DUENDE

Ursulina is a 14-year-old girl living with her uncle and aunt in Cali, Colombia. On the day of the Assumption of the Holy Virgin Mary, they were startled by the sight and sound of rocks and sticks falling in their yard with great noise. They thought at first that the neighbors were throwing them, but discovered that this was not the case. The commotion continued well into the night and kept them awake. They gathered some rocks to keep inside the house as legal evidence, which they later produced. In the morning they were astonished to find that the rocks outside the house had disappeared. The next night they heard a whistle that seemed to come from all directions at once; it sounded "lugubrious" and "tired." The aunt said it might be a *duende* (ghost), which made Ursulina fearful, because she had recently heard about a *duende* in a nearby town.

Soon they discovered that the whistle followed Ursulina wherever she went. Once, when the girl got close to the door, a very forceful knock was heard; later, Ursulina felt that somebody touched her face with clammy hands, and the whistle turned into a whispered "Sh sh sh sh. . . ." On the following morning, Ursulina was sent on an errand, and she felt her legs become heavy; she was almost unable to walk, and the distance to the store seemed enormous. She had the feeling that she was being accompanied by someone constantly, and that she was in an unfamiliar place.

Once, while having breakfast, Ursulina felt that someone with smooth and icy hands was embracing her, and then she felt the hands covering her eyes. She screamed in terror and called for help. Her aunt came and saw that Ursulina had something like an ointment of ashes and charcoal all over her face. Later that day, the girl was nauseated and vomited a good amount of toilet paper.

The *duende* centered his persecution on Ursulina; he began to cut locks of her hair and to pinch and scratch her arms and legs. Four days after the first incident, the *duende* appeared to Ursulina as a small black man wearing a huge hat, white shorts, black shirt, pointed boots, and long red socks. His feet were turned around, with heels in front and toes in back. He smiled at her, showing his big teeth; he called her and pointed to a little black doll he had with him. She felt as if a powerful force were pulling her upward. Then, she became dizzy and confused, failed to recognize people around her, and did not know where she was. The *duende* kept appearing, in a very gay mood; he danced and made fun of everybody. However, no one could see him but Ursulina. Once, he bit her on the hand and, later, on her right arm. When she prayed, he made fun of her. He knocked her crucifix from her hands and told her, "No matter how much they or you pray, I will never leave you, and you will be mine forever. Come on, let's go!" Some days later the *duende* grew in size. When Ursulina took a shower, the *duende* said with a grin, "Do you want me to rub you?" One day he squeezed her left breast with such strength that she fainted from pain. Another day he spit into her mouth and eyes, and the girl experienced a burning that lasted for days.

The *duende* changed shape frequently and sometimes appeared as a giant or a priest. Gradually he became bolder in his caressing; he touched Ursulina's legs and genitals while whispering, "Please come with me." Often he passed wind with great noise and then looked at Ursulina with a malicious grin. On one of these occasions, when his stench was unbearable, he asked her, "How do you like my perfume?" When Ursulina showed him her crucifix, he made fun of it and showed her, in turn, a makeshift crucifix with a black doll as Christ, which he pulled out of a can full of mud. When she went to church, he became a nuisance, whistling and pulling her hair, encouraging impudent acts, and trying to force her to leave the church with him.

Some days later, while a Protestant service was being conducted in Ursulina's house, a noise like the shuffling of feet was heard, becoming louder and louder. Then several women in the audience felt that their breasts and genitals were being touched and fondled. This was particularly embarrassing at the moment of saying the final prayers, when a prolonged and loud whistle ("like a locomotive's") was heard by everyone present. At that moment Ursulina screamed, "Stop it, stop it! I am not going with you. . . . Leave me alone!" Then she revealed that the *duende* came to her bed every night and raped her savagely, despite all her struggling. The whole audience was petrified.

Ursulina began to experience levitation. Her aunt and uncle saw the girl rising from her bed, touching the ceiling, and then falling again to the floor, as if a great force were pulling her upward and then letting her fall. One day this was particularly awesome, since every time she reached the ceiling, she was dropped on top of a trestle. The whole sequence resembled a ride on a "wild horse."

The family first approached the parish priest after Ursulina had been troubled by the *duende* at mass. The priest advised the family to go to the bishop and ask him to appoint an exorcist. The bishop sent two nuns to investigate the case and make a report. During their visit the *duende* displayed frantic activity, whistling, scratching, and hitting Ursulina, singing obscene songs, passing flatus, and making profane remarks about the visitors, who, in spite of not seeing or hearing him, were terrified by all the gesticulations and wild activity exhibited by the girl.

Ursulina was then taken to a spiritualist center, where she was instructed in the use of appropriate formulas to "talk with the spirit." She tried the method, but it had no effect on the *duende*. The director of the center gave her a special ring to wear, but the ring disappeared on the spot. Later she was instructed to write the *duende* notes asking him to leave her alone. To these he answered verbally, "The words in your letter are nice, but I cannot answer them, since I am a dove and you are flesh."

Disappointed by the ineffectiveness of the spiritualists, her family decided that Ursulina had to go to confession and receive Holy Communion. The family reports that then, "All hell broke loose." The *duende* dragged Ursulina by the hair through the house, whipped, scratched, and bit her all night long, and tormented her with threats and blasphemous language. The girl was in such a state the following morning that the priest refused to hear her confession and ordered her relatives to take her to the mental hospital.

Ursulina was brought to the hospital 1 month after the beginning of her troubles. She was found to be "well oriented" and "rather indifferent about her problem," describing auditory and visual hallucinations, as well as delusions of being "chased by a spirit." She was treated with an antipsychotic. An EEG showed episodic discharges, particularly prominent in the frontal-temporal area of the right hemisphere. This was interpreted as evidence of a possible brain lesion in this area. However, neurologic and X-ray examinations did not disclose any focal neurologic disorder, and the diagnosis of temporal lobe epilepsy was made. While in the hospital, Ursulina continued to see and hear the *duende* for 2 days, but not thereafter. She stayed in the hospital for 20 days.

Meanwhile, her relatives were astonished that everything was quiet at home now. They realized that Ursulina was the center of all the problems. However, they were reluctant to accept the idea that she suffered from a mental disorder, since they had actually witnessed so many strange things. They were willing to believe that the persecution by the spirit had led to mental derangement, but not the other way around. As soon as Ursulina recovered from her severe condition, she was taken out of the hospital and never returned to the outpatient department to keep a follow-up appointment.

Discussion of "El Duende"

A psychiatrist from Latin America provided the following information about the cultural context in which Ursulina's problems developed. Creatures such as the "ghost" are part of the mythology of most Latin American countries. The typical *duende* is a small, pot-bellied individual with a dark complexion, round face, flashing eyes, and large white teeth. He dresses eccentrically and in a very colorful way or occasionally is naked, but always wears a tall hat. His feet are turned around. He is agile and musical, plays jokes on his victims, is deceitful and mischievous, and is occasionally irritable and violent. He often falls in love with young women.

Religious as well as love-related events have been ascribed to the presence of the "ghost." Generally, his appearance is considered the result of a struggle between the victim and malignant forces. Hence, religious help is frequently sought, with requests for exorcism, blessings, and spiritual cures. Old formulas such as burning sulfur, placing holywater pots in rooms, aromatic fumes, and the crucial intervention of local healers, or *curanderos,* are used, with vigorous participation of the social group seemingly being a key ingredient in the therapy.

The concept of "poltergeist" describes phenomena such as rocks falling down, furniture being destroyed, and strange noises around the house, some of which Ursulina and her family experienced. Such phenomena have often been reported in several Latin American countries.

Ursulina had a variety of bizarre symptoms, including visual, auditory, tactile, and olfactory hallucinations (seeing, hearing, feeling, and smelling the *duende)* and delusional ideas about what was happening to her. In addition, she had a variety of physical symptoms (nausea, vomiting, heaviness in the limbs, and burning in the mouth and eyes). She also is described as experiencing "levitation" ("as if a great force were pulling her upward and then letting her fall"), which may have been the exaggerated way that her family described epileptic seizures she was having.

If we strictly apply the DSM-IV-TR criteria without considering the cultural context, the persistence of bizarre delusions and hallucinations, in the absence of a clearly established substance or medical condition that can account for the disturbance, leads to a diagnosis of Schizophreniform Disorder. This diagnosis is unsatisfactory for several reasons. First of all, virtually all of Ursulina's psychotic symptoms are exaggerations of beliefs that are shared by her family and neighbors. In fact, they claim to have observed many of the bizarre phenomena that she describes. Since, by definition, delusions are false beliefs that are not accepted by one's subculture, it is not even clear that Ursulina has delusions. Secondly, we suspect (but cannot prove) that some of her symptoms (the visual and olfactory hallucinations and the "levitation") may be due to temporal lobe epilepsy. Her bizarre symptoms may be a way in which she tries to make sense of the epileptic phenomena.

Forced to make a DSM-IV-TR diagnosis, we would acknowledge diagnostic uncertainty by noting, on Axis I, Psychotic Disorder Not Otherwise Specified (provisional diagnosis) (DSM-IV-TR, p. 343) and, on Axis III, complex partial seizures (temporal lobe epilepsy) (provisional diagnosis).

Follow-Up

Ursulina's problems began again soon after she left the hospital. She was taken to a brotherhood of spiritualists, where she gained prompt notoriety because of her keen "sensitivity." The leader of the group showed special interest in developing her abilities and teaching her to communicate with the "spirits." Later, Ursulina became the center of a cult and was given a prominent position in the group of spiritualists as an extraordinarily gifted "medium," under the name "Maria." She began to hold public seances during which she was able to go into a trance and make "astral trips." She visited several countries, the sun, the planets, and the stars.

As time went by, however, the spontaneous "trances" stopped altogether, and Ursulina felt herself free from persecution by "spirits." She gradually reduced the intensity of her spiritual activities, married, had a child, and, for all practical purposes, led an uneventful, "normal" life.

EVIL SPIRITS AND FUNERAL CARS

A 28-year-old woman from Surinam, South America (Dutch Guiana), now living in Amsterdam, is referred to a psychiatrist. Her social worker and her family doctor are worried because she sees funeral cars everywhere and says she wants to commit suicide. Moreover, sometimes she suddenly starts to tremble violently, her eyeballs roll upward, her arms and hands twist, and she utters strange words and no longer understands Dutch. After 5 minutes she regains consciousness, and it is possible to get in contact with her. She does not remember anything that happens during these attacks, but behaves as if she has undergone an exhausting experience.

The patient tells the psychiatrist that since she came to the Netherlands 7 years ago, she has been haunted four times by evil spirits, who push her "good spirits" aside and take over her body. Two of these spirits always come back during difficult periods and want her dead. One has the body of a frog, with a dog's head with horns; the other is a tall man with a white hat and white gloves. During these crises she also suffers from headache, back pain, abdominal pain, or chest pain. She also has sleeping problems and a lack of energy and appetite, and she broods. Occasionally she has "foam" in her mouth, which is an omen of death; at times she has "panting attacks."

At first the patient consulted her family doctor, who cured her panting attacks with a relaxation technique. She consulted two Surinamese diviners/healers in Amsterdam. A ritual was performed, after which her spirits were placated and all her complaints disappeared. These episodes were apparently connected with problems concerning her family in Surinam, who made her feel she was badly needed there, or with disputes with her siblings in the Netherlands.

Since her arrival in the Netherlands, the patient has worked at cleaning jobs and finally got a position in the linen room of a hospital. She became acquainted with a Dutchman working in the hospital; after she got pregnant, they decided to marry. Despite her taking birth-control pills meticulously after the delivery, she became pregnant again. Her request to work part time was initially refused. She made an appeal to the personnel manager, who gave her a part-time job. However, by that time relations with her own supervisor were so disturbed that she was dismissed. For the first time since her arrival in the Netherlands, she became economically dependent on her husband, who now forced her to justify all her expenses.

After the delivery of the unplanned baby, the patient again visited her family doctor, with a feeling of increasing fatigue in both arms, pain under her breasts, and pain behind her left breast, which at times radiated to her back. She felt too tired to take care of her children or to make love with her husband.

Now, 3 months later, the patient has pain everywhere, is frightened, cannot sleep, and feels feeble. She continually sees funeral cars following her, and she ruminates about killing herself. Treatment with haloperidol results in a heavy and dizzy sensation and has to be stopped after 1 day.

The patient tells the psychiatrist that she visited a Surinamese diviner and a Hindustani healer, who both told her that her soul had been robbed, that it was too late to do anything, and that she was going to die. Then her brother took her to a female diviner, a *lukuwoman*. This woman diagnosed her problem as the result of neglect of her ancestral spirits, who sought revenge; she gave the patient a bath with herbs, tore a white sheet into two parts over her body, smashed an egg on her head, and removed the mucus from her mouth, so that the evil spirits would leave her body. The treatment worked well. The patient felt much better, and could stand and walk again. The *lukuwoman* told her to go back to Surinam to strengthen her divining power by giving a family feast for the ancestral spirits. The patient also saw a Roman Catholic pastoral worker and a Rosicrucian.

The woman tells her psychiatrist that for the first time, the evil spirits are walking about her house. The spirits resemble gray-red nebulous beings, who off and on present as a red eye or as the aforementioned frog with the dog's head. At other times she sees auguries of death, such as a white floating sheet or the tall man with the white hat and white gloves. When she is scared, she cannot chase them away. She sees the cemetery where the funeral cars will take her; she hears the bell of her house chime; she cannot sleep because the frog changes into a little red ball with teeth that sucks her blood as soon as she goes to sleep. She eats the way she always has, but the spirits consume her, so that she has lost more than 22 pounds. Her menstruation has become irregular. Sometimes she feels that her body is changed and that she smells bad, like death itself.

The tall man with the white hat wants to have intercourse and sometimes lies upon her. Just when she dozes off, he tries to rape her. She wakes up, cannot move, and feels terribly scared. He presses heavily upon her heart (she indicates her breast bone) and sucks her nipples as if they were making love. He empties her breasts in the same way as a baby drinks milk. Her breasts have become totally flat; all that remains is a little piece of skin.

Once before, during one of her sick episodes, she had a similar experience. She had seen a diviner, who told her that somebody had cast a spell on her by sending a dwarf. Just when she was dozing off and her soul had left her body, the dwarf sat down heavily on her breast and tried to choke her by pressing her throat. But her soul was floating in the room and saw her body lying on the bed. Her soul told her, "They have got your heart; hear how it bounces." She thought she was going to die; and when the episode passed, she was so scared that she wanted to sleep in her husband's arms.

In addition to the evil spirits who pester her and who threaten to harm her children, the patient hears her ancestors' voices encouraging her to stand up.

Her husband explains to the psychiatrist that he will not participate in the therapy. Over the past few years they have spent an enormous amount of money on diviners. He is fed up with her stories about spirits, her insistence that he has to enter his house backward, and her interpretation of every draft in the house as the presence of spirits.

Discussion of "Evil Spirits and Funeral Cars"

This woman is referred to a psychiatrist primarily because of her talk of suicide. She has apparently been depressed since the birth of her child 3 months earlier. She also has the full syndrome of a Major Depressive Episode; in addition to her preoccupation with suicide, she has no energy (is too tired to take care of her children), cannot sleep, and has lost 22 pounds. The somatic delusions and hallucinations (her breasts have shrunk, her body smells like death) indicate Major Depressive Disorder (DSM-IV-TR, p. 375) Severe With Mood-Congruent Psychotic Features.

The unusual feature of this case is the patient's bizarre psychotic symptoms: she believes that the spirits want her dead, and she has visions of a whole assortment of weird creatures, some of whom wish her ill and others who are interested only in sex.

The Dutch psychiatrist who provided this case tells us that a member of her culture may have these experiences without being considered psychotic. The spirits walking around, sucking her blood; the funeral cars; and the tall man may be experienced as "visions." Whether such experiences should be considered as truly psychotic depends on the person's functioning when the visions are not present. In this case, such a judgment is difficult since, even apart from the visions, the patient has a Major Depressive Disorder With Mood-Congruent Psychotic Features.

There is insufficient information about her "panting attacks" to know whether they are full panic attacks, and we do not know how often they occur, so we cannot make an additional diagnosis of Panic Disorder.

Our diagnostic problems do not end here. This woman also has brief episodes during which she trembles violently, her eyeballs roll upward, and she twists, utters strange words, and no longer understands Dutch. Because there is no loss of consciousness, an epileptic seizure is most unlikely. She interprets these episodes as possession by spirits. We would see them as dissociative episodes that are not a normal part of a broadly accepted cultural or religious practice. The episodes do not meet the criteria for a diagnosis of a specific Dissociative Disorder. We would regard them as the trances of Dissociative Trance Disorder (DSM-IV-TR, p. 785), which is classified in

DSM-IV (and DSM-IV-TR) as Dissociative Disorder Not Otherwise Specified.

Finally, this patient has another kind of strange attack, occurring just when she falls asleep. She wakes up, cannot move, and feels terribly frightened. This would seem to be sleep paralysis, a benign neurologic phenomenon consisting of brief periods of inability to move or speak, usually occurring when awakening or, more rarely (as in this case), upon falling asleep. We would note it on Axis III.

Follow-Up

The psychiatrist saw this patient for eight 1½-hour sessions. He allowed her to go into a trance whenever her spirits wanted to speak, but he suggested that she could get control over her "possession." Together they discussed the personal meaning of her different spirits in Surinamese and West-African cosmology. After this, the trances stopped. She felt relieved that somebody finally understood her experiences and, unlike her Surinamese family, was not afraid of the spirits.

After four sessions (1 month later), she felt much better. However, her eating and sleeping problems continued, and she was given an antidepressant. One month later she felt healthy again. She left for Surinam, where, during a big family ritual celebration, her "spirits danced for hours." During this ceremony one of her ancestor spirits entered her body. She saw another Hindustani healer, who liberated her from this evil spirit. A year and a half later she reported that, since that time, she had felt entirely well.

CONTINENTAL EUROPE

Sleepless Housewife

Pam, a 28-year-old woman from the Bavarian countryside and the mother of two children, has been treated in a dermatology clinic for recurrent skin infections. She was referred to a psychiatric clinic 5 days after complaining to her dermatologist about insomnia, which started after she took her first dose of a new oral antibiotic, ofloxacin, that the dermatologist had prescribed.

Following her first sleepless night, Pam became unusually cheerful, social, and physically active. She played tennis for hours, saw friends she had not seen in years, and felt "tip-top." She awoke from only 1 hour of sleep feeling rested. After 3 days, she mentioned to her husband that "her thoughts were running away" and that "everything within her was vibrating." Two days later, the dermatologist, alarmed by her condition, discontinued the ofloxacin and prescribed an antianxiety drug, with instructions to increase the dose over the next 5 days, and made an appointment for her to be seen in the psychiatric clinic that same day.

Pam reported no psychiatric history for herself or any family member. Other than the ofloxacin, she had not taken any medications during the 4 weeks preceding her illness. Her medical history was unremarkable except for previous hypothyroidism, which had been successfully treated. All laboratory data and medical, gynecologic, and neurologic findings were within normal limits. The ECG, EEG, and a CT scan of the head were all normal.

For the next week the woman complained of "feeling all mixed up." On the one hand, she felt dysphoric and depressed and complained of loss of energy, indecisiveness, lack of interest, fatigue, and marked loss of appetite. On the other hand, she experienced racing thoughts, felt restless and irritable, and was unable to concentrate. Her affect was labile, alternating between episodes of unprovoked crying and laughing. She also had four panic attacks, one of them witnessed by her private physician, during which she was suddenly apprehensive, trembled, turned pale, was short of breath, had tachycardia, and almost fainted. On another occasion during a panic attack, she mentioned to her physician that she feared that "something evil had happened" and was worried that he "might be hiding something" from her.

By the tenth day after the beginning of her troubles, the patient had developed a typical depressive syndrome with a markedly depressive mood, loss of energy, loss of interest in her children, marked loss of appetite, insomnia, and pronounced psychomotor retardation. Two weeks later her depression seemed to lift shortly after she slept for several consecutive hours for the first time. Within a few days her mood was back to normal.

Discussion of "Sleepless Housewife"

This woman, who had no prior psychiatric history, developed a variety of manic symptoms (insomnia, elevated mood, racing thoughts, increased activity) immediately following taking a drug. Soon after stopping the drug, she developed various depressive symptoms (dysphoria, loss of energy, lack of appetite, and loss of interest) that intermingled with the manic symptoms. This was followed by a period with only depressive symptoms.

Because of the absence of a history of mood disturbance in the patient or in her family, and because of the close temporal relationship between taking the drug and the mood disturbance, it is reasonable to conclude that the drug was responsible for the manic and depressive disturbances. Therefore, in the absence of attentional disturbance suggesting a Delirium, we first make a diagnosis of Ofloxacin-Induced Mood Disorder (DSM-IV-TR, p. 409). Because the mood disorder has both manic and depressive features, we would note With Mixed Features.

We assume that the panic attacks, which lasted for 5 days, were also triggered by the drug. We could either list the additional diagnosis of Ofloxacin-Induced Anxiety Disorder With Panic Attacks (DSM-IV-TR, p. 483) or, more parsimoniously, just list the more prominent mood disorder.

It is reasonable to assume that the patient's paranoid ideation (the doctor is hiding something from her) is also a reaction to the drug. However, this feature does not seem marked enough to warrant an additional diagnosis.

VIVE LA FRANCE

Henri, a 21-year-old schoolteacher, is brought to the emergency room by the police on July 13th, the eve of the French *Fête Nationale* (Bastille Day). He had caused a commotion in the lobby of a hotel, molesting staff and patrons, opening other people's luggage, moving furniture and flowerpots, and asking people what they thought about the government, Colonel Qadhafi, and the Berlin wall, all this accompanied by shouts of "Vive la France!"

On admission, Henri is almost totally mute. He appears frightened and looks around the room in a suspicious manner. Suddenly he begins talking in a rambling way, declaring that people are not what they seem to be and that there are spies everywhere. He says that he is a spy himself, that his father was not his real father, that there are radiations everywhere, that he has a mission to accomplish, and that something either terrible or wonderful will happen. He then becomes euphoric as he confides that he can get hold of a lot of money and become as rich as the Rothschilds. Abruptly he begins to speak about his girlfriend, wonders where she is, starts to cry, and accuses himself of having transmitted an incurable disease to her.

Henri has no psychiatric history. According to his parents, he was perfectly "normal" up to the day before he was admitted to the hospital. He did not drink and had never been on drugs. He was liked by his pupils and respected by his colleagues. For the last 6 months he had had a steady girlfriend, whom he intended to marry at the end of the year. During the night of the 12th of July, he was unable to sleep, wandered around the house, and in the morning told his parents that the whole world was crazy. He asked a lot of bizarre questions, retired to his room, and refused to eat anything because he thought the food was full of "unnatural" ingredients. When his parents wanted to call a doctor, he left the house and disappeared.

Henri is transferred from the emergency room to the inpatient service. During the first week of hospitalization, his behavior keeps changing. He is oriented in time and space, but wonders whether the hospital is a "real" hospital and the doctors, "real" doctors. When asked about his job, he seems perplexed at the idea of being a schoolteacher, although he can give the address of the school where he was working. His speech is, for the most part, incomprehensible, because he either does not finish his sentences or shifts unpredictably from one subject to another.

At times Henri laughs and tries to talk to everyone who is nearby. At other times he is withdrawn, stays in his room, and cries. On yet other occasions he becomes agitated and anxious.

For several days he puts toilet paper in his ears to "keep the voices away," wears sunglasses to "avoid seeing things," and wears gloves to "prevent my hands from betraying me." He keeps away from radiators because radiations "block my mind, confuse my thoughts, and penetrate my body, giving me some kind of disease, possibly AIDS." He is afraid to sleep in his room and on several occasions takes his blankets and covers and tries to sleep in the middle of the corridor. He wakes up several times each night and falls asleep for 2 or 3 hours during the course of the day.

Results of the physical examination and all laboratory tests are negative. Henri is treated with a combination of two antipsychotic drugs. By the sixth week of his illness, all of his symptoms have disappeared and he is discharged on medication. He is seen once a week in the outpatient department for another month, during which the medication is progressively reduced and then stopped completely. Now, 2 months after the onset of his illness, he is considered "as before" by his family and colleagues. During the next year he is seen by a psychiatrist every 3 months and on each occasion is considered completely well.

Discussion of "Vive la France"

The significant features of this man's disorder are acute multiple delusions of rapidly changing content accompanied by symptoms of psychotic turmoil, including momentary shifts from elation to depression and fear, agitation to withdrawal, and pressure of speech to mutism. In addition, there are incoherence, hallucinations, and perplexity in the absence of disorientation. The disorder developed to its peak in less than 24 hours and resolved in a few weeks, with complete recovery within 2 months. There was no psychiatric history, and the onset of the disturbance was not preceded by a significant psychosocial stressor.

The psychiatrist who provided this case explained that the French classification of mental disorders led to a diagnosis of *Bouffée Délirante*. This diagnosis had its origin in the theories of the French psychiatrist Magnan. Current views correspond closely to the original description and emphasize 1) the acute onset of the disorder, which develops "like a bolt from the blue," in the absence of a psychosocial stressor; 2) the presence of unsystematized delusions of a polymorphic nature; 3) the presence of emotional turmoil, with intense and changing feelings of anxiety, happiness, or sadness; 4) the presence of perplexity, depersonalization, or derealization without impairment of consciousness; and 5) resolution of the disorder, with complete recovery within 2 months.

About two of three patients hospitalized in France with an acute psychosis are given an admission diagnosis of *Bouffée Délirante*.

Usually the diagnosis is changed at discharge—often to Schizophrenia if the patient has not fully recovered. The treatment described in this case is the usual treatment for *Bouffée Délirante*.

According to DSM-IV-TR, the differential diagnosis should include Brief Psychotic Disorder, Schizophreniform Disorder, Bipolar I Disorder, and Schizoaffective Disorder. There are many features suggesting a Manic Episode, such as the recurrent periods of euphoric mood, grandiosity, gregariousness, and overactivity. Although these periods are not sustained, one could argue that they alternate with depressive symptoms and thus constitute the picture of an episode with both manic and depressive features. However, according to DSM-IV-TR, Bipolar I Disorder, Mixed, requires that the patient has previously had at least one Major Depressive or Hypomanic or Manic Episode, which is not the case with Henri. Schizoaffective Disorder is ruled out because there is no period of 2 weeks or more of psychotic symptoms in the absence of prominent mood symptoms.

The presence of the characteristic symptoms of Schizophrenia (bizarre delusions and hallucinations) in an illness of greater than 1 month's, but less than 6 months', duration leads to a DSM-IV-TR diagnosis of Schizophreniform Disorder (DSM-IV-TR, p. 319). In addition, the disorder has all four of the indicators of With Good Prognostic Features: abrupt onset, confusion or perplexity, good premorbid functioning, and absence of blunted affect.

FORMER SOVIET UNION

CRIMES AGAINST THE STATE

In the fall of 1984, Gregor, a 40-year-old economist, is brought to the maximum security ward of the Moscow Central Institute for Forensic Psychiatry from the KGB prison. Four months earlier, while searching the house of a friend of Gregor's, the KGB agents discovered a book, written by Gregor, that was critical of the Soviet economic system. In this book Gregor defined himself as a "Marxist economist" and a patriot of his country. He used language indistinguishable from that of the "official" and "approved" concepts current in Soviet economic and political thought. However, the book was an impassioned argument for reform of the state economy in order to bring about greater prosperity and economic stability in the country.

Gregor was arrested and charged with "antigovernment propaganda and agitation harmful to the interests of the Socialist state." Because he was uncooperative during his detention, he has now been referred for a psychiatric evaluation by a KGB investigator, who writes in the referring document that "There are strong reasons to suspect that this detainee suffers from chronic mental illness, which is responsible for his behavior and has resulted in serious crimes against the state, with which he is charged."

The prisoner arrives in handcuffs, looking anxious and fearful. At the beginning of his admission report, the forensic psychiatrist takes note of "burning and penetrating eyes, and a Christlike beard."

During the interview the prisoner insists on his right to take notes and to write down the questions asked him; when this is denied, he refuses to participate in the evaluation interview. On the ward, surrounded by seriously ill offenders, he keeps to himself and is described as "withdrawn, with long staring spells, and persistent refusal to discuss his thoughts and feelings." The ward staff is puzzled by his "excessive attention" to food served in the hospital, and his concern that medication has been put into his food is described in ward notes as "paranoid."

By the end of the first week, the prisoner is demanding to see the medical director of the hospital; when the director obliges, the prisoner confronts him with an accusation of "corroborating in crimes against humanity." The doctor is reminded of the fate of the Nazi doctors during the Nuremberg Trials. The prisoner categorically denies the criminal nature of his activity and "claims" that he pursued his chosen profession in writing a book about the state economy.

From the information provided by the secret police investigator and summaries of treatment obtained from the local health center and the district mental health clinic, the forensic psychiatrist learns that the patient had a "stormy adolescence," during which he pursued, with abandon, the study of his country's history, literature, and art. He was described by his teachers as "stubborn, oppositional, and obsessed with his ideas." His principal wrote: "This young man is far too sensitive and intense for his age. He is negative about everything our country stands for, and his tastes in art and music are bizarre. However, he is a great mathematician, and with proper guidance and education, can be an asset to our country."

The records of the local draft board revealed that the prisoner was relieved from compulsory military duty because of a diagnosis of "psycho-neurosis" established by a psychiatrist at the district mental health clinic. The records from the clinic described a young man who was "moody, preoccupied with his interest in history and mathematics, precise and compulsive in his habits, with some excessive concern about his health." Apparently, the prisoner was seen at the mental health clinic only three times and never requested any treatment.

The forensic psychiatrist makes no attempt to contact, or interview by telephone, Gregor's wife, parents, or friends and colleagues (he is under strict orders not to reveal the prisoner's whereabouts because of the KGB's insistence on keeping Gregor incommunicado before the trial). Failing to do that, the forensic psychiatrist never learns that the prisoner was a "star student" in the department of economics of a leading state university, or that he was universally admired by his peers and faculty. Most of his professors later became his colleagues, when Gregor was invited to remain in the department to continue his research. The forensic psychiatrist also never learns that the prisoner has written several articles approved for publication in respected professional journals and that he has been married for 18 years, maintains numerous close and enduring friendships, and has adopted two children, after having been extensively interviewed by the state adoption agency before being approved as an adoptive parent. Finally, the forensic psychiatrist is also denied an opportunity to read Gregor's book, which presumably was a product of a disturbed mind.

By the end of the third week, the prisoner is forcibly given small doses of a neuroleptic. He becomes weak and apathetic and complains of dryness of the mouth, increased appetite, grogginess throughout the day, and an increasingly troublesome tremor. Each time the prisoner is given medication, he offers resistance. This is described in the record as "paranoid refusal to believe in the good intentions of the medical personnel, and inability to develop insight into his condition and his own needs."

When medication produces no change in the prisoner's attitude except for obvious side effects, it is discontinued. One week after this, the prisoner is looking more cheerful and finally agrees to cooperate with the expert committee, consisting of three forensic psychiatrists. When the committee sees the prisoner, none of its members has had a chance to read the manuscript that brought the man to the attention of the authorities. During the interview, the prisoner is attentive and guarded, and later he is described by one of the members as "hypervigilant, with obvious ideas of reference." The committee unanimously agrees on the diagnosis offered by the forensic psychiatrist, Sluggish Schizophrenia. (Sluggish Schizophrenia was considered by Soviet psychiatrists to be the mildest form of the continuous subtype of Schizophrenia. It is roughly equivalent to the concepts of "pseudoneurotic" and "pseudopsychopathic" Schizophrenia that were used by clinicians in the United States in previous decades. It was presumed to have a more favorable course than the other types of Schizophrenia.) The committee recommends compulsory psychiatric treatment for Gregor "because of his inability to have a critical attitude toward his own condition and circumstances and failure to cooperate with necessary medical treatment."

Discussion of "Crimes Against the State"

The Russian psychiatrist (now living in the United States) who provided this case suggests that the KGB investigator knew that the state would have considerable difficulty in prosecuting Gregor since it would have had to prove that he had a malicious intent to "undermine and harm the interests of the Socialist State." Because Gregor is articulate and persuasive, a public trial would have been embarrassing to the government. Knowing that Gregor had been given a psychiatric diagnosis that exempted him from the draft, the KGB investigator reasoned that a trial would be unnecessary and that the credibility of Gregor's ideas would be undermined if his behavior could be attributed to a mental disorder.

The forensic psychiatrist was given inadequate and biased information, had no access to his "patient's" family or colleagues, and had to deal with a frightened and unwilling man. Practicing within a social system with an extremely narrow range of "permissible" behavior and within a profession that uses an extraordinarily broad concept of Schizophrenia, the forensic psychiatrist could very well have been sincere in considering Gregor mentally ill. It is also possible that the psychiatrist was cynically using his power to make diagnoses, hospitalize, and treat in order to satisfy an implicit request from the KGB to take this "troublesome" man off their hands.

Whether or not the forensic psychiatrist actually believed that Gregor was ill, he probably justified his diagnosis as follows: The onset of Gregor's Schizophrenia was, as is usual in this illness, at the time of adolescent transition to adult life. He exhibited overvalued ideas, instability of mood, inappropriately intense and single-minded pursuit of interests unusual for boys of his age, and obsessive-compulsive personality traits. He developed a system of rationalized obsessive preoccupations with seeking reforms in Soviet society. His tragic world view is evidence of chronic dysphoria and anhedonia. His belief that he can make a contribution to the economic theory and well-being of his country is evidence of an overvalued idea that has progressed into a fantastic delusion of reform. His cautious attitude toward authorities and state-appointed physicians is an expression of paranoid and self-referential perception.

In contrast to the Soviet forensic psychiatrist, we see absolutely no justification for making a psychiatric diagnosis in Gregor's case. His difficulties are certainly a result of the interaction between his personality traits and an oppressive society. However, in a freer society these personality traits might not cause any particular difficulties—indeed, might even be rewarded.

FAR EAST

TIRED TECHNICIAN

Mr. Wu, a 36-year-old married technician, comes to an outpatient psychiatric clinic in Hunan, People's Republic of China, complaining of easy fatigability. He also has insomnia, and his ability to work has decreased because of persistent weakness and tension headaches.

These symptoms began about 12 years ago, without any evident cause. Mr. Wu noticed that he began to tire easily and felt weak after exerting any mental or physical effort. He also had difficulty falling asleep and awakened many times during the night. He felt that his mental energy was insufficient during the day. He could not read or watch television for more than half an hour without feeling weary. Though he could perform his occupational tasks, he had difficulty concentrating and his memory was poor. In the past 12 years he has hardly ever been free of these symptoms, but they fluctuate in intensity over time. When his condition is really bad, he feels distressed, irritable, and "nervous." It is not clear why he now comes for help.

Mr. Wu does not spontaneously complain about depression. However, when asked specifically about depressed mood, he says that sometimes he feels depressed and is unable to enjoy anything, which he attributes to his difficulty concentrating and his physical exhaustion. When he is feeling depressed, he experiences guilt, slowed thinking, appetite disturbance, and psychomotor retardation. The periods of depression never last more than 2 weeks and occur about five or six times a year.

Mr. Wu has gone to the local hospital on many occasions and has been treated with Chinese herbs and Western medicines. Once he went to see a psychiatrist, and an antidepressant was prescribed. All of these treatments were without effect.

Mr. Wu describes himself as an "introverted person" since puberty, always preferring to stay home by himself. He obtained above-average grades in school. After graduating from college, he was hired as a technician in a factory. At the present time he is still working at his job.

In the interview, Mr. Wu looks exhausted. There is no evidence of prominent anxiety or depression. Findings of a physical examination and laboratory tests are within normal limits.

Discussion of "Tired Technician"

Chinese-trained clinicians would have no difficulty in making a diagnosis of Mr. Wu's condition, since he has the characteristic features of Neurasthenia, one of the most commonly diagnosed disorders in the People's Republic of China. Mr. Wu expresses almost all of his complaints in terms of somatic symptoms. For many years he has not had the energy and strength to function adequately. He also complains of difficulty sleeping and headaches.

Although these symptoms, plus his poor concentration and memory, suggest a depressive syndrome, Mr. Wu denies persistent depression or anhedonia. Therefore, the diagnosis of Dysthymic Disorder, which a Western-trained clinician might consider, cannot be made. The relative rarity of Major Depressive Disorder and Dys-thymic Disorder in China is probably due to the Chinese use of physical symptoms as a metaphor for expressing unpleasant mood states, whereas in this country it is more common for patients to re-port unpleasant mood states. There is also evidence, however, that when Chinese patients with Neurasthenia are systematically inter-viewed about depressed mood, their symptoms usually meet the criteria for Major Depressive Disorder or Dysthymic Disorder. (For further discussion of the Chinese use of physical symptoms to ex-press dysphoria, see "Comrade Yen," p. 462).

We suspect that had a Western-trained clinician evaluated Mr. Wu, he or she might well have described him as appearing "de-pressed" rather than "exhausted" and would therefore have made a diagnosis of Depressive Disorder Not Otherwise Specified (DSM-IV-TR, p. 381), since the recurrent short-lived periods of depression correspond neither to Major Depressive Disorder nor to Dysthymic Disorder. However, if we accept the Chinese psychiatrist's description of Mr. Wu, then, according to DSM-IV-TR, his chronic physical complaints without any organic basis, and without a complaint of sus-tained depressed mood or anhedonia, indicate a diagnosis of Undif-ferentiated Somatoform Disorder (DSM-IV-TR, p. 492).

MENSTRUAL MADNESS

Mrs. Nee, a married 21-year-old woman, was hospitalized in the Hunan Province of the People's Republic of China, complaining of recurrent epi-sodes of "madness."

The first episode occurred when she was 15 years old, a year after her menarche. A week before her menses were expected, she began to have difficulty sleeping and became emotionally upset and irritable. She had palpitations and "hot flashes" in her face and extremities. When menstruation began, she suddenly started talking to herself in a rambling and incoherent way, saying, for example, "Make up mind, the sun in the West will down and the sun in the East will rise . . . you are one of my friends . . . ." She became aggressive, threw furniture around, and tore her clothes. Sometimes she laughed loudly and then abruptly began to cry. At night she was unable to fall asleep and jumped up and down on the bed. She was sexually seductive, grimaced, and ignored attempts to calm her down.

Eight days after the beginning of menstruation, she recovered, suddenly and completely, but remembered all the symptoms of the episode. In subsequent premenstrual and menstrual periods over the next several months, the same symptoms returned, and she was then referred to a local hospital. Upon examination the doctors found symptoms of autonomic nervous system and endocrine disturbances, including tachycardia, flushes, sweating, excessive menstrual flow, and secretion of milk. Eight days after the beginning of this menstrual period, she recovered completely, as before.

Mrs. Nee has had six to eight attacks of this kind each year, always beginning in the premenstrual period and persisting for about a week after the beginning of menstruation. In the intervals between menstruation, she shows no symptoms of emotional disturbance.

Treatment programs over the years have included an antipsychotic medication and electroconvulsive therapy, neither of which has helped.

Discussion of "Menstrual Madness"

The Chinese psychiatrist who submitted this case noted that the unofficial DSM-IV-TR diagnosis of Premenstrual Dysphoric Disorder was not appropriate since this woman's symptoms were most severe in the menstrual phase and did not remit until a week or more after menstruation began. In contrast, in Premenstrual Dysphoric Disorder, the symptoms are most marked in the late luteal phase and quickly remit when menstruation begins. Furthermore, the characteristic symptoms of Premenstrual Dysphoric Disorder are depressed mood, irritability, and anger, but do not include psychotic symptoms such as those in this case. Therefore, the Chinese psychiatrist made a diagnosis of Periodic Psychosis, a category that is not recognized by DSM-IV-TR even though there is a bit of literature describing brief psychotic episodes associated with the menstrual cycle. (It should be noted that the diagnosis of Premenstrual Dysphoric Disorder is not ruled out by the presence of psychotic symptoms; however, in this case the temporal pattern of symptoms is not consistent with the DSM-IV-TR criteria for that disorder.)

A possible diagnosis in this case is Psychotic Disorder Due to a
General Medical Condition since the psychotic symptoms are apparently etiologically related to the patient's menstrual cycle. However, this diagnosis requires prominent hallucinations or delusions,
which are not evident. Therefore, the only appropriate DSM-IV-TR
diagnosis is the residual category Psychotic Disorder Not Otherwise
Specified (DSM-IV-TR, p. 343), as the illness does not meet the criteria for any specific psychotic disorder.

Follow-Up

At her next menstrual period, Mrs. Nee's mental status was normal.
Following discharge, she was given maintenance estrogen and pro-
gesterone to reduce the intensity of the hormonal changes throughout the menstrual cycle. This treatment seemed to work, since at
the 9-month follow-up she was entirely well and had had no return
of her previous symptoms.

FRIGOPHOBIA

Mr. Lin is a separated 63-year-old former military officer and native of
Suchuang province in the People's Republic of China. Currently living in
Taiwan, he has long suffered from *pa-leng* (fear of cold).

One day in October 1952, when Mr. Lin had diarrhea after eating a
watermelon, he experienced a strange cold sensation on his abdomen.
This frightened him and caused him to visit an herb doctor, who told him
that watermelon and other fruits would cause deficiency of vitality. Mr.
Lin recalled that his father had warned him in his childhood that he
would eventually die of "cold" disease. To protect his abdomen and head
and to feel secure, he started to wear heat retainers such as blankets,
coats, towels, heavy clothes, and a hat. Eventually he wore all of these
heat retainers all day long, even on hot days. They weighed over 30 kilo-
grams (66 pounds).

He received treatment from the herb doctor based on the principle
of *shenn-kuei* (vital deficiency) for 6 months, but without any effect. He
then visited various internists and finally came to the psychiatric clinic in
March 1953. On arrival, he wore many clothes and blankets and a hat

and was in a panic state. He moved very slowly to avoid losing the warmth from his clothes.

Mr. Lin was given insulin subshock therapy for 3 months and was given electroconvulsive therapy 20 times; but he did not improve. In April 1954, he was admitted to the psychiatric ward and received prolonged sleep therapy for 3 weeks. He said that this therapy, which entailed absolute rest, was quite similar to *chin-tsuo* (quiet sitting), the Buddhist treatment that had cured his father. It was effective; subsequently, he discarded his heat retainers. On discharge he obtained a job in an insurance company as an advisor.

In 1957, Mr. Lin was again seized by fear of cold, without any obvious precipitating factor. He was readmitted, received prolonged sleep therapy again, and improved. The third admission was in June 1963. This time he was depressed about his mother's death on the mainland. Prolonged sleep therapy was once again effective. However, there was a relapse 2 months afterward. One more month of hospitalization was needed for a full course of sleep therapy and psychotherapy, which started in October 1963. The fifth and last hospitalization was from July 1965 to July 1980. None of the treatments were effective; his condition remained the same, with regression and social withdrawal. Finally, he was transferred to a veterans' hospital.

Mr. Lin was born in 1917, the second of four siblings and the only son in an old-fashioned scholar's family. His father was a *shiu-tsai* (scholar of the Ching Dynasty) and dominated the home. He paid much attention to his son because he was often ill, but brought him up very strictly. His mother, a typical, taciturn Chinese woman, loved him very much. However, his aunt, an unmarried enthusiastic Buddhist, bore most of the responsibility for the child's upbringing. He slept with her until he was 14. Neither his mother nor his aunt ever disciplined him. They did not let him get up at night, to prevent his catching cold. He wet his bed until he was 15.

The boy started masturbating, sometimes twice a day, when he was 15. When his father discovered this, he scolded him severely. At that time, his father also suffered from fear of cold on the abdomen and other emotional difficulties, which caused him to give up his job. Deeply steeped in traditional Chinese medicine, he then received a Buddhist therapy, *chin-tsuo* (quiet sitting).

Despite his poor records in school, which Mr. Lin attributed to his brain's being weakened by masturbation, he graduated from high school in 1935 and entered college to study politics. His father's affiliation with influential people facilitated his admission to a good school. Immediately after graduation from college, he became a high-ranking military officer—again, with his father's help.

In 1943, at the age of 26, Mr. Lin married a domineering woman, a college graduate 2 years older than himself. They had three children. He began to suffer from sexual difficulties and gained much weight. He gradually lost his sexual desire and frequently ejaculated prematurely.

In 1949, while still on the mainland, Mr. Lin was a director of a section of military supplies and transport and, in this capacity, had a good income. He moved to Taiwan in 1950, without his family, but accompanied by a girlfriend, an attractive dancer. He then lived with this girlfriend, surviving on his capital without working. Two years later, after most of his money had been spent, his girlfriend left him. He attributed her departure to his sexual inadequacy. He worried a good deal about his general lack of physical vitality. At about this time, he was informed that his father had been killed, his mother was seriously ill, and his wife had been forced to marry another man on the mainland. He became very depressed and soon had his first episode of fear of cold.

During his long hospitalizations, Mr. Lin has been described as "immature and overdependent" and "extremely rigid, demanding, and overpolite." He initially insisted that his illness was a physical defect that he had inherited from his father. Later he came to believe that it was related to *shenn-kuei* (vital deficiency) and loss of sexual power.

Discussion of "Frigophobia"

The Chinese psychiatrist who contributed this case noted that the clinic staff agreed on a diagnosis of *pa-leng,* an extreme form of a marked fear of cold. It represents a culture-bound disorder that is closely related to the traditional Chinese concepts of vitality and the *yin yang* principle. It is often associated with depression, Obsessive-Compulsive Disorder, or Histrionic Personality.

In order to make a DSM-IV-TR diagnosis, the first question to consider is whether Mr. Lin's experience of coldness is best understood as a delusion, a somatic hallucination, or merely preoccupation and anxiety about his physical condition. Delusions generally involve phenomena that are subject to consensual validation or disproof. Who is to say how cold Mr. Lin actually feels? We therefore prefer to regard his problem as chronic preoccupation with a physical symptom that cannot be explained by a known general medical condition or pathophysiologic mechanism. Thus, we make the diagnosis of Undifferentiated Somatoform Disorder (DSM-IV-TR, p. 492), recognizing that this particular presentation of the disorder may be seen only in China, because of its compatibility with Chinese cosmology.

There are several references in the case to long-standing personality problems, and one might speculate on the role that identification with his father played in the development of Mr. Lin's disturbance. However, there is insufficient information to make a specific personality disorder diagnosis.

HOT-TEMPERED ELDER

A 70-year-old Beijing housewife, Mrs. Chen, is brought to the clinic by her husband. According to him, her sons, and her sons' wives, her behavior at home has gradually and increasingly become "abnormal" over the past 10 years. They all suspect that she has some "nervous illness," despite the fact that she remains quite normal in her contact with neighbors and friends and is energetic in the care of her house and unchanged in her loving relations with her many grandchildren.

The patient had married at 19 and had lived with her husband's extended family for several decades. She had been a meek, docile, deferential, and industrious housewife of the younger generation and a considerate, kind, and modest member of her peer group. She never became angry or complained about anything. She had been regarded by the entire family as virtuous, showing good sense and reason, although her husband's mother was quite strict and hypercritical toward her. Her husband's parents had died one after the other about 20 years ago. After that, Mrs. Chen became the housekeeper and authority of the family.

The family dates the patient's change in personality as beginning about 10 years previously. She has become increasingly domineering and dogmatic, always speaking in a commanding tone to everyone in the family. If any family member fails to obey her, she flares up, pouring out a stream of abuse and shouting at the top of her voice. In recent months the house has become more crowded as her youngest son's bride has come to live with the family and her second son and his wife have had a new baby. The rearrangement of rooms was not in accordance with Mrs. Chen's wishes, and she complains bitterly and incessantly to any family members who will listen. The whole family suffers from her imperviousness to reason and her loud complaining.

Mrs. Chen is in good physical health. There are no signs of intellectual impairment. Her memory is good, and no psychotic symptoms are observed. The consulting psychiatrist found it easy to make contact with her. She did not deny being a "hot-tempered elder," but touched upon the "quarrels" lightly, saying that the younger members of her family were "disobedient and concerned only about themselves."

Discussion of "Hot-Tempered Elder"

We had many questions for the Chinese psychiatrist who provided this case and offered the unofficial diagnosis of morbid development of personality in later life. First, we wondered if there might be cultural reasons to expect this kind of personality change in an older person. We were told that it is the cultural tradition in China for the young to "be obedient and heed what an elder says . . . and that the eldest woman of the family is the matriarch in dealing with the household affairs while her retired husband has practically no right to interfere." Therefore, there is cultural support for the eldest woman to take over the household in a way that would have been considered inappropriate when she was younger.

Given this cultural context, we asked if the family regarded her change of personality as pathological, and were told that her case was so extreme that the family members all suspected that she had some "nervous illness." Finally, we wondered if the personality change might be caused by frontal-lobe damage or some other chronic organic mental disorder. We were told that findings of a thorough neurological examination were negative.

With all this information, we prefer the Chinese psychiatrist's diagnosis to anything that is available in DSM-IV-TR. In DSM-IV-TR, Personality Disorders are defined as beginning by early adulthood, and the only other personality disturbance that is recognized is Personality Change Due to a General Medical Condition, which is not supported by Mrs. Chen's physical and neurological examination.

COMRADE YEN[*]

Comrade Yen, a 40-year-old teacher in a rural town in China, was interviewed in 1982. She is intelligent, articulate, and deeply depressed. She sits immobile on the wooden stool opposite us, looking fixedly at the floor. Her black hair, wound tightly in a bun, is streaked with white; her handsome, high-cheekboned face is deeply lined with crow's feet radiating outward from each eye. She slowly recounts for us the story of her chronic headaches.

> There are several sources. Before the Cultural Revolution [approximately 1966–1976] I was outgoing, active, and had high self-regard. As a teenager I had been secretary of the local Communist Youth League. I dreamed of advanced education and a career with the Party. My family and friends all expected great achievements. I had ambition and high goals. Then, during the Cultural Revolution, I was severely criticized. I had to leave my position in the Youth League. I went to the distant countryside to a very poor place. I couldn't adjust to the conditions. The work was too hard; there was too little to eat. Bad smells were everywhere, and nothing was clean. Terrible living conditions!

All of this was made worse by the realization that Comrade Yen's career aspirations were no longer tenable, that even a return to an urban environment was unlikely. The daughter of intellectuals, with several generations of professionals in the family, Comrade Yen felt deeply the lost opportunity for a university education and career in the Communist Party, sources of social mobility in China. Cut off from family and friends, books and newspapers, yet not well accepted, at least initially, by the peasants among whom she lived, she became aloof and solitary.

---

[*]From Kleinman A: *Social Origins of Distress and Disease: Neurasthenia, Depression and Pain in Modern China*. New Haven, CT, Yale University Press, 1986.

As the Cultural Revolution accelerated, Comrade Yen occasionally bore the brunt of self-criticism sessions. On one occasion she was denied an injection by a nurse at a rural county hospital, who accused her of being a "stinking intellectual." She began to experience a change in personality. She constantly felt demoralized; and instead of her former optimism, she felt a hopelessness that generalized to all aspects of her life. Comrade Yen expected only the worst to happen. She became introverted and sensitive to what she perceived as the rejecting and critical eyes of peasants and cadres. She first began to depreciate her goals, then herself.

Hesitant where she had once been assertive, lacking confidence where she once had radiated it, Comrade Yen regarded herself as inadequate and coped by further narrowing her behavioral field and already limited options. She stayed to herself. Eventually she obtained a post as a primary-school teacher in a rural town. When her native abilities became apparent to her fellow teachers, they wanted to elect her the principal; but Comrade Yen declined because she feared the responsibility and did not want to expose herself again to a situation in which she might well fail and suffer further losses.

Comrade Yen married a native of the region who is presently a peasant but was previously a cadre in a mine. They live apart, and it is clear she prefers it this way. He resides with a distant production team, while she lives in the small commune town. They have three children, two adolescent sons who live with their father and one daughter who still lives at home with her mother. Comrade Yen is angry that her husband has not been rehabilitated and given back his post as a cadre. It is aggravating to her that her husband has given up, declaring that he will never regain his former status. This is a chronic source of frustration, another difficulty about which she feels nothing can be done.

Comrade Yen's third source of anger is her daughter. "I really did not want to have her. I wanted to be alone. We already had enough children. When I was very pregnant, I hit myself several times quite hard against the wall, hoping I might abort. But my husband wanted a child, and I could not decide on an abortion at the hospital. Thus, I blamed myself when I gave birth to a baby girl with a withered arm. I felt I caused it." The daughter grew up to be beautiful and very bright, an outstanding student. But her mother grieved for her because of her deformity. "In China normal people don't marry cripples. Even though she can do everything—cook, clean, play sports—I knew she would have trouble marrying."

At this point in our interview, the patient silently cried, her gaze fixed on the cement floor beneath the table separating us. Her husband, who had accompanied her, looked much older than Comrade Yen. He was wide-eyed at being in a provincial capital he had visited only a few times before. His coarse peasant features contrasted with his wife's more refined face, but he joined her in weeping openly when she continued on about their daughter:

> There is no hope for her. Even though she is one of the best students in the senior middle school, she cannot take the examination to go to the university. Her school principal and the secretary of the local branch of the party decided that only completely healthy, normal children can take the examination. We appealed to the county authorities, but they upheld the decision. Nothing can be done. Our daughter will live at home and do what work she can.

There followed several minutes during which the patient could not go on, but sobbed and wept. Finally, she told us how she and her husband had arranged for their daughter to meet another "cripple" in a nearby town. But her daughter decided she would not marry someone else who was deformed; she preferred to remain single.

Comrade Yen shared her complete hopelessness with us. Often she thinks it would be preferable to be dead. Her headaches keep her to herself. She cannot face any more "stress"; it is too upsetting. "My health is too uncertain. I cannot do too much. I think only of my headaches, not of the future or the past." Comrade Yen severely restricts her world. She withdraws from all but essential responsibilities. She cannot plan any outing "because of bad influences on my health: the weather, the noise, the crowds . . . ."

Because of her feelings of inadequacy, failure, hopelessness, and despair, Comrade Yen has limited her life to school and dormitory room. Only on occasional weekends does she visit her husband. Her daughter stays with her. They appear to be like two recluses, each grieving about somewhat different losses. Comrade Yen's world is now that of pain: experiencing her hurt, waiting for it, fearing it, talking about it, and blaming her problems on it. It is the pain (and related complaints) that legitimizes her withdrawal at work and in family life and sanctions her isolation, her demoralization and depression. Her chronic pain is an unavailing expression of her multiple losses. Before we departed, she sent us a letter:

> I feel always sad about being ill for such a long time. I feel headaches, dizziness, don't like to talk, take no pleasure in things. My head and eyes feel

swollen. My hair is falling out. My thinking has slowed down. Symptoms are worse when I am with others, better when I am alone. Whenever I do anything, I have no confidence. I think because of the disease I have lost my youth and much time and everything. I grieve for my lost health. I must work a lot every day just like the others, but I have no hope in what lies ahead. I think there is nothing you can do.

Discussion of "Comrade Yen"

[The following discussion was prepared by Dr. Arthur Kleinman, who submitted this case.]

Comrade Yen was one of more than 150 cases with the diagnosis of Neurasthenia whom I studied in 1980 and 1983 in the outpatient psychiatry clinic of the Hunan Medical College. Her case, like the others I studied, was referred by the clinic's psychiatrists to a research team consisting of several Chinese psychiatrist trainees in a postdoctoral research training program, my wife, who is a China scholar, and me. We interviewed Comrade Yen and our other subjects for 2 to 3 hours. This interview was repeated 5 weeks later, and again at 3-year follow-ups (in both of which Comrade Yen declined to take part).

Comrade Yen is quite representative of the group we studied and of patients in China's psychiatric clinics generally. Her symptoms can be traced to a major social source of stress, the turmoil of the Cultural Revolution. Her initial illness was an episode of Major Depressive Disorder (DSM-IV-TR, p. 375), which was neither recognized nor appropriately treated. Over time she suffered several recurrences of Major Depressive Disorder that never fully remitted. Had she been diagnosed during one of these periods, the diagnosis would be qualified as In Partial Remission to account for the chronic demoralization between episodes.

During periods of depression, her chief complaints have been physical symptoms of headaches, dizziness, and lack of energy. Although she looks depressed, neither she nor her doctors focus on dysphoria or any other emotion. This is in keeping with traditional cultural norms that orient Chinese to regard emotional display as unseemly, stigmatize any behavior suggesting mental illness, authorize a disabled role only for physical complaints, and provide an elaborate and subtle somatic semantic system for expressing psychosomatic and social problems. Moreover, headaches and dizziness and a weakness-exhaustion cluster of complaints have long held salience in Chinese culture as signs of real disease requiring Chinese medical treatment and deserving all of the benefits of the sick role.

During the Cultural Revolution—China's decade-long historical whirlwind—many people under great social pressure, especially those with personal vulnerability, were diagnosed as having Neurasthenia. At present, although this cross-cultural difference in diagnostic styles is still true, psychiatrists in China increasingly diagnose patients like Comrade Yen as cases of Depressive or Anxiety Disorders.

FEAR OF THINKING ALOUD

Ms. Mura, a 48-year-old unmarried woman in Tokyo, consults a psychiatrist with the complaint that she is "thinking aloud unconsciously and hurting the feelings of other people around me." She lives with her 78-year-old mother; her 43-year-old unmarried brother, a bank employee; and her 37-year-old unmarried sister, who is a government clerk. When she spoke to her sister about her problem, her sister assured her that no one at home hears her speaking her thoughts out loud. However, Ms. Mura insists that she often does and that her sister is a "foggy head" and other family members are unobservant.

Five years ago, Ms. Mura's brother started to talk to himself while bathing at home. This annoyed her, and she worried that she might someday do the same thing. Three years later, she began to feel that she was expressing her thoughts aloud without realizing it. She feared that other people's feelings were hurt when they heard her critical thoughts being spoken aloud.

She says she is never aware of thinking aloud or of speaking ill of others. When questioned about how she knows that this is actually happening, she says that she has received several telephone calls during which no one spoke. She is sure they were made by somebody who knows her habit of thinking aloud and who has attempted to evoke her habit while she was holding the phone receiver. When a new bill-collector appeared a few weeks ago, she concluded that the previous collector had heard her think ill of him, even though she had no memory of this. When a store clerk smiled at her yesterday, she considered it a response to her thinking ill of the store when she had passed by some days ago.

Ms. Mura believes that her habit of thinking aloud is known to everybody in her neighborhood. She hesitates to go out shopping, fearing that people will avoid her or look back or turn their heads away from her. Whenever she leaves the house, she believes that her neighbors come out of their homes and stand at their gates or on the street, watching her and saying she is a "queer woman."

Ms. Mura had an apparently unremarkable childhood. She graduated from high school with a good record. She worked for many years, first as an assistant teacher at a primary school, then as a cartographer and in various clerical jobs. For the last few years she has stayed at home doing housework and sometimes has taken part-time jobs.

She describes herself as always having been reserved, prudent, conscientious, and tender in sentiment. She was never overly sociable, but has had some close friends. She has been sensitive to the feelings of others and always desired the acceptance of those around her.

During the interview Ms. Mura's mood is appropriately sad. When she speaks of her habit of thinking aloud, she has tears in her soft eyes. She says she would rather die than live with such pain and misery.

Discussion of "Fear of Thinking Aloud"

This patient is seriously distressed by her belief that she must have hurt the feelings of other people around her by unconsciously thinking ill of them aloud. She interprets various trivial actions and behaviors of other people as responses to her unintended malicious messages spoken to them while she was "thinking aloud." She believes this in spite of her sister's reassurance that she never thinks aloud at home.

This clinical picture is not rare in Japan, where it is called *Taijin-kyofu,* which can be translated as "fear of other people" or "anthropophobia." In this disorder, the predominant disturbance is an unrealistic interpretation of trivial actions and behaviors of people around the patient, leading to the preoccupation or belief that the patient is causing unpleasant feelings in the other people. In mild cases patients are aware that their fears are excessive and unreasonable.

Patients with *Taijin-kyofu* complain of varying worries, such as fear of body odor (*Taishu-kyofu*), in which the patient believes that he or she emits rank odors from the body, often from the axilla, mouth, anus, or genital area; fear of glancing (*Shisen-kyofu*), in which the patient believes that he or she glances at other people unintentionally and gives them unpleasant feelings; fear of blushing (*Sekimen-kyofu*), in which the patient is fearful about blushing in front of others; fear of ugly facial expressions (*Shubou-kyofu*), such as grinning, or showing the whites of the eyes; or fear of thinking aloud (*Dokugo-kyofu*). In Japan, *Taijin-kyofu* is usually considered a type of neurotic disorder appearing in a person with a "sensitive personality."

In diagnosing Ms. Mura, the first judgment that must be made is whether her belief that she offends people by "thinking aloud" is a delusion, an overvalued idea, or only an unrealistic fear. It seems clear that in this case we are dealing with a delusion, since not only has she conviction in this unfounded idea but it markedly influences her behavior. Since this is the only psychotic symptom, the next issue is whether the delusion is bizarre, that is, involves a phenomenon that the person's culture would regard as totally implausible. This is clearly not the case, since it is possible to speak one's thoughts aloud inadvertently. Therefore, Schizophrenia is ruled out and the diagnosis of Delusional Disorder, Unspecified Type, is appropriate (DSM-IV-TR, p. 329).

Whereas some of the delusions associated with *Taijin-kyofu* are observed in the United States (for example, delusions of having a bad odor), Ms. Mura's delusion that she has inadvertently offended other people is virtually never seen and seems to be culture-specific and an expression of the extreme concern with issues of shame found in Japanese culture.

INDIA

FITS

Mrs. Chatterjee, a 26-year-old patient, attends a clinic in New Delhi, India, with complaints of "fits" for the last 4 years. The "fits" are always sudden in onset and usually last 30–60 minutes. A few minutes before a fit begins, she knows that it is imminent, and she usually goes to bed. During the fits she becomes unresponsive and rigid throughout her body, with bizarre and thrashing movements of the extremities. Her eyes close and her jaw is clenched, and she froths at the mouth. She frequently cries and sometimes shouts abuses. She is never incontinent of urine or feces, nor does she bite her tongue. After a "fit" she claims to have no memory of it.

These episodes recur about once or twice a month. She functions well in between the episodes and reports no prominent depressive or anxiety symptoms.

Both the patient and her family believe that her "fits" are evidence of a physical illness and are not under her control. However, they recognize that the fits often occur following some stressor, such as arguments with family members or friends.

Mrs. Chatterjee comes from a middle-class urban family. She has been married for 5 years to a clerk in a government office. They have two children. Her mother-in-law and father-in-law live with the family, and this has sometimes led to conflicts.

She is described by her family as being somewhat immature but "quite social" and good company. She is self-centered, she craves attention from others, and she often reacts with irritability and anger if her wishes are not immediately fulfilled. She handles routine household tasks well.

On physical examination, Mrs. Chatterjee was found to have mild anemia but was otherwise healthy. A mental status examination did not reveal any abnormality in her speech, thought, orientation, perception, or intellectual functions. She did not display any sustained mood change, and her memory was normal. An electroencephalogram showed no seizure activity. A skull X-ray was also normal.

Discussion of "Fits"

The Indian psychiatrist who contributed this case made a diagnosis of Hysteria. He noted that this kind of presentation is quite common in India, Pakistan, and neighboring countries; in fact, Hysteria is diagnosed in 5%–8% of all patients seen in the psychiatric unit of his general hospital.

The predominant symptom resembles an epileptic seizure; however, the absence of such typical features of neurologic seizures as incontinence and biting of the tongue strongly suggests that a neurologic condition or general medical condition cannot explain the seizures. This is further substantiated by the normal electroencephalogram.

We see no evidence of intentional feigning of the symptoms, as in Factitious Disorder With Physical Symptoms. Because the predominant symptom suggests a physical disorder (epilepsy), there is no evidence that the seizures are culturally sanctioned behaviors, and the symptoms seem to recur in response to stressful situations, we diagnose Conversion Disorder With Seizures or Convulsions (DSM-IV-TR, p. 498). However, we would not quarrel with a clinician who diagnosed a Dissociative Disorder Not Otherwise Specified, viewing the "fits" as a disturbance of the normally integrative functions of memory and consciousness.

Follow-Up

The patient was treated, with her husband, in family sessions over the next 2 months. The couple was taught that the patient's fits were not evidence of a serious physical illness. In addition, the husband was urged to take a more active role in handling problems that arose between the patient and her in-laws and to pay more attention to the patient in general, but not during her fits. The couple stopped therapy after 2 months, during which time the patient had no more fits.

POLYNESIA

CULTURAL HEALING

A 26-year-old Polynesian female bus driver was brought to the emergency room of a hospital in New Zealand following an incident in which the bus she was driving knocked the arm of a pedestrian, resulting in a loud thump against the bus but not injuring the pedestrian. The bus driver was brought to the emergency room by witnesses to the accident who said she was in a state of "emotional shock." When seen by the emergency-room doctor, she had an unfocused stare and was holding up one finger on each hand and softly repeating "One, killed" very slowly. She would not respond to questions, but did not resist passive movement of her arms. She seemed to be preoccupied rather than depressed, suspicious, or anxious.

Six weeks before the accident, the patient had married a European man. Three years earlier she had left her Polynesian husband, with whom she had two children, ages 9 and 5 years. She had joint custody of the two children; but her new husband was moving to a job in a different city, and she was fearful about the changes in custody arrangements that this might cause. Her family was pressuring her to return to her home islands with her new husband, but financing this posed further problems, particularly as she felt her job was threatened because of some disciplinary proceedings at her workplace. She viewed these as portents of misfortune for her family.

The patient came from a "high-born" Pacific Island family and had come to New Zealand 10 years previously. Before the incident she had a happy, friendly, outgoing disposition, had many friends, and was regarded as a conscientious worker by her employers.

In the emergency room, the patient's mental state improved slightly over several hours. She then spoke in a slow, monotonous tone, expressing fears of coming to further harm. She was responsive to reassurance and showed no evidence of delusions or hallucinations. She was released to her husband's care; but the next day he found her hiding under a blanket, clutching a kitchen knife, and in her previous mute state. He brought her back to the hospital, where she was given an antianxiety drug and an attempt was made to get her to talk about her problems. This resulted in only transient improvement.

Because her symptoms had a clear relationship to the accident, her Polynesian relatives encouraged her husband to take her to a cultural healer, who gave her massage and a drink. She refused the latter, bit the glass, and broke it. The healer interpreted this as indicating that she was possessed by the ghost of her Polynesian ex-father-in-law, who had recently died and who was (allegedly) angry that she had deserted his son. (When next seen at the hospital, the patient acknowledged that she saw some resemblance between the man involved in the accident and her father-in-law.) Within a few hours after visiting the healer, all of the patient's symptoms disappeared.

Discussion of "Cultural Healing"

The psychiatrist who contributed this case noted that similar kinds of cases are seen in psychiatric units of general hospitals in New Zealand in approximately 1 of every 100 admissions. He suspects that many such patients never come to the hospital and that this woman came primarily because her episode occurred in a public place.

This case would appear to be an example of Dissociative Trance Disorder (DSM-IV-TR, p. 785), which is listed as Dissociative Disorder Not Otherwise Specified because, when examined, the patient seemed to be in a "trance" state, with narrowing of awareness of her immediate surroundings and development of stereotyped behaviors or movements seemingly beyond her control. It is less clear what to make of her extreme fearfulness (hiding under a blanket clutching a kitchen knife) and her belief that there had been portents of her misfortune. We give her the benefit of the doubt and do not add a diagnosis of psychosis.

Follow-Up

Ten days after her recovery following her visit to the healer, the thought that she might be responsible for causing a car or bus accident kept intruding into the patient's mind (an obsession?). She became terrified of going near a bus and was twice stopped by the traffic police for driving too slowly and with excessive caution. Her family brought her back to the hospital, where she was treated with an intensive behavioral program consisting of relaxation training

> and graded exposure to buses. Within 2 weeks she had totally recovered, and was still well 1 year later.

SCANDINAVIA

FACTORY WORKER

Jorgen, a married 35-year-old factory worker in Oslo, has asked for a psychiatric consultation because of pressure from his wife. Together they have had some joint sessions of marital counseling, in which the main problem has been identified as his difficulty in expressing any feelings. For example, he hardly ever talks to his wife about anything other than tasks that need to be done. When they make love, his wife feels that he is mechanical and does it without any tenderness. The marriage counselor suggested that he be seen in individual psychotherapy. Jorgen acknowledges general dissatisfaction with his life and admits that his wife's complaints may be justified. Her complaints about him have increased considerably since she had a passionate affair with another man and began her own psychotherapy about a year ago.

During the two evaluation sessions, Jorgen is timid and hesitant and seldom makes eye contact with the psychiatrist. His posture is stiff, and he is quite formal. He tells his story slowly and in great detail, with few gestures or expressions of emotion.

He is the only child of working-class parents. His father was abroad as a sailor for a year when Jorgen was 3 years old, during which time he lived with his mother and her parents. He remembers feeling uncomfortable when his father returned. During his childhood he believed that his parents did not love him. They gave him food, shelter, clothes, and money, but took no interest in him emotionally. He is still bitter because of this and has little contact with them now.

Although he was intellectually bright in elementary school, he recalls being scolded by his teachers because he was noisy and domineering in class. Gradually, he became more silent and timid at school. His favorite sport was sailing a small boat. He did a lot of racing, but, he says, "For some reason I was always second best." He had a few friends and dated occasionally.

Jorgen did well in high school and college and later studied science at the university. While he was finishing his physics thesis, he got an assistantship as a science teacher at a senior high school in the upper-class part of the city. The students there made fun of his accent. He became quite anxious and tense because of this and had to leave the job. While at the university he had been politically active in the Marxist party. Partly because of party ideology and partly because of the above-mentioned teaching experience, he left the university without finishing his thesis.

He started to work on an assembly line in a big factory. He tried to influence the other workers politically and had moderate success. His fellow workers understood that he was intelligent and chose him to negotiate with the board of directors concerning working conditions. He became quite anxious in this situation. He felt "fuzzy" in his head and was unable to make his points except when he specifically could point to laws and agreements.

Although he was preoccupied with sex and wanted a close relationship with a girl, he rarely dated. In his relations with girls he was shy, passive, and helpless. When he was in his mid-20s, he met his future wife, a nurse, who was also shy. They married after 1 year, although their sexual adjustment was poor. It seemed that the relationship helped both of them overcome their loneliness. His wife seemed to tolerate the lack of intimacy in their marriage and their poor sex life, until her affair and her own psychotherapy. Her increasing demands on him caused Jorgen to realize that he was emotionally inhibited, and he discovered that a few drinks made him feel freer. He developed a pattern of taking a couple of drinks each night, but denies that this has ever caused any problems.

Discussion of "Factory Worker"

The Norwegian psychiatrist who contributed this case notes that in his country such a patient would be given the diagnosis of character neurosis, a term used to describe "inhibitions of the personality" that restrict the person's enjoyment of life and the use of his abilities and talents. Restrictions in the expression of love, intimacy, and

anger and the competitive display of one's talents are common, as
in this case. People given this diagnosis often have a rigid posture
and inhibition of spontaneous use of their bodies and may present
themselves to others as formal, reserved, and lacking vitality. "A
patient with a character neurosis drives through life with the
brakes on."

The clinical picture seen in this Norwegian patient is no different
from that seen in many patients receiving outpatient psychotherapy
in the United States. Some traits are characteristic of several personality disorders (Obsessive-Compulsive, Dependent, and Avoidant),
but the full diagnostic criteria are not met for any one disorder. It is
nevertheless apparent that this man does suffer from a pervasive
pattern of inflexible and maladaptive behavior that has caused him
significant functional impairment. Therefore, we diagnose Personality Disorder Not Otherwise Specified (DSM-IV-TR, p. 729).

THE LUMBERMAN

A Norwegian lumberman was admitted to the psychiatric ward of a hospital shortly after starting his required military duty at the age of 20. During
the first week after his arrival at the military base, he thought the other re-
cruits looked at him in a strange way. He watched the people around him
in order to see whether they were out "to get" him. He heard voices calling
his name several times. He became increasingly suspicious and after another week had to be admitted to the Psychiatric Department at the University of Oslo. There he was guarded, scowling, skeptical, and depressed.
He gave the impression of being very shy and inhibited. His psychotic
symptoms disappeared rapidly when he was treated with an antipsychotic
drug. However, he had difficulties in adjusting to hospital life. Transfer to a
long-term mental hospital was considered; but after 3 months, a decision
was made to discharge him to his home in the forest. He was subsequently
judged unfit to return to military service and was struck from the military
lists.

The patient, the eldest of five siblings, was the son of a farm laborer
in one of the valleys of Norway. His father was an intemperate drinker
who became angry and brutal when drunk. The family was very poor,

and there were constant quarrels between the parents. As a child, the patient was inhibited and fearful and often ran into the woods when troubled. He had academic difficulties and barely passed elementary school.

When the patient became older, he preferred to spend most of his time in the woods, where he worked as a lumberman from the age of 15. He had his own horse, lived in a log cabin, and disliked being with people. He sometimes took part in the youth dances in the village. Although never a heavy drinker, he often got into fights in the village when he had a drink or two. At the age of 16, he began to keep company with a girl 1 year his junior who sometimes kept house for him in the woods. They eventually became engaged.

Discussion of "The Lumberman"

The Norwegian psychiatrist who provided this case made the Scandinavian diagnosis of Reactive Psychosis, Paranoid Type. The patient displays the typical features of the disorder: reaction to extreme stress that exacerbates underlying psychological conflicts, in which the prognosis for full recovery is very good. In order to label a psychosis reactive, the psychic trauma must be considered of such significance that the psychosis would not have appeared in its absence. There must be a temporal connection between the trauma and the onset of the psychosis, and the content of the psychotic symptoms must reflect the traumatic experience. In this case, for an extremely shy and isolated man, military service was a much more serious stressor than for an ordinary person of the same age.

According to DSM-IV-TR, the differential diagnosis would be between Delusional Disorder and Brief Psychotic Disorder. The nonbizarre delusion that he was being persecuted suggests Delusional Disorder, Persecutory Type; but Delusional Disorder requires a duration of at least 1 month, and this patient apparently recovered from his psychotic symptoms within a few weeks. Therefore, our diagnosis would be Brief Psychotic Disorder (DSM-IV-TR, p. 332), since this diagnosis applies to psychotic illnesses of at least 1 day but no more than 1 month, with eventual full return to premorbid functioning, as in this case. The importance of the stressor could be indicated on Axis IV.

Although the lumberman has had a tendency toward social isolation and difficulties with peers as an adolescent, there is insufficient information to justify a Personality Disorder diagnosis. Therefore, we shall simply note the presence of schizoid personality traits on Axis II.

Follow-Up

The patient was reinterviewed by hospital personnel at 4 years, 7 years, and 23 years after his admission. He has had no recurrences of any psychotic symptoms and has been fully employed since 6 months after he left the hospital. He married the young woman to whom he was engaged, and at the last follow-up, he had two grown children.

After leaving the hospital, the patient worked for 2 years in a factory, and then as a lumberman. For the last 20 years, he has managed a small business, which he has run well. He has been happy at work and in his family life. He has made an effort to overcome his tendency toward isolation and has several friends. Among other duties, he has been chairman of a sheep-rearing association in the county. He is well liked in the village.

The patient believes that his natural tendency is to be socially isolated and that his disorder was connected with the fact that in the military situation, he was forced to deal with other people.

Chapter 5

Historical Cases

EMIL KRAEPELIN (1856–1926)

Kraepelin, a professor of psychiatry in Germany, provided the basis for modern classification of mental disorders. He used the natural history of the illness—its onset, course, and outcome—and its clinical picture as the basis for classification. Thus, he differentiated Maniacal-Depressive Insanity from Dementia Praecox (later renamed Schizophrenia by Bleuler). He subdivided Dementia Praecox into three types: catatonic, hebephrenic, and paranoid.

Kraepelin's major textbook was first published in 1883 and went into nine editions. The following cases are taken verbatim from his Lectures in Clinical Psychiatry.* *They have provided generations of clinicians with detailed illustrations of his diagnostic concepts.*

MUSIC STUDENT

You see before you a student of music, aged nineteen, who has been ill for about a year. The highly gifted patient, without any tangible cause, while studying music, became depressed, felt ill at ease and lonely, made all manner of plans, which he always gave up, for changing his place of residence and his profession, for he could come to no fixed resolutions. During a visit to Munich, he felt as if people in the street had something to say to him, and as if he were talked about everywhere. He heard an offensive remark at an inn at the next table, which he answered rudely. Next day

---

*From Kraepelin E: *Lectures in Clinical Psychiatry* (1904). Translated by Johnstone TP. New York, Hafner Publishing, 1968. "Music Student," p. 74; "Schoolmaster," p. 262; "Wicked Young Lady," p. 265; "The Innkeeper," p. 97; "Stately Gentlemen," p. 140; "The Widow," p. 157; "The Farmer," p. 4; "Oberrealschul Student," p. 77; "The Suffering Lady," p. 252; "Onanistic Student," p. 21; "Factory Girl," p. 83.

he was seized with the apprehension that his remark might be taken as *lèse majesté*. He heard that students asked for him at the door, and he left Munich posthaste with every precautionary measure, because he thought himself accompanied and followed on the way. Since then he overheard people in the street who threatened to shoot him, and to set fire to his house, and on that account he burned no light in his room. In the streets voices pointed out the way he ought to go so as to avoid being shot. Behind doors, windows, hedges, pursuers seemed everywhere to lurk. He also heard long conversations of not very flattering purport as to his person. In consequence of this, he withdrew altogether from society, but yet behaved in such an ordinary way that his relatives, whom he visited, did not notice his delusions. At last the many mocking calls which he heard at every turn provoked the thought of shooting himself.

After about 6 months he felt more free, "comfortable, enterprising, and cheerful," began to talk a lot, compose, criticized everything, concocted great schemes, and was insubordinate to his teacher. The voices still continued, and he recognized in them the whisperings of master spirits. Hallucinations of sight now became very marked. The patient saw Beethoven's image radiant with joy at his genius; saw Goethe, whom he had abused, in a threatening attitude; masked men and ideal female forms floated through his room. He saw lightning and glorious brilliancy of colors, which he interpreted partly as the flowing out of his great genius, partly as attestations of applause from the dead.

He regarded himself as the Messiah, preached openly against prostitution, wished to enter into an ideal connection with a female student of music, whom he sought for in strange houses, composed the "Great Song of Love," and on account of this priceless work was brought to the hospital by those who envied him, as he said.

The patient is quite collected, and gives connected information as to his personal circumstances. He is clear as to time and place, but betrays himself by judging his position falsely, inasmuch as he takes us for hypnotizers, who wish to try experiments with him. He does not look upon himself as ill; at the most as somewhat nervously overexcited. Through diplomatic questions we learn that all people know his thoughts; if he writes, the words are repeated before the door. In the creaking of boards, in the whistle of the train, he hears calls, exhortations, orders, threats. Christ appears to him in the night, or a golden figure as the spirit of his father; coloured signs of special meaning are given through the window. In prolonged conversation the patient very quickly loses the thread, and produces finally a succession of fine phrases, which wind up unexpectedly with some facetious question. His mood is arrogant, conceited, generally condescending, occasionally transitorily irritated or apprehensive. The patient speaks much and willingly, talks aloud to himself, and marches boisterously up and down the ward, interests himself more than is desirable in his fellow patients, seeking to cheer them and to manage them. He is very busy, too, with letter-writing and composing, but only produces furtive, carelessly jotted down written work, with numerous marginal notes.

Kraepelin's Diagnosis: Maniacal-Depressive Insanity

Discussion of "Music Student"

There are two phases of this illness. In the first, the patient is described as "depressed" and indecisive (". . . he could come to no fixed resolutions") and as having suicidal ideas (". . . thought of shooting himself"). We suspect that this was a Major Depressive Episode; but we do not have enough information about other depressive symptoms, such as loss of appetite and sleep disturbance, to make a firm diagnosis.

The psychotic features during this period consisted of mood-incongruent persecutory delusions and hallucinations; they apparently had no relation to typical depressive themes such as deserved punishment, personal inadequacy, or guilt. There were persecutory delusions (e.g., "Behind doors, windows, hedges, pursuers seemed everywhere to lurk") and hallucinations (e.g., "He . . . heard long conversations of not very flattering purport as to his person"). There were ideas of reference (e.g., "He heard that students asked for him at the door, and he left Munich posthaste with every precautionary measure, because he thought himself accompanied and followed on the way").

Currently the patient is clearly in a Manic Episode (DSM-IV-TR, p. 362). There is an elevated mood with grandiosity (e.g., "He regarded himself as the Messiah . . ."), hyperactivity (e.g., he "marches boisterously up and down the ward . . ."), overtalkativeness, and poor judgment (e.g., he "interests himself more than is desirable in his fellow patients, seeking to cheer them and to manage them"). There is a suggestion of loose associations and, possibly, flight of ideas (e.g., "In prolonged conversation the patient very quickly loses the thread, and produces finally a succession of fine phrases, which wind up unexpectedly with some facetious question"). Most of his psychotic features are mood-congruent in that they are associated with typical manic themes of inflated worth, knowledge, and identity. Hallucinations (e.g., "The patient saw Beethoven's image radiant with joy at his genius") and delusions (e.g., he "composed the 'Great Song of Love,' and on account of this priceless work was brought to the hospital by those who envied him") are present. In addition, there are illusions (e.g., "In the creaking of boards, in the whistle of the train, he hears calls, exhortations, orders, threats").

It is interesting to note the presence of certain psychotic symptoms such as possible thought-broadcasting (e.g., "all people know his thoughts; if he writes, the words are repeated before the door"). Even though many clinicians have regarded such symptoms as indicative of Schizophrenia, neither Kraepelin nor DSM-IV-TR regards these as incompatible with a Mood Disorder.

If, during the first phase of the illness, the patient had psychotic symptoms in the absence of a full depressive syndrome, then the diagnosis would be Schizoaffective Disorder, Bipolar Type. Since we suspect that he probably had a full depressive syndrome, we would diagnose Bipolar I Disorder, Most Recent Episode Manic, Severe With Psychotic Features (Mood-Congruent) (DSM-IV-TR, p. 389).

THE SCHOOLMASTER

First you see a schoolmaster, aged 31, who came to the hospital of his own accord 4 weeks ago in order to be treated here. The patient was, in fact, violently agitated when he had to come here, sank down on his bed, and said that the discussion in the hospital would cost him his life. He begged to be allowed to sit in the hall before the lecture began, so that he could see the audience come in gradually, as he could not face a number of people so suddenly.

The patient is quite collected, clear, and well-ordered in his statements. He says that one of his sisters suffers in the same way as himself.

He traces the beginning of his illness back to about 11 years ago. Being a clever lad, he became a schoolmaster, and had to do a great deal of mental work to qualify. Gradually he began to fear that he had a serious disease, and was going to die of heart apoplexy. All the assurances and examinations of his doctor could not convince him. For this reason he suddenly left his appointment and went home one day 7 years ago, being afraid that he would die shortly. After this he consulted every possible doctor, and took long holidays repeatedly, always recovering a little, but invariably finding that his fears returned speedily. These were gradually reinforced by the fear of gatherings of people. He was unable to cross large squares or go through wide streets by himself. He avoided using the railway for fear of collisions and derailments, and he would not travel in a boat lest it might capsize. He was seized with apprehension on bridges and when skating, and at last the apprehension of apprehension itself caused palpitations and oppression on all sorts of occasions. He did not improve after his marriage 3 years ago. He was domesticated, good-natured, and manageable, only "too soft." On the way here, when he had finally made up his mind to place himself in our hands, he trembled with deadly fear.

The patient describes himself as a chicken-hearted fellow, who, in spite of good mental ability, has always been afraid of all sorts of diseases—consumption, heart apoplexy, and the like. He knows that these anxieties are morbid, yet cannot free himself from them. This apprehensiveness came out in a very marked way while he was under observation in the hospital. He worried about every remedy, whether it was baths, packs, or medicine, being afraid it would be too strong for him, and have a weakening effect. He always wished to have a warder within call in case he got agitated. The sight of other patients disturbed him greatly; and when he went for a walk in the garden with the door shut, he was tormented by the fear of not being able to get out of it in case anything happened. At last he would hardly venture in front of the house, and always had to have the door open behind him so that he could take refuge indoors in case of necessity. He begged to have a little bottle of "blue electricity" that he had brought with him to give him confidence. Sometimes he was seized with violent palpitation of the heart while he was sitting down. Some little acne spots gave him so much alarm that he could neither go for a walk nor sleep. It struck him that his look had got very gloomy, and he thought it was the beginning of a mental disturbance which would certainly seize upon him while he was here.

Kraepelin's Diagnosis: Insanity of Irrepressible Ideas

Discussion of "The Schoolmaster"

The patient demonstrates three significant diagnostic features. First of all, there is a morbid preoccupation with a fear of having a serious physical disease (e.g., "he began to fear that he had a serious disease, and was going to die of heart apoplexy. All the assurances and examinations of his doctor could not convince him"). This, in the absence of a general medical condition that can account for the disturbance, justifies the diagnosis of Hypochondriasis (DSM-IV-TR, p. 507).

Secondly, there is a strong suggestion of recurrent panic attacks (e.g., "Sometimes he was seized with violent palpitation of the heart while he was sitting down. . . . He trembled with deadly fear"). Perhaps because Kraepelin did not recognize recurrent panic attacks as a distinct clinical syndrome, there is no mention of other characteristic symptoms such as shortness of breath, dizziness, and sweating, but we suspect these symptoms were also present.

Finally, there is an irrational avoidance of being in public places (e.g., "He was unable to cross large squares or go through wide streets by himself. . . . He was seized with apprehension on bridges"). This suggests Agoraphobia (i.e., anxiety about being in places or situations from which escape might be difficult [or embarrassing] in the event of developing paniclike symptoms). Most likely the recurrent panic attacks led to the Agoraphobia, indicating the diagnosis of Panic Disorder With Agoraphobia (DSM-IV-TR, p. 441).

Some clinicians might wish to make the additional diagnosis of a Specific Phobia to account for the fear and avoidance of trains and boats, because the patient attributes his anxiety to concern that an accident might occur rather than to the possibility that he might be incapacitated while alone (part of Agoraphobia). We do not add this diagnosis because we are not sure that he is markedly distressed by this fear or that it causes significant impairment in social or occupational functioning.

WICKED YOUNG LADY

A young lady, aged 26 . . . The slightly built, ill-nourished, sickly looking girl has an expression of pain and trouble. Her hands and fingers are always in slight movement, reflecting her mental restlessness. She is quite collected and clear, but only gives monosyllabic answers. . . . She was constitutionally healthy herself, lively, and cheerful, but fell ill 10 years ago of chronic inflammation of the tarsal joint, which brought her under medical treatment for a year. Even now walking is made difficult and slightly painful by the stiffness of the joint. In answer to our questions, the patient says that she is not insane, but only a wicked person who would be sent to the devil if people knew how continually she sins. She does not deserve to be well treated, and she cannot bear that people should look on her as an invalid, when in reality she is only pretending. It is impossible to get any details from her, as she evades every attempt to extract information. We can only learn that she has been to confession unworthily, and so could find no rest, even if she went to the end of the world. She must go away, anywhere, only not to her home, where she has lied and deceived. She cannot stay here either, as people are far too good to her.

So far as we know this state of depression has developed quite gradually in the last year or two. It struck the patient's relations that her mood changed quickly and abruptly. She occasionally expressed religious doubts, on account of which she was sent to the priest, and also to a place of pilgrimage. But this only produced an aggravation of her condition each time. The restlessness increased, and the patient's sleep and appetite became worse and worse, her strength gradually becoming very much reduced in consequence. She felt burdened with grievous sins, of which she could not properly repent, and so was fallen into the power of the devil. She had neither wishes nor will; everything had become indifferent to her. Her whole previous life, with all her transgressions, stood out clearly before her, so that she was surprised at her own memory. She could not help brooding and having unclean thoughts, which broke her heart. Hence she worked feverishly, just to avoid thinking, although everything was very difficult for her.

After great reluctance, she has informed me of the purport of her tormenting thoughts. She was almost continually haunted by ideas associated with the reproductive organs of the opposite sex, which need not be detailed here. Thoughts of this kind, concerned in different ways with the same object, persecute her unceasingly without her being able to ignore them. Hence she says that she must really wish to have such thoughts; she must find pleasure in them, or they would not come. It is very difficult to divert the patient's mind from her painful self-torture; she always returns to it. She is quite unable to read, or to occupy herself mentally in any other way, as these sexual ideas attach themselves, by the most remarkable connections, to her course of thought, however remote it may be. In her general thinking the patient is clumsy and slow. She has always to overcome great disinclination, even when she has to write a simple letter. She generally obeys the doctor's orders, but has a number of peculiarities. The baths give her pains; meat is not good for her; she must follow certain paths in her whole way of life if she is not to grow worse. No physical disturbances have appeared except stiffness, swelling, and pain in the left instep, and a tendency to constipation, which has existed for many years. She sleeps badly.

Kraepelin's Diagnosis: Maniacal-Depressive Insanity

Discussion of "Wicked Young Lady"

What apparently disturbs this patient most are the sexual ideas that force themselves into her awareness against her will. As Kraepelin notes in his discussion of the case, even though she says that she must really "wish" to have such ideas, it is clear that she has a strong desire to be freed from her tormenting thoughts, but cannot refrain from them. These thoughts have all the characteristics of obsessions, or what Kraepelin referred to as "irrepressible ideas": The thoughts are recurrent and persistent. She recognizes them as products of her own mind and unsuccessfully attempts to suppress them. Because the obsessions cause her marked distress, a diagnosis of Obsessive-Compulsive Disorder (DSM-IV-TR, p. 462) is warranted.

In addition to the Obsessive-Compulsive Disorder, the patient has an episode of illness that meets the criteria for Major Depressive Disorder, Single Episode (DSM-IV-TR, p. 375). In addition to the depressed mood there are guilt, disturbed sleep, decreased appetite and energy (i.e., "sleep and appetite became worse and worse, her strength gradually becoming very much reduced"), loss of interest (e.g., "She had neither wishes nor will; everything had become indifferent to her"), difficulty concentrating, and, possibly, psychomotor agitation (e.g., her "restlessness").

The patient's guilt is of psychotic proportions—she believes that she has "fallen into the power of the devil." This delusion is mood-congruent in that it involves the theme of guilt and deserved punishment. Therefore, we would add Severe With Psychotic Features to the diagnosis of Major Depressive Disorder.

Do the prominent obsessions justify a separate diagnosis in addition to the diagnosis of Major Depressive Disorder? As Kraepelin noted, "A single symptom, however characteristic it may be, never justifies a definite diagnosis by itself, and only the whole picture can ever be decisive of the clinical hypothesis." DSM-III, following Kraepelin's approach, instructed the clinician to make only one diagnosis, assuming that the obsessions were best understood as an associated feature of the Major Depressive Disorder. In DSM-III-R and in DSM-IV (and DSM-IV-TR), this hierarchic relationship has been suspended, and the clinician is instructed to make both diagnoses if the content of the obsessions differs from the content of the depressive thoughts associated with Major Depressive Disorder.

THE INNKEEPER

The innkeeper, aged 34, whom I am bringing before you today was admitted to the hospital only an hour ago. He understands the questions put to him, but cannot quite hear some of them, and gives a rather absent-minded impression. He states his name and age correctly. . . . Yet he does not know the doctors, calls them by the names of his acquaintances, and thinks he has been here for 2 or 3 days. It must be the Crown Hotel, or, rather, the "mad hospital." He does not know the date.

He moves about in his chair, looks round him a great deal, starts slightly several times, and keeps on playing with his hands. Suddenly he gets up, and begs to be allowed to play the piano for a little at once. He sits down again immediately, on persuasion, but then wants to go away "to tell them something else that he has forgotten." He gradually gets more and more excited, saying that his fate is sealed; he must leave the world now; they might telegraph to his wife that her husband is lying at the point of death. We learn, by questioning him, that he is going to be executed by electricity, and also that he will be shot. "The picture is not clearly painted," he says; "Every moment someone stands now here, now there, waiting for me with a revolver. When I open my eyes, they vanish." He says that a stinking fluid has been injected into his head and both his toes, which causes the pictures one takes for reality; that is the work of an international society, which makes away with those "who fell into misfortune innocently through false steps." With this he looks eagerly at the window, where he sees houses and trees vanishing and reappearing. With slight pressure on his eyes, he sees first sparks, then a hare, a picture, a head, a washstand-set, a half-moon, and a human head, first dully and then in colours. If you show him a speck on the floor, he tries to pick it up, saying that it is a piece of money. If you shut his hand and ask him what you have given him, he keeps his fingers carefully closed, and guesses that it is a lead-pencil or a piece of India rubber. The patient's mood is half apprehensive and half amused. His head is much flushed, and his pulse is small, weak, and rather hurried. His face is bloated and his eyes are watery. His breath smells strongly of alcohol and acetone. His tongue is thickly furred, and trembles when he puts it out, and his outspread fingers show strong, jerky tremors. The knee-reflexes are somewhat exaggerated.

Our patient has drunk hard since he was 13 years old. . . . At last, by his own account, he drank 6 or 7 litres of wine a day and 5 or 6 stomachic bitters, while he took hardly any food but soup. Some weeks ago he had occasional hallucinations of sight—mice, rats, beetles, and rabbits. He mistook people at times, and came into his inn in his shirt. His condition has grown worse during the last few days.

Kraepelin's Diagnosis: Delirium Tremens

Discussion of "The Innkeeper"

This is a classic case of what traditionally has been called Delirium Tremens. In DSM-IV-TR it is called Alcohol Withdrawal Delirium (DSM-IV-TR, p. 146) to differentiate it from Delirium caused by withdrawal from other drugs, such as sedatives or hypnotics.

The delirium is evidenced by the onset, over a short period of time, of multiple signs of cognitive impairment. There is reduced ability to maintain attention to external stimuli (e.g., "He understands the questions put to him, but cannot quite hear some of them, and gives a rather absentminded impression . . . begs to be allowed to play the piano . . . looks eagerly at the window. . . ."). There are disorientation (e.g., "he does not know the doctors . . . [or] the date"), and rambling speech.

In addition, the patient displays several features that are often seen in a delirium due to withdrawal from alcohol: perceptual disturbances (e.g., "he sees houses and trees vanishing and reappearing [hallucinations]. . . . If you show him a speck on the floor, he tries to pick it up, saying that it is a piece of money" [illusions]), increased psychomotor activity (e.g., "He moves about in his chair . . . and keeps on playing with his hands"), autonomic hyperactivity (e.g., "His head is much flushed, and his pulse is small, weak, and rather hurried"), and, finally, persecutory delusions (e.g., "he is going to be executed by electricity").

Although the case description makes no mention of a recent reduction in alcohol ingestion, it is reasonable to assume that the delirium resulted from alcohol withdrawal in a person who has been dependent on alcohol for a long period of time. Therefore, we would add the diagnosis of Alcohol Dependence (DSM-IV-TR, p. 213).

STATELY GENTLEMAN

The stately gentleman, aged 62, who presents himself before us with a certain courtly dignity, with his carefully tended moustache, his eyeglasses, and his well-fitting if perhaps somewhat shabby attire, gives quite the impression of a man of the world. He is somewhat testy at first because he has to allow himself to be questioned before the young gentlemen, but soon enters into a long, connected conversation in a quiet and positive manner. We learn from him that as a young man he went to America, and there went through many vicissitudes, finally settling in Quito, where as a merchant he made a small fortune. With this he returned home 21 years ago, but on the dissolving of his business connections he was done out of considerable sums. At home he lived at first on his money, spending his time in amusements, reading the newspaper, playing billiards, going for walks, and sitting about in cafes. At the same time he occupied himself with all sorts of schemes from which he hoped for recognition and profit. Thus, he submitted to the leading Minister the plan (with a map) whereby Germany could lay claim to a lot of still unpossessed land. . . . A short time after that same Minister travelled to Berlin, and now began the German Colonial Policy, without . . . due thanks falling to the lot of the real originator. . . . Then our patient drew up a plan for the cultivation of cinchona and cacao in our colonies; he also made several inventions for the better connection of railway metals, by which the jolting, an important cause of derailment, would be done away with. Finally, he applied for a number of situations which seemed suited to him, including that of the consulship at Quito, but had always only failures to record.

He was enticed into a district asylum, under the false pretext that he would be given a post, and there he assisted in the management till it became evident to him that they had no intention of paying him for his services. When, on that account, he tried hard for other situations, they sent him, also under false pretenses, to the hospital, where he is now illegally detained. That, he concluded with bitterness, was the thanks which the Fatherland bestowed upon him for his services.

[He] then relates, little by little, that a woman whom he calls by the nickname Bulldog, and who was the daughter of the English Consul at Quito, had persecuted him for 23 or 24 years with her plans for marriage, and sought in every way to cross his steps in order to reduce him to submission. Even in America things ultimately never went as he wished, and a hundred stuffed birds had, out of spite, been stolen from him by means of a skeleton key; everywhere he noticed the frauds of the Bulldog and her accomplices. "If people do everything differently from what I should have wished, there must be something more than meets the eye." The half-crazy American also travelled home after him, had insinuated herself into this neighborhood, had the impudence to dress herself up in man's clothes, and to force marriage by preventing him from finding a post, and by these means brought him to want. This artful person had approached him under various names, though he had always told her that one did not win a man's love through such chicanery. He would perhaps be the richest man in California if the Bulldog had not prevented it. She was also to blame for his being brought to the asylum. "Who else, then, could it possibly be?" Both at home and abroad he was eternally meeting her. . . . All objections that one raises to these ideas are received by the patient in a superior, incredulous manner, and glance off from his steadfast conviction without leaving the slightest impression.

Kraepelin's Diagnosis: Paranoia

Discussion of "Stately Gentleman"

This is a classic example of the traditional diagnosis of Paranoia, and what in DSM-IV-TR is called Delusional Disorder (DSM-IV-TR, p. 329). The patient demonstrates an elaborate system of persecutory delusions: his contributions to German foreign policy are not acknowledged; he is employed by the district asylum—without pay; he is pursued by the "Bulldog," who dresses in men's clothes and prevents him from obtaining employment. As is frequently the case in patients with a Delusional Disorder, there is grandiosity. For example, his ideas were incorporated into German colonial policy; he would "perhaps be the richest man in California if the Bulldog had not prevented it."

This condition is distinguished from Schizophrenia, Paranoid Type, by the absence of bizarre delusions (i.e., delusions that are patently absurd), hallucinations, or disorganized speech. Furthermore, whereas in Schizophrenia continued deterioration in social functioning is common, in Delusional Disorder it is generally absent, as in this case. In the traditional concept of paranoia, the illness has an insidious onset and a chronic course of many years, as is true in this patient. All such cases fall within the more inclusive DSM-IV-TR category of Delusional Disorder, which does not require an insidious onset and requires a duration of only 1 month. Because the predominant theme in this case involves delusions of being malevolently treated, the Delusional Disorder is further specified as Persecutory Type.

THE WIDOW

The widow, aged 35, whom I will now bring before you . . . gives full information about her life in answer to our questions, knows where she is, can tell the date and the year, and gives proof of satisfactory school knowledge. It is noteworthy that she does not look at her questioner, and speaks in a low and peculiar, sugary, affected tone. When you touch on her illness, she is reserved at first, and says that she is quite well, but she soon begins to express a number of remarkable ideas of persecution. For many years she has heard voices, which insult her and cast suspicion on her chastity. They mention a number of names she knows, and tell her she will be stripped and abused. The voices are very distinct, and, in her opinion, they must be carried by a telescope or a machine from her home. Her thoughts are dictated to her; she is obliged to think them, and hears them repeated after her. She is interrupted in her work, and has all kinds of uncomfortable sensations in her body, to which something is "done." In particular, her "mother parts" are turned inside out, and people send a pain through her back, lay ice-water on her heart, squeeze her neck, injure her spine, and violate her. There are also hallucinations of sight—black figures and the altered appearance of people—but these are far less frequent. She cannot exactly say who carries on all the influencing, or for what object it is done. Sometimes it is the people from her home, and sometimes the doctors of an asylum where she was before who have taken something out of her body.

The patient makes these extraordinary complaints without showing much emotion. She cries a little, but then describes her morbid experiences again with secret satisfaction and even an erotic bias. She demands her discharge, but is easily consoled, and does not trouble at all about her position and her future. Her use of numerous strained and hardly intelligible phrases is very striking. She is ill-treated "flail-wise," "utterance-wise," "terror-wise"; she is "a picture of misery in angel's form," and "a defrauded mamma and housewife of sense of order." They have "altered her form of emotion." She is "persecuted by a secret insect from the District Office." Her former history shows that she has been ill for nearly 10 years. The disease developed gradually. About a year after the death of her husband, by whom she has two children, she became apprehensive, slept badly, heard loud talking in her room at night, and thought that she was being robbed of her means and persecuted by people from Frankfort, where she had formerly lived. Four years ago she spent a year in an asylum. She thought she found the "Frankforters" there, noticed poison in the food, heard voices, and felt influences. After her discharge she brought accusations against the doctors of having mutilated her while she was there. She now thought them to be her persecutors, and openly abused the public authorities for failing to protect her, so she had to be admitted to this hospital two months ago. Here she made the same complaints day after day, without showing much excitement, and wrote long-winded letters full of senseless and unvarying abuse about the persecution from which she suffered, to her relations, the asylum doctors, and the authorities. She did not occupy herself in any way, held no intercourse with her fellow patients, and avoided every attempt to influence her.

Kraepelin's Diagnosis:
Dementia Praecox, Paranoid

Discussion of "The Widow"

This patient demonstrates numerous characteristic symptoms of Schizophrenia. The most conspicuous are bizarre persecutory delusions (e.g., "voices . . . must be carried by a telescope or a machine from her home. Her thoughts are dictated to her; she is obliged to think them"; she said she was "persecuted by a secret insect from the District Office"), some of which are also somatic (e.g., "her 'mother parts' are turned inside out"). She also has persecutory hallucinations (e.g., "she has heard voices, which insult her and cast suspicion on her chastity"). Her speech is at times incoherent (e.g., "she is . . . 'a defrauded mamma and housewife of sense of order'"), with neologisms (e.g., "flail-wise," "utterance-wise," "terror-wise"). Her affect is both flat (e.g., "The patient makes these extraordinary complaints without showing much emotion") and inappropriate (e.g., "She . . . describes her morbid experiences again with secret satisfaction and even with an erotic bias").

In addition, common associated features of Schizophrenia are described: apathy (e.g., she "does not trouble at all about her position and her future"), lack of insight (e.g., she "says that she is quite well"), and social withdrawal (e.g., she "held no intercourse with her fellow patients").

These characteristic symptoms, the marked impairment in multiple areas of functioning, in the absence of a significant mood disturbance, justify the DSM-IV-TR diagnosis of Schizophrenia (DSM-IV-TR, p. 312). The 10-year duration, apparently without periods of remission, indicates that the course has been Continuous. The type would be noted as Undifferentiated (DSM-IV-TR, p. 316), since the presence of flat affect rules out the Paranoid Type, and the characteristic features of the Catatonic and the Disorganized Types are not present.

THE FARMER

I will place before you a farmer, aged 59, who was admitted to the hospital a year ago. The patient looks much older than he really is, principally owing to the loss of teeth from his upper jaw. He not only understands our questions without any difficulty, but answers them relevantly and correctly; can tell where he is and how long he has been here; knows the doctors; and can give the date and the day of the week. His expression is dejected. The corners of his mouth are rather drawn down, and his eyebrows drawn together. . . . On being questioned about his illness, he breaks into lamentations, saying that he did not tell the whole truth on his admission, but concealed the fact that he had fallen into sin in his youth and practiced uncleanness with himself; everything he did was wrong. "I am so apprehensive, so wretched; I cannot lie still for anxiety. O God, if I had only not transgressed so grievously!" He has been ill for over a year. . . . It began with stomachache and head troubles, and he could not work any longer. "There was no impulse left." He can get no rest now, and fancies silly things, as if someone were in the room. Once it seemed to him that he had seen the Evil One: perhaps he would be carried off. . . . As a boy, he had taken apples and nuts. "Conscience has said that that is not right; conscience has only awakened just now in my illness." He had also played with a cow, and by himself. "I reproach myself for that now." It seemed to him that he had fallen away from God. . . . His appetite is bad, and he has no stools. He cannot sleep. "If the mind does not sleep, all sorts of thoughts come." He fastened his neckerchief to strangle himself, but he was not really in earnest. Three sisters and a brother were ill too. The sisters were not so bad; they soon recovered. "A brother has made away with himself through apprehension."

The patient tells us this in broken sentences, interrupted by wailing and groaning. In all other respects, he behaves naturally, does whatever he is told, and only begs us not to let him be dragged away—"There is terrible apprehension in my heart." Except for a little trembling of the outspread fingers and slightly arrhythmic action of the heart, we find no striking disturbances at the physical examination. As for the patient's former history, he is married, and has four healthy children, while three are dead. The illness began gradually 7 or 8 months before his admission, without any assignable cause. Loss of appetite and dyspepsia appeared first, and then ideas of sin. . . .

Kraepelin's Diagnosis: Melancholia

Discussion of "The Farmer"

This patient is clearly suffering from a Major Depressive Disorder, Single Episode (DSM-IV-TR, p. 375). There is a pervasive depressed mood (e.g., "I am so apprehensive, so wretched"; "his expression is dejected"). In addition there are the typical associated features: loss of interest (e.g., "There was no impulse left"), self-reproach for earlier sexual activities (e.g., "He had also played with a cow, and by himself"), insomnia, poor appetite, weight loss, thoughts of suicide, and excessive guilt. There is a suggestion of a hallucination (e.g., "Once it seemed to him that he had seen the Evil One"); however, in the context of his culture, this may not have great pathological significance. Similarly, in the context of his culture, it is difficult to decide if his guilt is of delusional proportions. Therefore, we would qualify the Major Depressive Episode as Severe Without Psychotic Features.

With additional information, the Major Depressive Episode would probably also meet the criteria for With Melancholic Features. The loss of interest would appear to be pervasive. It seems likely that his severely depressed mood is unresponsive to environmental events. In addition, there are several other characteristic features of melancholia: marked psychomotor agitation (e.g., "I cannot lie still for anxiety"), significant anorexia, weight loss, and excessive guilt (e.g., "I am so . . . wretched . . . if only I had not transgressed so griev-ously!"). We do not know about other characteristic melancholic features such as whether his depression is regularly worse in the morning and whether he has early morning awakening.

OBERREALSCHUL STUDENT

The patient I will show you today has almost to be carried into the room, as he walks in a straddling fashion on the outside of his feet. On coming in, he throws off his slippers, sings a hymn loudly, and then cries twice (in English), "My father, my real father!" He is 18 years old, and a pupil of the Oberrealschul [high school], tall, and rather strongly built, but with a pale complexion, on which there is very often a transient flush. The patient sits with his eyes shut, and pays no attention to his surroundings. He does not look up even when he is spoken to, but he answers, beginning in a low voice, and gradually screaming louder and louder. When asked where he is, he says, "You want to know that too; I tell you who is being measured and is measured and shall be measured. I know all that, and could tell you, but I do not want to." When asked his name, he screams, "What is your name? What does he shut? He shuts his eyes. What does he hear? He does not understand; he understands not. How? Who? Where? When? What does he mean? When I tell him to look, he does not look properly. You there, just look! What is it? What is the matter? Attend; he attends not. I say, What is it, then? Why do you give me no answer? Are you getting impudent again? How can you be so impudent? I'm coming! I'll show you! You don't turn whore for me. You mustn't be smart either; you're an impudent, lousy fellow, an impudent, lousy fellow as stupid as a hog. Such an impudent, shameless, miserable, lousy fellow I've never met with. Is he beginning again? You understand nothing at all—nothing at all; nothing at all does he understand. If you follow me now, he won't follow, will not follow. Are you getting still more impudent? Are you getting impudent still more? How they attend, they do attend," and so on. At the end he scolds in quite inarticulate sounds.

The patient understands perfectly, and has introduced many phrases he has heard before into his speech, without once looking up. He speaks in an affected way, now babbling like a child, now lisping and stammering, sings suddenly in the middle of what he is saying, and grimaces. He carries out orders in an extraordinary fashion, gives his hand with the fist clenched, goes to the blackboard when he is asked, but, instead of writing his name, suddenly knocks down a lamp, and throws the chalk among the audience. He makes all kinds of senseless movements, pushes the table away, crosses his arms, and turns round on his axis, chair and all, or sits balancing, with his legs crossed and his hands on his head. Catalepsy can also be made out. When he is to go away, he will not get up, has to be pushed, and calls out loudly, "Good-morning, gentlemen; it has not pleased me."

. . . The patient himself was always quiet and very industrious, but of moderate mental endowment. Seven months ago, during the holidays, he suddenly began to learn in a quite senseless way, and then became confused, thought he was laughed at for being dirty, and washed himself all day long, was afraid his effects would be taken, broke the windows, seemed to hear voices, attacked his mother without any cause, became wet and dirty in his habits, and would not speak a word. In the hospital he was almost dumb, was cataleptic, gave his hand stiffly and jerkily, and almost entirely refused to eat. His expression was generally indifferent, though sometimes cheerful, and visits from his relations made no impression at all on him.

The patient understood quite well what was taking place around him, but as a rule he did not obey orders; indeed, he sometimes did the exact opposite of what was wanted. Thus, he shut his eyes when his pupils were mentioned, covered his face with his handkerchief if you wished to see it, and drew his hand back when he ought to have stretched it out. He was often dirty, and also smeared feces about, and rolled them into little balls—a sign diagnostic of great emotional dullness. After refusing food for a long time, he suddenly asked for Swiss cheese and then for chocolate, and devoured them both greedily. From this we can plainly see the senseless and impulsive nature of his refusal of food. Once he laid his outstretched leg on the next bed, and remained in that position when the bed was moved away. In the seventh month of the illness the patient began to be excited, after having sung occasionally during the period of dumbness. In the middle of the night he threw away his bedding, rocked rhythmically up and down on the bedstead, and screamed incessantly, "Now, I want to know where my brother is." Since then he has been in a continual state of excitement, is destructive and abusive, and talks in a confused way. He briefly informed his relations, from whom he takes the eatables they bring when they come to see him, without talking to them much, that he was going to travel by Gibraltar to the Cameroons and by Constantinople to Bucharest.

Kraepelin's Diagnosis: Catatonic Excitement

Discussion of "Oberrealschul Student"

In the absence of any known general medical condition that could account for the disturbance, the combination of disorganized speech and catatonic behavior (stupor and excitement) clearly indicates the diagnosis of Schizophrenia (DSM-IV-TR, p. 312). The diagnosis is further confirmed by the history of onset of symptoms 7 months previously, with a clear deterioration in functioning. Although the hyperactivity, confused speech, and irritability might suggest a Manic Episode, there is no description of a period with a persistent elevated, expansive, or irritable mood. Although the patient often is irritable and even violent, his mood seems to fluctuate unpredictably. In contrast, when irritability is seen in mania, it usually is a response to frustration of grandiosity or hyperactivity.

Although delusions and hallucinations have been present, the most prominent and persistent features are the disorganization of speech and behavior. The patient's frequent incoherence and grossly disorganized behavior are characteristic of the Disorganized Type of Schizophrenia. However, there are also numerous prominent examples of classic catatonic behavior: he exhibits negativism (e.g., refuses to do what is asked of him or does the opposite), catatonic excitement (e.g., excessive motor activity that is purposeless and not influenced by external stimuli), and posturing (e.g., kept his leg in an awkward position). In DSM-IV-TR, the Disorganized Type is not diagnosed if the clinical picture is dominated by catatonic symptoms, which represent more specific forms of disorganized behavior.

THE SUFFERING LADY

The young lady, aged 30, carefully dressed in black, who comes into the hall with short, shuffling steps, leaning on the nurse, and sinks into a chair as if exhausted, gives you the impression that she is ill. She is of slender build, her features are pale and rather painfully drawn, and her eyes are cast down. Her small, manicured fingers play nervously with a handkerchief. The patient answers the questions addressed to her in a low, tired voice, without looking up, and we find that she is quite clear about time, place, and her surroundings. After a few minutes, her eyes suddenly become convulsively shut, her head sinks forward, and she seems to have fallen into a deep sleep. Her arms have grown quite limp, and fall down as if palsied when you try to lift them. She has ceased to answer, and if you try to raise her eyelids, her eyes suddenly rotate upwards. Needlepricks only produce a slight shudder. But sprinkling with cold water is followed by a deep sigh; the patient starts up, opens her eyes, looks round her with surprise, and gradually comes to herself. She says that she has just had one of her sleeping attacks, from which she has suffered for 7 years. They come on quite irregularly, often many in one day, and last from a few minutes to half an hour.

Concerning the history of her life, the patient tells us that . . . she was educated in convent schools, and passed the examination for teachers. As a young girl, she inhaled a great deal of chloroform, which she was able to get secretly, for toothache. She also suffered from headaches, until they were relieved by the removal of growths from the nose. She very readily became delirious in feverish illnesses. Thirteen years ago she took a place as governess in Holland, but soon began to be ill, and has passed the last 7 years in different hospitals, except for a short interval when she was in a situation in Moravia.

It would appear from the statements of her relations and doctors that the patient has suffered from the most varied ailments, and been through the most remarkable courses of treatment. For violent abdominal pains and disturbances of menstruation, ascribed to stenosis of the cervical canal and retroflection of the uterus, recourse was had 5 years ago to the excision of the wedge supposed to cause the obstruction, and the introduction of a pessary. At a later period loss of voice and a contraction of the right forearm and the left thigh set in, and were treated with massage, electricity, bandaging, and stretching under an anaesthetic. Heart oppression and spasmodic breathing also appeared, with quickly passing disablements of various sets of muscles, disturbances of urination, diarrhea, and unpleasant sensations, now in one and now in another part of the body, but particularly headaches. Extraordinarily strong and sudden changes of mood were observed at the same time, with introspection and complaints of want of consideration in those about her and in her relations, although the latter had made the greatest sacrifices. Brine baths, Russian baths, pine-needle baths, electricity, country air, summer resorts, and finally, residence on the Riviera—everything was tried, generally with only a brief improvement or with none at all.

The immediate cause of the patient being brought to the hospital was the increase in the "sleeping attacks" 2 years ago. They came on at last even when the patient was standing, and might continue for an hour. The patient did not fall down, but simply leaned against something. The attacks continued in the hospital, and spasmodic breathing was also observed, which could be influenced by suggestion.

After spending 8 months here, the patient went away at first to her sister's. But after a few months she had to be taken to another asylum, where she stayed about a year, and then, after a short time spent with her family, came back to us.

During her present residence here, so-called "great attacks" have appeared, in addition to her previous troubles. We will try to produce such an attack by pressure on the very sensitive left ovarian region. After 1 or 2 minutes of moderately strong pressure, during which the patient shows sharp pain, her expression alters. She throws herself to and fro with her eyes shut, and screams to us loudly, generally in French, not to touch her. "You must not do anything to me, you hound, *cochon, cochon!*" She cries for help, pushes with her hands, and twists herself as if she were trying to escape from a sexual assault. Whenever she is touched, the excitement increases. Her whole body is strongly bent backwards. Suddenly the picture changes, and the patient begs piteously not to be cursed, and laments and sobs aloud. This condition, too, is very soon put an end to by sprinkling with cold water. The patient shudders, wakes with a deep sigh, and looks fixedly round, only making a tired, senseless impression. She cannot explain what has happened.

The physical examination of the patient shows no particular disturbances at present, except the abnormalities already mentioned. There is only a well-marked weakness, in consequence of which she often keeps to her bed or lies about. All her movements are limp and feeble, but there is no actual disablement anywhere. She often sleeps very badly. At times she wanders about in the night, wakes the nurses, and sends for the doctor. Her appetite is very poor, but she has a habit of nibbling between her meals at all kinds of cakes, fruit and jam, which are sent at her request, by her relations.

With her growing expertness in illness, the emotional sympathies of the patient are more and more confined to the selfish furthering of her own wishes. She tries ruthlessly to extort the most careful attention from those around her, obliges the doctor to occupy himself with her by day or night on the slightest occasion, is extremely sensitive to any supposed neglect, is jealous if preference is shown to other patients, and tries to make the attendants give in to her by complaints, accusations, and temper outbursts. The sacrifices made by others, more especially by her family, are regarded quite as a matter of course, and her occasional prodigality of thanks only serves to pave the way for new demands. To secure the sympathy of those around her, she has recourse to more and more forcible descriptions of her physical and mental torments, histrionic exaggeration of her attacks, and the effective elucidation of her personal character. She calls herself the abandoned, the outcast, and in mysterious hints makes confession of horrible, delightful experiences and failings, which she will confide only to the discreet bosom of her very best friend, the doctor.

Kraepelin's Diagnosis: Hysterical Insanity

Discussion of "The Suffering Lady"

Although Somatization Disorder (DSM-IV-TR, p. 490) was a new diagnostic category in DSM-III, this nineteenth-century case is a classic example of the disorder. There is a history of many physical symptoms and complaints, not adequately explained by a physical disorder or injury, that go back to the patient's adolescence. The DSM-IV-TR criteria for the disorder require unexplained symptoms in four areas: pain (four symptoms), gastrointestinal (two symptoms), sexual/reproductive (one symptom), and pseudoneurologic (one symptom). There are many references to multiple vague pain and gastrointestinal symptoms. She has had many pseudoneurologic (conversion) symptoms: loss of voice, seizures, trouble walking, and muscle weakness. There is reference to "disturbances of menstruation." As is commonly the case, genuine physical problems coexist but are hardly adequate to explain the myriad physical complaints.

The "sleeping attacks" represent periods of dissociation—that is, temporary alterations of consciousness not due to a substance or general medical condition—although in this case they are better thought of as pseudoneurologic symptoms of Somatization Disorder. Thus, the additional diagnosis of a Dissociative Disorder Not Otherwise Specified is not made.

Kraepelin's description of the way in which this woman relates to others is based on his observations of her current condition; however, it is reasonable to assume that it is characteristic of her long-term functioning. The vivid portrayal of the patient as someone who is self-centered, expresses emotion with exaggeration, displays rapidly shifting and shallow expression of emotions, and needs to be the center of attention is sufficient evidence for an additional diagnosis of Histrionic Personality Disorder (DSM-IV-TR, p. 714). Several features of Narcissistic Personality Disorder are also present: a sense of the uniqueness of her problems, entitlement, and interpersonal exploitation—but not the five symptoms required for a diagnosis. Nevertheless, we would have no quarrel with an additional provisional diagnosis of Narcissistic Personality

Disorder (DSM-IV-TR, p. 717) based on the suspicion that the patient might well have fantasies of ideal love with "her very best
friend, the doctor."

ONANISTIC STUDENT

You have before you today a strongly built and well-nourished man,
aged 21, who entered the hospital a few weeks ago. He sits quietly looking
in front of him, and does not raise his eyes when he is spoken to, but evidently understands all our questions very well, for he answers quite relevantly, though only slowly and often only after repeated questioning.
From his brief remarks, made in a low tone, we gather that he thinks he is
ill, without getting any more precise information about the nature of the illness and its symptoms. The patient attributes his malady to the onanism he
has practiced since he was 10 years old. He thinks that he has thus incurred
the guilt of a sin against the sixth commandment, has very much reduced
his power of working, has made himself feel languid and miserable, and
has become a hypochondriac. Thus, as the result of reading certain books,
he imagined that he had a rupture and suffered from wasting of the spinal
cord, neither of which was the case. He would not associate with his com-
rades any longer, because he thought they saw the results of his vice and
made fun of him. The patient makes all these statements in an indifferent
tone, without looking up or troubling about his surroundings. His expression betrays no emotion; he only laughs for a moment now and then.
There is occasional wrinkling of the forehead or facial spasm. Round the
mouth and nose a fine, changing twitching is constantly observed.

The patient gives us a correct account of his past experiences. His
knowledge speaks for the high degree of his education; indeed, he was
ready to enter the University a year ago. He also knows where he is and
how long he has been here, but he is only very imperfectly acquainted
with the names of the people round him, and says that he has never
asked about them. He can only give a very meager account of the general events of the last year. In answer to our questions, he declares that
he is ready to remain in the hospital for the present. He would certainly
prefer it if he could enter a profession, but he cannot say what he would
like to take up. . . . The patient makes his statements slowly and in
monosyllables, not because his wish to answer meets with overpowering

hindrances, but because he feels no desire to speak at all. He certainly hears and understands what is said to him very well, but he does not take the trouble to attend to it. He pays no heed, and answers whatever occurs to him without thinking. No visible effort of the will is to be noticed. All his movements are languid and expressionless, but are made without hindrance or trouble. There is no sign of emotional dejection, such as one would expect from the nature of his talk, and the patient remains quite dull throughout, experiencing neither fear nor hope nor desires. He is not at all deeply affected by what goes on before him, although he understands it without actual difficulty. It is all the same to him who appears or disappears where he is, or who talks to him and takes care of him, and he does not even once ask their names.

He broods, staring in front of him with expressionless features, over which a vacant smile occasionally plays, or at the best turns over the leaves of a book for a moment, apparently speechless, and not troubling about anything. Even when he has visitors, he sits without showing any interest, does not ask about what is happening at home, hardly even greets his parents, and goes back indifferently to the ward. He can hardly be induced to write a letter, and says that he has nothing to write about. But he occasionally composes a letter to the doctor, expressing all kinds of distorted, half-formed ideas, with a peculiar and silly play on words, in very fair style, but with little connection. He begs for "a little more allegro in the treatment," and "liberationary movement with a view to the widening of the horizon," will "ergo extort some wit in lectures," and "nota bene for God's sake only does not wish to be combined with the club of the harmless." "Professional work is the balm of life."

The development of the illness has been quite gradual. Our patient . . . did not go to school till he was 7 years old, as he was a delicate child and spoke badly, but when he did he learned quite well. He was considered to be a reserved and stubborn child. Having practiced onanism at a very early age, he became more and more solitary in the last few years, and thought that he was laughed at by his brothers and sisters, and shut out from society because of his ugliness. For this reason he could not bear a looking-glass in his room. After passing the written examination on leaving school, a year ago, he gave up the viva voce, because he could not work any longer. He cried a great deal, masturbated much, ran about aimlessly, played in a senseless way on the piano, and began to write observations "On the Nerve-play of life," which he cannot get on with. He was incapable of any kind of work, even physical, felt "done for," asked for a revolver, ate Swedish matches to destroy himself, and lost all affection for his family. From time to time he became excited and troublesome, and shouted out of the window at night. In the hospital, too, a state of excitement lasting for several days was observed, in which he chattered in a confused way, made faces, ran about at full speed, wrote disconnected scraps of composition, and crossed and recrossed them with flourishes and unmeaning combinations of letters. After this a state of tranquility ensued, in which he could give absolutely no account of his extraordinary behavior.

Kraepelin's Diagnosis: Dementia Praecox (Insanity of Adolescence)

Discussion of "Onanistic Student"

The most prominent features of the illness are delusions of guilt (e.g., his onanism has caused his illness), persecutory delusions (e.g., "he thought [his comrades] saw the results of his vice and made fun of him"), incoherence, and flat and inappropriate affect (e.g., "His expression betrays no emotion; he only laughs for a moment now and then"). These features, the absence of a general medical condition that could account for the disturbance, and the chronic nature of the illness establish the diagnosis of Schizophrenia (DSM-IV-TR, p. 312).

If this patient were seen at the time that he "chattered in a confused way, made faces, ran about at full speed," the appropriate subtype might be Catatonic or Disorganized. At the point at which he was presented by Kraepelin, he was neither frequently incoherent nor excited; therefore, the appropriate subtype is Undifferentiated (DSM-IV-TR, p. 316).

The initial description of the patient might lead some clinicians to consider the possibility of a Major Depressive Episode: psychomotor retardation, delusions of guilt, and hypochondriacal preoccupation are present. However, as Kraepelin later notes, "There is no sign of emotional dejection, such as one would expect from the nature of his talk."

FACTORY GIRL

The factory girl, aged 32, who now comes into the room with an awkward and very deep curtsy, presents an entirely different aspect from the last patient. She declines to sit down to talk to us, thanks us for the "honor," goes up and down with affected, waddling steps, and begins to declaim and recite verses, and to interpolate witty remarks in our discussion of her condition. Her name is what the parson christened her, and she is as old as her little finger. She knows her position, the date, where she is, and the people around her, and can give the most exact information about her past experiences. She does not consider herself insane. She often interweaves her disconnected talk with scraps of bad French and senselessly altered quotations, such as "Ingratitude is the world's praise"; "Many hands, many minds." She rides single phrases to death in uninterrupted repetition— "Devil's dung on the soul's foot, the soul's foot in devil's dung." She often uses very strange and almost incomprehensible compound words and phrases.

Her mood is silly, cheerful, sometimes erotic, and then again irritable. She takes pleasure in the most indecent sexual allusions, and occasionally in outbursts of the wildest abuse. She does not obey orders, and refuses to give her hand on the ground that they are her hands. She will not write, and pertly refuses to do anything she is asked. She chatters continually, and will not let anyone get in a word. Her speech is extremely laboured. She cuts the separate syllables sharply asunder, accentuates the final syllables sharply, pronounces *g* like *k,* and *d* like *t,* talks like a child, in imperfectly formed sentences, distorts words, inserts senseless expletives and strangely formed words, and constantly changes the subject. All her movements and gestures are clumsy, angular, and stiff, and are very lavishly employed, but monotonous; she hops about, bends down, claps her hands and makes faces. She has ornamented her clothes in an extraordinary way with embroidery and crochet-work of startingly bright wool. From her talk it appears that she looks on herself as the mistress of the house; she pays the nurses and appoints them, and will get herself better doctors. Moreover, she complains of being exposed to sexual assaults, and says that her lungs, heart, and liver have been taken out. She says she is engaged to a doctor in the asylum where she was before. She tells her name with the prefix "von." She also seems to have heard voices, but will only make evasive statements about them.

The patient . . . was considered very selfish and obstinate . . . from her youth up. She was first a servant girl and then a factory hand, had two illegitimate children, and then aborted once. About 6 months later, 2 years ago now, she saw gray men and women's heads, and heard knocking and voices which called abusive words to her. Later on she wrote a love-letter to the proprietor of her factory, and was dismissed and picked up helpless on the street. When taken to an asylum, she was quiet and collected at first, but soon had brief attacks of the most violent excitement, during which she undressed herself completely, hit out round her in a senseless way, and bit. Later on she showed a repellent, discontented disposition and a tendency to stereotypism and impulsive actions. When she was brought here a year and a quarter ago she presented the same picture as now in all essential features. It should perhaps be added that she showed echopraxis, followed the same track—a figure of eight, for instance—for hours in the garden, and was very refractory. For a long time she had to be kept quite alone in the garden and in her room, because, though quite collected and free from great emotional excitement, she was very dangerous to the other patients.

Kraepelin's Diagnosis: Catatonic Excitement

Discussion of "Factory Girl"

This case indicates how difficult it is to distinguish the excitement seen in the Catatonic Type of Schizophrenia from that seen in a Manic Episode. This woman has many symptoms that suggest the manic syndrome. Her mood is described as alternately silly, cheerful, and irritable. There are pressure of speech (e.g., "She chatters continually, and will not let anyone get in a word") and hyperactivity (e.g., "she hops about, bends down, claps her hands"). She is also grandiose (e.g., "she looks on herself as the mistress of the house; she pays the nurses and appoints them") and sexually provocative.

We are told that for some unspecified period before the excitement began, there were persecutory hallucinations, apparently not accompanied by any disturbance in mood. Assuming that this period was longer than 2 weeks, according to DSM-IV-TR this would rule out the diagnosis of Bipolar I Disorder and would suggest the diagnosis of Schizoaffective Disorder or Schizophrenia. Whether the diagnosis of Schizophrenia is made depends on the duration of the mood syndrome in relation to the total duration of the active and residual periods. If the mood syndrome is relatively brief, the diagnosis is Schizophrenia; if not, it is Schizoaffective Disorder. Since we are told that this patient is pretty much the same now as she has been for the year that she has been in the hospital, we would conclude that the manic syndrome has not been brief and diagnose Schizoaffective Disorder, Bipolar Type (DSM-IV-TR, p. 323). An important implication now for such a diagnosis is that it would suggest the advisability of a trial of lithium therapy.

Kraepelin notes the primary disturbance as one of behavior rather than mood. He emphasizes the negativism (e.g., "She does not obey orders . . . and pertly refuses to do anything she is asked"), stereotypism (e.g., "she . . . followed the same track—a figure of eight, for instance—for hours in the garden"), and mannerisms (e.g., "All her movements and gestures are clumsy, angular, and stiff, and are very lavishly employed"). These features, plus the "attacks of the most violent excitement," disorganized speech, and lack of any deep emotion, led him to make a diagnosis of Catatonic Excitement, which he believed was a form of what we now call Schizophrenia.

Many clinicians (particularly those trained before DSM-III) would agree with Kraepelin's diagnosis of Schizophrenia because they would question the description of the patient's excitement as a manic syndrome, considering the mood to be more shallow and silly than elevated or expansive. They would also point to the incoherence, grossly disorganized behavior, hallucinations, and inappropriate affect in an illness that has lasted continually for more than 2 years (unusual in Bipolar I Disorder) and that represents a distinct change from the patient's usual level of functioning.

Catatonic symptoms, if not due to a general medical condition or substance, used to be regarded as pathognomonic of Schizophrenia. It is now recognized that catatonic symptoms may also be seen in a manic syndrome (as in this case, we think) and in a Manic Episode of Bipolar I Disorder (see "A Praying Athlete," p. 209).

EUGEN BLEULER (1857–1939)

Bleuler, a Swiss psychiatrist, coined the term Schizophrenia *to describe what he considered to be the fundamental disturbance—a splitting of the psychic functions that, in extreme cases, leads to disorganization of the personality. Whereas Kraepelin by and large limited himself to describing the clinical picture and course of the illness, Bleuler attempted to understand the underlying psychopathologic process as well. He differed from Kraepelin in maintaining that deterioration was not characteristic of the illness. He added a subtype, Simple, which he believed occurred as frequently as the other subtypes, although it was rarely seen in hospitals.*

The following case is taken verbatim from a translation of his major work, Dementia Praecox or the Group of Schizophrenias.[*]

DOMESTIC TYRANT

A normal, intelligent girl marries at 20 and lives happily for more than 5 years. Very gradually she becomes irritable, gesticulates while talking, her peculiarities continue to increase; she cannot keep a servant anymore; she is constantly quarreling with her neighbors. Within her own family group, she has developed into an unbearable domestic tyrant who knows no duties, only rights. She is unable to manage the household or do the housework anymore because she makes all kinds of silly, stupid, and useless purchases and is proving herself utterly impractical. During the many years in which she is in the hospital, she exhibits the same behavior only in increasing measure, so that it is only possible to keep her either in her own room or outdoors where there are very few people. However, after some 10 years of hospitalization, she can be released although she still causes trouble by her gossiping and disagreeableness. She complains continually of some vague nervous troubles because, as she says, she was not properly treated in the hospital. Yet she is entirely indifferent to important things such as her relations to her family, etc. She has no love for her children. She is incapable of pulling herself together although she knows quite well that she could have a very decent life if she were less of a nag and a scold. There were no traces of paranoid or catatonic symptoms.

---

[*] Bleuler E: *Dementia Praecox or the Group of Schizophrenias,* first published in 1911.

Bleuler's Diagnosis: Simple Schizophrenia

Discussion of "Domestic Tyrant"

According to the information available, this woman functioned well until she was 25. She then developed a progressively incapacitating illness characterized by poor judgment, irritability, and indifference to others. No psychotic symptoms, disorders of mood, or symptoms suggesting a dementia are described. This peculiar picture corresponds to no DSM-IV-TR Axis I disorder! Many of the features of her illness suggest a severe Personality Disorder, but Bleuler's description of her as living "happily" until her illness began at age 25 suggests a distinct change in functioning. This is inconsistent with the concept of a Personality Disorder, since manifestations of a Personality Disorder are generally recognizable by adolescence or earlier. We are therefore left with the rather unsatisfying but accurate diagnosis of Unspecified Mental Disorder (Nonpsychotic) (DSM-IV-TR, p. 743).

Bleuler was able to diagnose this patient as having Schizophrenia because he emphasized the "primary symptoms" (e.g., disturbances of association and affect, ambivalence, and autism) and did not require, as does DSM-IV-TR, the presence of psychotic symptoms, such as delusions or hallucinations. We suspect that a clinician interviewing this patient today would uncover either evidence of some period with psychotic symptoms, suggesting Schizophrenia, or an earlier onset, suggesting a severe Personality Disorder, or perhaps both.

ALOIS ALZHEIMER (1864–1915)

Alzheimer was a German neuropathologist who investigated the relationship between anatomic changes in the brain and mental disorder. In 1907 he described a deceased patient from the insane asylum in Frankfurt am Main whose nervous system had been given to him for investigation because the patient presented with an unusual clinical picture that could not be categorized under any of the known diseases.

PERPLEXED WOMAN[*]

A woman, 51 years old, showed jealousy toward her husband as the first noticeable sign of the disease. Soon a rapidly increasing loss of memory could be noticed. She could not find her way around in her own apartment. She carried objects back and forth and hid them. At times she would think that someone wanted to kill her and would begin shrieking loudly.

In the institution her entire behavior bore the stamp of utter perplexity. She was totally disoriented to time and place. Occasionally she stated that she could not understand and did not know her way around. At times she greeted the doctor like a visitor, and excused herself for not having finished her work; at times she shrieked loudly that he wanted to cut her, or repulsed him with indignation, saying that she feared from him something against her chastity. Periodically she was totally delirious, dragged her bedding around, called her husband and her daughter, and seemed to have auditory hallucinations. Frequently, she shrieked with a dreadful voice for many hours.

Because of her inability to comprehend the situation, she always cried out loudly as soon as someone tried to examine her. Only through repeated attempts was it possible finally to ascertain anything.

Her ability to remember was severely disturbed. If one pointed to objects, she named most of them correctly, but immediately afterwards she would forget everything again. When reading, she went from one line into another, reading the letters or reading with a senseless emphasis. When writing, she repeated individual syllables several times, left out others, and quickly became stranded. When talking, she frequently used perplexing phrases and some paraphrastic expressions (milk-pourer instead of cup). Sometimes one noticed her getting stuck. Some questions she obviously did not comprehend. She seemed no longer to understand the use of some objects. Her gait was not impaired. She could use both hands equally well. Her patellar reflexes were present. Her pupils reacted. Somewhat rigid radial arteries; no enlargement of cardiac dullness; no albumin.

During her subsequent course, the phenomena that were interpreted as focal symptoms were at times more noticeable and at times less noticeable. But always they were only slight. The generalized dementia

[*]From Wilkins RH, Brody IA: "Alzheimer's Disease." *Archives of Neurology* 21:109–110, 1969.

progressed however. After 4½ years of the disease, death occurred. At the end, the patient was completely stuporous; she lay in her bed with her legs drawn up under her, and in spite of all precautions she acquired decubitus ulcers.

Alzheimer's Diagnosis: A Peculiar Disease of the Cerebral Cortex

Discussion of "Perplexed Woman"

The first sign of the illness was apparently delusional jealousy. Persecutory delusions, and possibly auditory hallucinations, developed later. However, the more significant disturbance is the gradual development of a progressive Dementia with marked impairment in immediate and recent memory, disorientation to time and place, and many signs of disturbed higher cortical functioning. For example, her use of "paraphrastic expressions (milk-pourer instead of cup)" indicates aphasia, and her inability to understand the use of some objects indicates agnosia.

Alzheimer refers to her as periodically being "totally delirious," although he may have been referring more to periods of agitation and excitement than to a disturbance of consciousness, which is a requirement for the DSM-IV-TR concept of Delirium.

The evidence of a Dementia with insidious onset and a generally progressive deteriorating course, plus the exclusion of all other specific causes of the Dementia, indicates Dementia of the Alzheimer's Type (DSM-IV-TR, p. 157). Because the illness began before the patient was 65, With Early Onset is noted, and because of the prominent behavioral disturbance (e.g., agitation), the subtype With Behavioral Disturbance is noted. Furthermore, Psychotic Disorder Due to Alzheimer's Disease, With Delusions, is also diagnosed because of the delusional jealousy.

The historical significance of this case is that it was the first one in which microscopic examination of the brain revealed the characteristic histopathologic changes of what has become known as Alzheimer's disease: senile plaques, neurofibrillary tangles, and granulovacuolar degeneration of neurons. The neurologic disorder Alzheimer's disease is recorded on Axis III.

JOSEF BREUER (1842–1925)

Breuer was a Viennese physician who collaborated with Freud in using hypnosis to treat patients with hysteria. The case of "Anna O." was abstracted from Breuer and Freud's Studies in Hysteria.[*] *Anna O. was treated and her case reported by Breuer. It was the case that suggested to Freud the possibility of a "talking cure"—later known as psychoanalysis.*

ANNA O.

Anna O. was the only daughter of a wealthy Viennese Jewish family. She became ill when she was 21, in 1880.

> Up to the onset of the disease, the patient showed no sign of nervousness, not even during pubescence. She had a keen, intuitive intellect, a craving for psychic fodder, which she did not, however, receive after she left school. She was endowed with a sensitiveness for poetry and fantasy, which was, however, controlled by a very strong and critical mind. . . . Her will was energetic, impenetrable and persevering, sometimes mounting to selfishness; it relinquished its aim only out of kindness and for the sake of others. . . . Her moods always showed a slight tendency to an excess of merriment or sadness, which made her more or less temperamental. . . . With her puritanically minded family, this girl of overflowing mental vitality led a most monotonous existence.

She spent hours daydreaming, making up fanciful plots in what she called her "private theatre." She was at times so engrossed in fantasy that she did not hear when people spoke to her.

In July 1880, her father, whom she admired and "loved passionately," developed tuberculosis. From July through November Anna was his night nurse, sitting up with him every night, observing his pain and deterioration, with the knowledge that he would not recover.

Her own health eventually began to decline:

> [S]he became very weak, anemic, and evinced a disgust for nourishment, so that despite her marked reluctance, it was found necessary to take her away from the sick man. The main reason for this step was a

---

[*] From Breuer J, Freud S: *Studies in Hysteria* (1895). Translated by Brill AA. Boston, MA, Beacon Press, 1937, p. 14.

very intensive cough about which I [Breuer] was first consulted. I found that she had a typical nervous cough. Soon, there also developed a striking need for rest, distinctly noticeable in the afternoon hours, which merged in the evening into a sleep-like state, followed by strong excitement. . . . From the eleventh of December until the first of April the patient remained bedridden.

In rapid succession there seemingly developed a series of new and severe disturbances.

Left-sided occipital pain; convergent strabismus (diplopia), which was markedly aggravated through excitement. She complained that the wall was falling over (obliquus affection). Profound analyzable visual disturbances, paresis of the anterior muscles of the throat, to the extent that the head could finally be moved only if the patient pressed it backward between her raised shoulders and then moved her whole back. Contractures and anesthesia of the right upper extremity, and somewhat later of the right lower extremity. . . .

It was in this condition that I took the patient under treatment, and I soon became convinced that we were confronted with a severe psychic alteration. There were two entirely separate states of consciousness, which alternated very frequently and spontaneously, moving further apart during the course of the disease. In one of them she knew her environment, was sad and anxious, but relatively normal; in the other, she hallucinated, was "naughty"—i.e., she scolded, threw the pillows at people whenever and to what extent her contractures enabled her to, and tore with her movable fingers the buttons from the covers and underwear, etc. If anything had been changed in the room during this phase, if someone entered, or went out, she then complained that she was lacking in time, and observed the gap in the lapse of her conscious ideas. . . . In very clear moments she complained of the deep darkness in her head, that she could not think, that she was going blind and deaf, and that she had two egos, her real and an evil one, which forced her to evil things, etc. . . . there appeared a deep, functional disorganization of her speech. At first, it was noticed that she missed words; gradually, when this increased, her language was devoid of all grammar, all syntax, to the extent that the whole conjugation of verbs was wrong. . . . In the further course of this development she missed words almost continuously, and searched for them laboriously in four or five languages, so that one could hardly understand her. . . . She spoke only English and understood nothing that was told her in German. The people about her were forced to speak English. . . . There then followed 2 weeks of complete mutism. Continuous effort to speak elicited no sound.

About ten days after her father died, a consultant was called in, whom she ignored as completely as all strangers, while I demonstrated to him her peculiarities. . . . It was a real "negative hallucination," which has so often been reproduced experimentally since then. He finally succeeded in attracting her attention by blowing smoke into her face. She then suddenly saw a stranger, rushed to the door, grabbed the key, but fell to the floor unconscious. This was followed by a short outburst of anger, and then by a severe attack of anxiety, which I could calm only with a great deal of effort.

The family was afraid Anna would jump from the window, so she was removed from her third-floor apartment to a country house, where for 3 days "she remained sleepless, took no nourishment, and was full of suicidal ideas." She also broke windows, etc., and evinced hallucinations [of black snakes, death's heads, etc.] without *absences* [dissociated periods].

Breuer treated Anna by asking her, under hypnosis, to talk about her symptoms, a technique she referred to as "chimney sweeping." As the treatment proceeded, she had longer periods of lucidity and began to lose her symptoms. After 18 months of treatment, as Anna prepared to spend the summer in her country home, Breuer pronounced her well and said he would no longer be seeing her. That evening he was called back to the house, where he found Anna thrashing around in her bed, going through an imaginary childbirth. She insisted that the baby was Breuer's. He managed to calm her by hypnotizing her. According to Ernest Jones, Breuer then "fled the house in a cold sweat" and never saw her again.

Anna remained ill intermittently over the next 6 years, spending considerable time in a sanatorium, where she apparently became addicted to morphine. She was often fairly well in the daytime, but still suffered from hallucinatory states toward evening.

By 30 she had apparently completely recovered and moved to Frankfort with her mother. There she became a feminist leader and social worker. She established an institution for "wayward girls" and spoke out against the devaluation of women that she believed was inherent in orthodox Judaism.

Anna never married, but was said to be an attractive and passionate woman who gathered admirers wherever she went. She had no recurrences of her illness and never spoke about it—in fact, she apparently asked her relatives not to speak of it to anyone. In her later years her attitude toward psychoanalysis was clearly negative, and she became quite angry at the suggestion that one of her "girls" be psychoanalyzed.

Anna died at 77 of abdominal cancer.

Breuer's Diagnosis: Hysteria

Discussion of "Anna O."

Anna O. presents a clinical picture that was apparently seen with some frequency in consulting rooms in the Victorian period. We doubt that many clinicians at the present time see patients quite like Anna O. For this reason, DSM-IV-TR does not have a single category that would encompass the variety of symptoms and the often chronic course that correspond to the traditional concept of Hysteria. Anna O. is therefore a diagnostic enigma for today's clinician.

Anna becomes depressed after her father's death: "she remained sleepless, took no nourishment, and was full of suicidal ideas." We are reluctant to make a diagnosis of a Major Depressive Episode since this severe condition apparently lasted only a few days.

The most striking feature of Anna's illness, and the reason for Breuer's being called in on the case, was the numerous physical symptoms: cough, left-sided occipital pain, convergent strabismus, visual disturbance, weakness of throat muscles, contractures, and anesthesia of the extremities. If we assume that Breuer had correctly ruled out a general medical condition as the cause of these symptoms, they indicate a Conversion Disorder (DSM-IV-TR, p. 498).

Her "sleep-like state[s]," going through an imaginary childbirth, and alternating states of consciousness all indicate a Dissociative Disorder; but since the description does not correspond to any of the specific DSM-IV-TR Dissociative Disorders, the diagnosis must be Dissociative Disorder Not Otherwise Specified (DSM-IV-TR, p. 532).

Anna had many other symptoms that suggest a psychotic disorder—disorganized speech (e.g., "her language was devoid of all grammar, all syntax, to the extent that the whole conjugation of verbs was wrong"), hallucinations (e.g., of black snakes and death's heads), and possible delusions (e.g., she complained that she "had two egos, her real and an evil one, which forced her to do evil things"). Because of these seemingly psychotic symptoms, rigid use of the DSM-IV-TR criteria might lead to a diagnosis of Schizophrenia. However, this diagnosis fails to capture the essence of Anna O.'s illness. The problem is that DSM-IV-TR does not recognize "hysterical" psychotic symptoms, with the exception of the category Factitious Disorder with Psychological Symptoms. Did Anna O. intentionally produce her symptoms, as in a Factitious Disorder? Certainly Breuer and Freud did not think so. We also doubt that Anna O. "decided" to produce her various symptoms.

If forced to give a DSM-IV-TR diagnosis that would account for these "psychotic" symptoms, we would add Psychotic Disorder Not Otherwise Specified (DSM-IV-TR, p. 343), thereby indicating the unusual nature of her psychotic disorder. Admittedly, the approach taken here fragments Anna O.'s illness into several different diagnoses, each of which describes a different phase.

SIGMUND FREUD (1856–1939)

Sigmund Freud, the originator of psychoanalysis, attempted to explain the mechanisms by which unconscious conflicts result in the clinical manifestations of psychopathology. The cases that follow have been edited to focus on the descriptive features rather than on the psychodynamic explanations of the symptoms. These cases, first published between 1909 and 1911, were abstracted from Volume 3 of Freud's collected papers.

LITTLE HANS

Little Hans's parents were friends and early followers of Freud who had agreed to bring up their first child with "no more coercion than might be absolutely necessary for maintaining good behavior. And, as the child developed into a cheerful, good-natured, and lively little boy, the experiment of letting him grow up and express himself without being intimidated went on satisfactorily."

Freud asked Hans's father to collect observations on the sexual life of his child and received frequent letters reporting on Hans, beginning just before his third birthday. All went well until Hans was nearly 5, at which time Freud received the following letter from his father:

My dear Professor, I am sending you a little more about Hans—but this

---

*From *The Collected Papers of Sigmund Freud,* Vol 3. Edited by Jones E. Translated by Strachey J, Strachey A. New York, Basic Books, 1959. "Little Hans," p. 149; "The Rat Man," p. 296; "Dr. Schreber," p. 390.

time, I am sorry to say, material for a case history. As you will see, during the last few days he has developed a nervous disorder, which has made my wife and me most uneasy, because we have not been able to find any means of dissipating it. . . . No doubt the ground was prepared by sexual over-excitation due to his mother's tenderness; but I am not able to specify the actual exciting cause. He is afraid *that a horse will bite him in the street,* and this fear seems somehow to be connected with his having been frightened by a large penis. . . . I cannot see what to make of it. Has he seen an exhibitionist somewhere? Or is the whole thing simply connected with his mother? It is not very pleasant for us that he should begin setting us problems so early. Apart from his being afraid of going into the street and from his being depressed in the evening, he is in other respects the same Hans, as bright and cheerful as ever.

It was some months later that Hans remembered an incident that had, in fact, occurred just before his symptoms began. He had been walking with his mother and had been frightened when a large horse pulling a bus had fallen down and kicked its feet around violently.

The first evidence of the disturbance was noticed in early January (1908): "Hans woke up one morning in tears. Asked why he was crying, he said to his mother: 'When I was asleep I thought you were gone and I had no Mummy to cuddle with.'" Several days later, on January 7,

[Hans] went to the Stadtpark with his nursemaid as usual. In the street he began to cry and asked to be taken home, saying that he wanted to "cuddle" with his Mummy. At home he was asked why he had refused to go any further and had cried, but he would not say. Till the evening he was cheerful, as usual. But in the evening he grew visibly frightened; he cried and could not be separated from his mother, and wanted to "cuddle" with her again. Then he grew cheerful again and slept well.

On January 8 my wife decided to go out with him herself, so as to see what was wrong with him. They went to Schonbrunn, where he always likes going. Again he began to cry, did not want to start, and was frightened. In the end he did go, but was visibly frightened in the street. On the way back from Schonbrunn he said to his mother, after much internal struggling: "I was afraid a horse would bite me." (He had, in fact, become uneasy at Schonbrunn when he saw a horse.) In the evening he seemed to have had another attack similar to that of the previous evening, and to have wanted to be "cuddled." He was calmed down. He said, crying: "I know I shall have to go for a walk again tomorrow." And later: "The horse'll come into the room."

On Freud's instructions, Hans's father had some discussion with the little boy about his desire to be taken into his mother's bed and his excessive interest in "widdlers"—his own and everyone else's.

There ensued a fairly quiet period during which Hans could be persuaded to walk in the park, but felt compelled to look at the horses: "I have to look at horses, and then I'm frightened."

After 2 weeks in bed with influenza, and then a tonsillectomy, his phobia became much worse. "He goes out on to the balcony, it is true, but not for a walk. As soon as he gets to the street door he hurriedly turns round."

In late March, with some persuasion, he consented to go to the zoo with his father. There he was afraid of the large animals but not the small ones and would not even look at the elephant or the giraffe. "During the next few days it seemed as though his fears had again somewhat increased. He hardly ventured out of the front door, to which he was taken after luncheon."

It was during this period that there was much discussion between father and son about Hans's masturbation, about the nature of the female sexual apparatus, and about Hans's desire to get into bed and "cuddle" with his mother.

Freud had one session with Hans, during which he made a connection between the white horses that Hans was particularly afraid of and Hans's father, and explained to Hans that he was afraid of his father "precisely because he was so fond of his mother."

In subsequent weeks Hans alluded to his fear that his mother and father would go away and leave him.

Over a period of some months, Hans's symptoms disappeared, and he became closer to his father. Freud saw Hans only once again, when he was "a strapping youth of nineteen" who "suffered from no troubles or inhibitions." He had no memory of the anxiety, the phobia, or the analysis.

Freud's Diagnosis: Phobia

Discussion of "Little Hans"

There can be little doubt that Hans has a phobia. He has a persistent excessive fear of and compelling desire to avoid horses. Since the dreaded object does not involve a fear of having a panic attack, of being in situations or public places from which escape is impossible, or of being in social situations with the possibility of public humiliation or embarrassment, this is a Specific Phobia (DSM-IV-TR, p. 449).

There are other important features. Hans has nightmares about being separated from his mother ("When I was asleep I thought you [his mother] were gone and I had no Mummy to cuddle with"). In the evenings, when anticipating going to bed, he is extremely distressed, perhaps to the point of panic, and cannot be separated from his mother. Finally, he has an unrealistic fear that his parents will "go away and leave him." These are all expressions of excessive anxiety concerning separation from his parents and together support the additional diagnosis of Separation Anxiety Disorder (DSM-IV-TR, p. 125).

THE RAT MAN

A youngish man of university education introduced himself to [Freud] with the statement that he had suffered from obsessions ever since his childhood, but with particular intensity for the last 4 years. The chief features of his disorder were *fears* that something might happen to two people of whom he was very fond—his father and a lady whom he admired. Besides this he was aware of *compulsive impulses*—such as an impulse, for instance, to cut his throat with a razor; and further he produced *prohibitions,* sometimes in connection with quite unimportant things. He had wasted years, he told me, in fighting against these ideas of his, and in this way had lost much ground in the course of his life. He had tried various treatments, but none had been of any use to him.

The experience that precipitated this patient's first visit to Freud occurred when he was on maneuvers with a military unit. An officer had described to him a form of torture in which the prisoner was tied up, a pot of rats was turned upside down on his buttocks, and the rats bored their way into his anus. He reported: "At that moment the idea flashed through my mind *that this was happening to a person very dear to me"* (in fact, to the lady he loved, and to his father, who had actually died 9 years before). When the officer had spoken of this ghastly punishment, and the obsessions had come into his head, he had warded them off by employing a particular "formula." He said to himself, "But," accompanied by a gesture of repudiation, and then, "Whatever are you thinking of?"

> That evening, he continued, the same Captain had handed him a packet that had arrived by the post and had said: "Lt. A. has paid the charges for you. You must pay him back." . . . At that instant, however, a "sanction" had taken shape in his mind, namely, *that he was not to pay back the money* or it would happen—(that is, the fantasy about the rats would come true as regards his father and the lady). And immediately, in accordance with a type of procedure with which he was familiar [to make sure the fantasy would not come true], there had arisen a command in the shape of a vow: "You must pay back the 3.8 crowns to Lt. A.". He had said these words to himself almost half aloud.

The necessity of obeying his vow sent him on a complicated journey during which he went in search of Lt. A. He discovered that Lt. A. was not, in fact, the one who had paid the charges. He therefore devised numerous complicated schemes in order to follow the exact wording of his vow (that is, pay back the 3.8 crowns to Lt. A.) even though it was now clear that he did not owe the money to Lt. A.

The first instances of obsessive thoughts had occurred when the patient was 6 or 7. As he grew older, they waxed and waned, but they had now persisted since his father's death. Freud describes the "exciting cause" of his incapacitation as follows:

After his father's death the patient's mother proposed that he marry a wealthy cousin, thus ensuring

> a business connection with the firm [that] would offer him a brilliant opening in his profession. This family plan stirred up in him a conflict as to whether he should remain faithful to the lady he loved in spite of her poverty, or whether he should follow in his father's footsteps and marry the lovely, rich, and well-connected girl who had been assigned to him. And he resolved his conflict, which was in fact one between his love and the persisting influence of his father's wishes, by falling ill; or, to put it more correctly, by falling ill he avoided the task of resolving it in real life. . . . the chief result of this illness was an obstinate incapacity for work, which allowed him to postpone the completion of his education for years.

Freud relates numerous examples of his patient's obsessions and compulsions in relation to his "lady":

[A]s they were sitting together during a thunderstorm, he was obsessed, he could not tell why, with the necessity for counting up to 40 or 50 between each flash of lightning and its accompanying thunder-clap. On the day of [the lady's] departure he knocked his foot against a stone lying in the road, and was *obliged* to put it out of the way by the side of the road, because the idea struck him that her carriage would be driving along the same road in a few hours' time and might come to grief against this stone. But a few minutes later it occurred to him that this was absurd, and he was *obliged* to go back and replace the stone in its original position in the middle of the road. After her departure he became a prey to an *obsession for understanding,* which made him a curse to all his companions. He forced himself to understand the precise meaning of every syllable that was addressed to him, as though he might otherwise be missing some priceless treasure. Accordingly he kept asking: "What was it you said just then?" And after it had been repeated to him he could not help thinking it had sounded different the first time, so he remained dissatisfied.

Freud's analysis focused on the patient's ambivalence toward his father and his lady, originating in his precocious and intense sexuality and early feelings of rage against his father—both of which had been severely repressed. The rat symbol led Freud and his patient through a series of associations that included anal eroticism, the patient's having been beaten by his father at age 4 for biting someone, the father's early problems with gambling [in German a gambler is a *Spielratte* [or "play-rat"], the infantile notion of anal birth, and the patient's own real childhood experience of having worms. After a year of analysis, the patient was cured of his symptoms and, in Freud's words, "the rat delirium disappeared."

Freud's Diagnosis: Obsessive-Compulsive Neurosis

Discussion of "The Rat Man"

The Rat Man is plagued by both obsessions and compulsions. The obsessions are recurrent, persistent ideas (e.g., that something terrible will happen to his sweetheart), impulses (e.g., to cut his throat), and images (e.g., that a rat is boring into the anus of his father). He experiences them as intrusive and inappropriate (ego-dystonic) and evolves complicated formulas in an effort to neutralize them (e.g., "He said to himself: 'But,' accompanied by a gesture of repudiation, and then, 'Whatever are you thinking of?'"). He recognizes that the obsessions are products of his own mind.

The compulsions are repetitive, purposeful behaviors that are performed according to certain rules and are designed to prevent some dreaded future event (e.g., he had to remove a stone from the road so that his sweetheart's carriage would not "come to grief against this stone"). As with the obsessions, he recognizes that the behavior is unreasonable, in that it is not connected in a realistic way with what it is designed to prevent. In addition, he derives no pleasure from carrying out the compulsion, other than the release of tension.

Minor obsessions and compulsions that do not cause significant distress or interfere with social or role functioning do not warrant a diagnosis. However, the Rat Man has "wasted years . . . in fighting against these ideas." Thus, a diagnosis of Obsessive-Compulsive Disorder (DSM-IV-TR, p. 462) is indicated. Obsessive-Compulsive Disorder is often seen in people with Obsessive-Compulsive Personality Disorder. However, in this case there is no description of the patient's personality functioning, apart from the symptoms of his Obsessive-Compulsive Disorder.

DR. SCHREBER

In 1903, a German judge, Dr. Daniel Paul Schreber, published his own case history, translated as *Memoirs of a Neurotic*. Freud made his analytic interpretations of the connection between unconscious homosexuality and paranoia on the basis of this document and a report prepared by Dr. Schreber's physician for a mental competency hearing. Freud quotes at length from both.

All we know about Dr. Schreber's first illness, in 1884, is that it was diagnosed as an "attack of severe hypochondria," from which he recovered completely after 6 months, and he returned to his wife and his judicial position. It is unclear how old he was at this time; but since he was already married and had some status in his profession, he cannot have been very young. Subsequent to this illness he was elected to a high judicial position.

The second illness, in 1893, began with the idea that he was to be transformed into a woman. In Dr. Schreber's words,

> A conspiracy against me was brought to a head. . . . Its object was to contrive that, when once my nervous complaint had been recognized as incurable or assumed to be so, I should be handed over to a certain person in a particular manner. Thus my soul was to be delivered up to him, but my body. . . . was to be transformed into a female body, and as such surrendered to the person in question with a view to sexual abuse, and was then simply to be "left where it was"—that is to say, no doubt, abandoned to corruption.

Dr. Weber, the director of the Sonnenstein Sanatorium in which Schreber was a patient, described his condition as follows:

> He was chiefly troubled by hypochondriacal ideas, complained that he had softening of the brain, that he would soon be dead, etc. But ideas of persecution were already finding their way into the clinical picture, based upon sensorial illusions which, however, seemed only to appear sporadically at first, while simultaneously a high degree of hyperaesthesia was observable—great sensitiveness to light and noise. Later, the visual and auditory illusions became much more frequent. . . . He believed that he was dead and decomposing, that he was suffering from the plague; he asserted that his body was being handled in all kinds of revolting ways; and, as he himself declares, to this day, he went through worse horrors than any one could have imagined, and all on behalf of a sacred cause. The patient was so much occupied with these pathological phenomena that he was inaccessible to any other impression and would sit perfectly rigid and motionless for hours. . . . On the other hand, they tortured him to such a degree that he longed for death. He made repeated attempts at drowning himself in his bath, and asked to be given the cyanide of potassium that was intended for him. His delusional ideas gradually assumed a mystical and religious character; he was in direct communication with God, he was the plaything of devils, he saw "miraculous apparitions," he heard "holy music," and in the end he even came to believe that he was living in another world.

It may be added that there were certain people by whom he thought he was being persecuted and injured and upon whom he poured abuse. The most prominent of these was his former physician, Flechsig, whom he called a "soul-murderer." The voices he heard during this period mocked him and jeered at him.

Over the next few years there was a gradual change in Dr. Schreber's condition, as his distress about being transformed into a "strumpet" developed into a conviction that it was all part of a divine plan and that he had a mission to redeem the world. In Schreber's words:

> Now, however, I became clearly aware that the order of things imperatively demanded my emasculation, whether I personally liked it or not, and that no *reasonable* course lay open to me but to reconcile myself to the thought of being transformed into a woman. The further consequence of my emasculation could, of course, only be my impregnation ... by divine rays to the end that a new race of men might be created.

And, Schreber elaborates,

> The *only thing* which could appear unreasonable in the eyes of other people is the fact, already touched upon in the expert's report, that I am sometimes to be found, standing before the mirror or elsewhere, with the upper portion of my body partly bared, and wearing sundry feminine adornments, such as ribbons, trumpery necklaces and the like. This only occurs, I may add, when I am by myself, and never, at least so far as I am able to avoid it, in the presence of other people.

Dr. Weber, in a report dated 1900, described Schreber's changed condition as follows:

> Since for the last 9 months Herr President Schreber has taken his meals daily at my family board, I have had the most ample opportunities of conversing with him on every imaginable topic. Whatever the subject was that came up for discussion (apart, of course, from his delusional ideas), whether it concerned events in the field of administration and law, or of politics, or of art, or of literature, or of social life—in short, whatever the topic, Dr. Schreber gave evidence of a lively interest, a well-informed mind, a good memory and sound judgment; his ethical outlook, moreover, was one which it was impossible not to endorse. So, too, in his lighter talk with the ladies of the party, he was both courteous and affable, and if he touched upon matters in a more humorous vein, he invariably displayed tact and decorum. Never once, during these innocent talks round the dining-table, did he introduce subjects which would more properly have been raised at a medical consultation.

Dr. Schreber made numerous appeals to regain his liberty. In Freud's words:

He did not in the least disavow his delusion or make any secret of his intention of publishing [his memoirs]. On the contrary, he dwelt upon the importance of his ideas to religious thought, and upon their invulnerability to the attacks of modern science; but at the same time, he laid stress upon the absolute harmlessness of the actions, which, as he was aware, his delusions obliged him to perform. Such, indeed, were his acumen and the cogency of his logic that finally, and in spite of his being an acknowledged paranoiac, his efforts were crowned with success. In July 1902 Dr. Schreber's civil rights were restored.

Freud's Diagnosis: Dementia Paranoides

Discussion of "Dr. Schreber"

Dr. Schreber's illness is characterized by bizarre delusions (i.e., involving a phenomenon that the person's culture would regard as totally implausible), which begin as persecutory (e.g., that he will be transformed into a woman, with a view to sexual abuse) and later become somatic (e.g., he complains that he has softening of the brain), nihilistic (e.g., he feels he is dead and decomposing), religious (e.g., he states he is in direct communication with God), and, finally, grandiose (e.g., he feels he has a mission to redeem the world). What Dr. Weber refers to as "hypochondriacal ideas" are, in fact, somatic delusions. This leads one to suspect that the original illness, diagnosed as "an attack of severe hypochondria," also involved somatic delusions. The delusions are accompanied by auditory hallucinations (e.g., holy music), visual hallucinations (e.g., seeing miraculous apparitions), and, probably, tactile hallucinations as well (e.g., his experience that his body was being handled in all kinds of revolting ways). His sitting "rigid and motionless for hours" suggests catatonic stupor (i.e., marked decrease in reactivity to the environment and reduction in spontaneous movements and activity). The same behavior might suggest depressive stupor; but, apart from the suicidal ideas, there is no other reference to characteristic depressive symptoms.

Although the predominant psychotic symptoms are paranoid delusions, the diagnosis of Delusional Disorder is not made because of prominent hallucinations and the bizarre nature of the delusions. The presence of bizarre delusions and prominent hallucinations, with functioning in many areas that is markedly below the highest level achieved before the onset of the disturbance, suggests a diagnosis of Schizophrenia (DSM-IV-TR, p. 312). The prominent persecutory delusions and hallucinations, in the absence of either disorganized speech or behavior, flat or inappropriate affect, or current catatonic behavior, indicate the Paranoid Type (DSM-IV-TR, p. 314).

JACOB S. KASANIN (1897–1946)

Kasanin provided a bridge between Schizophrenia and Affective Disorder by first proposing, in 1933, the term Schizoaffective. *According to Kasanin, this disorder occurs in "fairly young individuals, quite well integrated socially, who suddenly blow up in a dramatic psychosis and present a clinical picture which may be called either schizophrenic or affective, and in whom the differential diagnosis is extremely difficult." The following cases have been adapted from his article "The Acute Schizoaffective Psychoses."*

SUSPICIOUS WIFE

S.R., female, white, married, age 25, admitted to the hospital February 25, 1932.

Diagnosis: dementia praecox.

Chief complaint: The patient was sent to a psychiatric hospital from the [city] hospital where she was restless, excited and showed a "schizophrenic reaction type."

Personal history: The patient was always an active, energetic, industrious person. She was ambitious, full of life, was very much interested in her house and held several positions after marriage. She was extremely affectionate, demonstrative and romantic . . . . The patient has one child, a boy of 6 years, to whom she was extremely devoted.

From Kasanin J: "The Acute Schizoaffective Psychoses." *American Journal of Psychiatry* 13:97–126, 1933.

Present illness: [Six months before admission] when the little boy began to attend school, the patient felt that she ought to escort him to school. Her husband [a policeman] ridiculed her anxiety about the boy. She became upset and told the husband that if anything ever happened to the boy, she would be through with him. [A month before admission] a policeman in their neighborhood committed suicide. The husband came home, told his wife about the incident, and said that such work would drive anybody to suicide. This seemed to have affected the patient, and she became depressed afterward. When the husband asked the patient about the cause of her depression, she told him that somebody was coming between them and complained about the interference of his parents. . . . The patient cried a good deal and [a week later] she said that her heart was bad and that she was going to die. [A few days] later she became very upset, said something was going to happen in the house, said the peddler who came to the door was going to hurt her and had a feeling that the chimney was going to fall down and kill her. She said that her house was a house of ill omen. . . . [Five days before admission] the patient suddenly got up in the middle of the night, dressed, packed her suitcase, and said that she was going to her parents. The husband helped his wife to do it. Immediately on her arrival at her father's home, the patient commenced to accuse her father and mother of being in league to influence her husband against her. She stayed there that day, and the next night the sleeplessness was repeated. She got up and went into her brother's room. She accused him of intending to poison her husband and that he was trying to come between them. Suddenly she left the house, called up the police and asked them to come to her parents' house and rescue her, as something dreadful was going to happen. The husband succeeded in preventing the police from coming, and took her over to the city hospital.

When the husband came to see the patient at the city hospital, she accused him of trying to wean the boy away from her and complained of all kinds of peculiar noises in the hospital. She felt that the other patients in the ward were discussing her affairs, swore at her, said that her husband was unfaithful to her and that he was going to steal the boy away from her. The other patients also said that her husband was "four in one," intimating that he was of mixed blood and part Negro. She thought that these voices were "rayed" from someone who was in a trance in one of the other rooms. When her husband visited her at the hospital he appeared "funny"—his eyes were glassy and had a peculiar staring expression in them.

[She was then transferred to a psychiatric hospital.] She said that she felt sad, unhappy and depressed. The intellectual functions were intact. She expressed a large number of ideas, revolving around her relationship to her husband. She complained that there was a good deal of interference in their home life. She also felt that she was going to be harmed, thought that her husband was going to shoot her rather than shoot himself. She said that when she was at the city hospital, she heard her name being called out over the loud speaker. She denied any hallucinations in the psychiatric hospital. She also said that while at the city hospital she smelled many and various odors. [Two weeks after admission] she was transferred to a state hospital. There she was sullen, morose and made very little attempt to get interested in the ward. She was mildly depressed and was quite embarrassed when asked about her illness. She spoke freely about her illness and said that while she was in the psychopathic hospital she saw "studies" of her husband from childhood to manhood. She saw him as a boy, a sailor, and a police officer. She said that she had had many somatic sensations before she came to the hospital and had "funny impressions which seem to spell danger." She could not help but feel that something dreadful was going to happen to her child, and that her husband would blame her if anything happened to him. She had the suspicion that her husband was unfaithful to her, and that he had begun to take "dope," as he seemed very dull and stupid. She intimated that her gastric symptoms may have been due to poison. Within a few weeks the patient changed a great deal. She began to laugh, appeared happy, talked very freely and spoke a great deal about "radio hypnotism," to which she attributed all her troubles.

[She was discharged after 2 months, and at a 6-month follow-up] appeared perfectly well, resumed her care of the house and got a job in a department store during the Christmas rush. [Two years later] she, herself, analyzed the whole situation and described the conditions which led to her breakdown. . . . The patient [had] moved into a new house which she bought with her own savings. She had a great deal of work to do putting the house in order, as it was an old house. . . . She was troubled by the fact that the furnace was not working properly and she could smell gas in the house. She lost her appetite, could not sleep and felt very bad. . . . Things did not go very well with her personal life. Her husband loved and adored her, but he was under the influence of his mother, who disliked the patient. One night while she was in bed, she saw three bright stars from her window. She could not fall asleep. The stars were bright red in color. She did close her eyes, but when she opened them again, the stars would still be there. She felt that something terrible was going to happen.

A review of the family situation brought out the fact that there was a real foundation for some of the patient's beliefs. Both her family and her husband's family were doing everything possible to estrange the patient and her husband. . . . The patient said that the psychosis was a good thing, as somehow it has helped to straighten out the various tangles in her life, and gave her courage, confidence in herself. The patient is doing very well now and handles unusually well affairs that are just as complicated as they were before.

Kasanin's Diagnosis: Schizoaffective Schizophrenia

Discussion of "Suspicious Wife"

This patient apparently recovered completely less than 4 months after the onset of the first definite symptoms (i.e., after the suicide of her husband's friend). Her illness is characterized by depressed mood and a variety of changing persecutory delusions, some of which are bizarre. In addition, there are auditory hallucinations (or at least illusions) with a persecutory content, and problems with appetite and sleep and thoughts of her own death.

The patient is frequently described as depressed and unhappy, although the persistence of a prominent depressed mood is not established. In fact, within a few weeks "She began to laugh, appeared happy, talked very freely and spoke a great deal about 'radio hypnotism,' to which she attributed all of her troubles." This indicates that even if there were a sustained depressed mood and the associated symptoms of the depressive syndrome, the psychotic symptoms apparently are present when she is no longer depressed. For this reason, the criteria for a Major Depressive Episode are not met, and the differential diagnosis is thus between Schizoaffective Disorder and Schizophreniform Disorder. Because there is no specific evidence of the full depressive syndrome, we prefer the diagnosis of Schizophreniform Disorder (DSM-IV-TR, p. 319), a disorder with all of the characteristics of Schizophrenia except that the duration is at least 1 month but less than 6 months. We specify With Good Prognostic Features because of the onset of psychotic symptoms within 4 weeks of the first noticeable change in the patient's behavior, her good premorbid functioning, and the absence of flat or blunted affect.

MAGNET MAN

E.F., male, age 20, single laborer, white, [was] admitted to the hospital March 15, 1929.

Diagnosis: dementia praecox.

Chief complaint: The patient was sent to the hospital by his family because about 2 weeks before admission he became overactive, exhibited queer behavior, and spoke a great deal about his theories of life. Finally he became so excited that he was taken to the outpatient department, from which he was referred to the hospital.

Personal history: The patient did well in the various positions in which he was employed. . . . He was a model employee but very quiet and shy. . . . As far as his personality is concerned, he was quite an average young man. . . . His outside interests were mostly athletic. He took part in several sports and played baseball with amateur groups. . . . Several months prior to admission he fell in love with a girl who worked in the same factory where he worked and told his family about it. He wanted to bring the girl to the house, but his mother told him he was too young to go out with girls. Although the patient spoke about having dates with the girl, she told her foreman that their acquaintance was very casual.

Present illness: Two weeks before admission, the co-workers in the factory noticed that the patient began to talk a great deal and that he began to sing very loudly. Quite suddenly he declared that he was going on the stage or else would join a professional baseball team. The same behavior was observed at home. He sent a telegram to a Boston baseball team, which was at that time playing in the South, asking the manager for a position. He told his family that he was going to make a great deal of money and they should finance him for the trip. He slept very poorly and was very restless at night. A week before admission, he went to one of the Harvard physicians and offered him his body for scientific purpose. The latter referred him to the hospital. He was quite excited for several days and spoke a great deal about scientific experiments on his brain and the cure of insanity. Finally he was brought to the outpatient clinic. . . .

For several days the patient was quite active and restless, but responded very well to frequent baths. He was very cooperative and talked freely to the physician. He took a fair amount of interest in the ward routine and was friendly with other patients. His speech was relevant, but at times incoherent, and he spoke about a great many things. The patient spoke a great deal about his philosophy of life, giving several variants of his theory of personal magnetism.

For some time the patient has had a conflict over auto-eroticism which he has practiced since childhood. He also had sex relations with a 9-year-old girl when he was of the same age, and it disturbed him. The conflict was intensified by the fact that he was quite religious. He saw a girl a year ago and fell in love with her, but it took him a long time before he was introduced to her. Finally he asked her for a date, about 4 months ago. She refused. He felt bad, but he asked again 3 months ago, and she told him she was going to the beach with her parents. He finally got a date about a week prior to his admission to the hospital; they went to her house after the movies, and they "got to loving on the sofa." He felt magnetism go over him when he kissed her, and when he passed his hand over her hair, he "felt the flow of magnetism just like in a wet dream."

He began speculating about causes of this and thought he had made a new discovery. The patient said that he was able to solve all his conflicts by this discovery. He found that the brain controlled the fluid that traveled throughout the whole body and could be drawn from mouth, teeth, roof of the mouth, lips and nose, if touched. This fluid would travel throughout the whole body, producing a magnetic feeling passing over him, the same as a sexual act. . . . Not only did he get this magnetic feeling when he touched an animate object, but an inanimate object as well. When in church he felt that the holy images might be alive and that God was in communication with him. He stated that when he expectorated, the saliva was equivalent to spermatic fluid. . . . [He felt this power came to him from God.] The patient said that he could see God if he closed his eyes. He could see God moving about, saw Him moving His fingers and saw His features. He saw God sitting on the throne, pointing His fingers and controlling the movement of the world. God never talked to him. At one time he saw God mold clay and blow the breath of life into it.

Clinical course: Within a few days the patient became quiet and cooperative, but still insisted on elaborating his ideas. Commitment to a state institution was recommended; but 9 days after the patient entered the hospital, he was taken home by his family. Within a few weeks he joined one of the branches of the governmental service and has been doing very well in his field of service.

Kasanin's Diagnosis: Schizoaffective Schizophrenia

Discussion of "Magnet Man"

This brief illness is characterized by elevated and expansive mood, pressure of speech, grandiosity, and hyperactivity. The patient is described as sleeping "very poorly" and being "very restless at night." We assume that this represents the characteristic decreased need for sleep seen in a Manic Episode. In addition, there are many delusions, all of them involving grandiose themes, and hallucinations of God. Thus, his psychotic symptoms are all congruent with his elevated mood.

Kasanin undoubtedly made a diagnosis of Schizoaffective Schizophrenia because he believed that the prominent bizarre delusions were incompatible with a diagnosis of mania; but in recent years, in this country, the concept of mania has broadened. Hence, beginning with DSM-III, even the most bizarre delusions do not necessarily exclude a diagnosis of mania. Because of the rather clear evidence of the full manic syndrome and no evidence that the psychotic symptoms were present at a time when there was no mood disturbance, the diagnosis in this case is Bipolar I Disorder (DSM-IV-TR, p. 388). Because this is the first Manic Episode and there is no history of a Major Depressive Episode, the diagnosis is further qualified as Single Manic Episode. Finally, the specification of Severe With Mood-Congruent Psychotic Features is noted.

PAUL HOCH (1902–1964) AND
PHILIP POLATIN (1905–1980)

*Drs. Hoch and Polatin, from the New York State Psychiatric Institute, pro-
posed in 1949 the concept of Pseudoneurotic Schizophrenia. According to
them, this diagnosis applies to patients who have "the basic mechanisms
of schizophrenia" yet, because of their "subtle" manifestations, "there is
no way to demonstrate it clinically." Many of the patients in question had
been analyzed "for a considerable period of time; and the suspicion [had]
never been raised that they were not psychoneurotic." The following case
is adapted from their article "Pseudoneurotic Forms of Schizophrenia."*

FEARFUL GIRL

S.s. is a 21-year-old girl who was hospitalized because she had not improved after a year of outpatient psychotherapy.

> On admission, she stated, "I have fears of food; I have fears of something
> happening to my family; I cannot sleep; I get depressed; I become tense,
> anxious and agitated."

She was cooperative and pleasant, gave a coherent and reasonably
complete history, and denied delusions or hallucinations (although she
had sometimes been afraid that she might someday have hallucinations).
Her affect was labile, with a shallow quality.

> At times she speaks of feeling very hopeless and of feeling that suicide is
> the only answer in the end; but usually she does not appear to feel this
> way, and more often seems rather to enjoy the uniqueness that she feels
> her illness possesses. Occasionally a really depressing thought will strike
> her; at such times she will appear truly depressed, with ready tears and a
> more convincing attitude of despair. Ideas suggesting irreparable organic
> damage or deficits in the field of emotional experience seem most capa-
> ble of provoking these markedly depressed moods, which are usually
> short-lived.

From Hoch P, Polatin P: "Pseudoneurotic Forms of Schizophrenia." *Psychiatric
Quarterly* 23:248–276, 1949.

S.S. dates the beginning of her illness to a night in her 15th year when she overheard her parents having intercourse. She became sexually aroused and describes

> feeling there was something wrong with me, like I was going up in an elevator, and I thought it would never go away; I thought maybe I couldn't experience any sexual feeling. Soon afterward, the word *fuck* was popping in my mind and kept going over and over, and not for a minute could I get it out of my thoughts. A couple of months later it was still going over in my mind, and then I told myself, "Why should you think such a word like that, that you cannot tell to anyone, if they asked you what is wrong," so I changed it to *worry*. . . . I don't know how I ever got through school. Ever since I was 15, *worry* kept rotating in my mind continually. I got so I couldn't swallow; I couldn't eat. Food did not agree with me because I was worried. The word *fuck* made me feel nauseated; I couldn't sleep. I would lie there with agitation, with the idea of the word going over and over.

Since that time, she has had a number of similar preoccupations—the fear that she would someday be so concerned about the cleanliness of food that she would be able to eat only kosher food; the fear that she would come to believe in Christ and thus upset her orthodox Jewish family; the worry that she might upset her sisters so much that they would become insane. She also had some compulsions, such as having to turn off the light six times each night and having to leave her shoes in a parallel line when she went to bed; but these were not elaborate or time consuming.

She has had many crushes on boys, but no sexual relationships. She has stated, in an amobarbital interview, that she does not know whether she is male or female, that she fears she cannot lead a normal life or be happy. She appears to have had no close girlfriends, but to have been intensely and ambivalently involved with her extended family.

S.S. finished high school and a 1-year business course and was able to work as a clerk until a year ago, when she came home from work with a dazed appearance and refused to talk to anyone, saying "You wouldn't understand." It was at that time that she was referred for outpatient treatment. She spent the year at home, doing very little except trying to "understand" her illness.

On the ward she is described as careless and listless, staying in bed all day, with no initiative. "She manifests a belief in thought magic and also shows a fluctuating appraisal of reality and, at times, depersonalization."

Hoch and Polatin's Diagnosis: Pseudoneurotic Schizophrenia

Discussion of "Fearful Girl"

This woman suffers from a variety of symptoms: morbid fears of possible future events, labile but "shallow" affect, obsessions (e.g., thinking about the words *fuck* and *worry*), compulsions (e.g., turning off the light and lining up her shoes), identity disturbance (e.g., that she might be male or become a Christian), difficulties in interpersonal relations (e.g., she had no close girlfriends), magical thinking, depersonalization, and markedly impaired functioning (e.g., spending the last year at home thinking about her illness). Undoubtedly, this plethora of chronically disabling symptoms was a major factor in Hoch and Polatin's diagnosis of Schizophrenia. However, the absence of delusions, hallucinations, flat affect, and disorganized speech or behavior rules out a DSM-IV-TR diagnosis of Schizophrenia.

An Axis I diagnosis of Obsessive-Compulsive Disorder (DSM-IV-TR, p. 462) is justified by the prominence of the obsessions and compulsions and the degree of distress and interference in functioning they cause the patient. She probably does not recognize the morbid fears as inappropriate, and they are therefore ego-syntonic rather than true obsessions. However, they are best understood as an associated feature of the Obsessive-Compulsive Disorder.

The Axis I diagnosis does not account for the patient's chronic maladaptive pattern of relating to and thinking about her environment and herself. Some of her symptoms are characteristic of Borderline Personality Disorder: identity disturbance and affective instability. Others are characteristic of Schizotypal Personality Disorder (e.g., her magical thinking, her having no close friends, her shallow affect). It is likely that other features of these disorders were present, although not noted. In the absence of positive evidence that the criteria for these specific personality disorders are met, a diagnosis of Personality Disorder Not Otherwise Specified (DSM-IV-TR, p. 729) is appropriate.

ALBERT HOFMANN (1906–   )

Dr. Hofmann, a chemist working in a large Swiss pharmaceutical company, had been studying the synthesis of various natural ergot alkaloids. In April 1943 he described the following experiences.[*]

DR. HOFMANN

Last Friday, April 16, 1943, I was forced to stop my work in the laboratory in the middle of the afternoon and to go home, as I was seized by a peculiar restlessness associated with a sensation of mild dizziness. On arriving home, I lay down and sank into a kind of drunkenness, which was not unpleasant and which was characterized by extreme activity of imagination. As I lay in a dazed condition with my eyes closed (I experienced daylight as disagreeably bright) there surged upon me an uninterrupted stream of fantastic images of extraordinary plasticity and vividness and accompanied by an intense, kaleidoscope-like play of colors. This condition gradually passed off after about 2 hours.

Dr. Hofmann suspected that his strange experiences were the result of accidentally ingesting the drug that he had been working on. Three days later he conducted an experiment on himself by taking the smallest dose of the substance that he believed could be expected to have any effect. After 40 minutes, in his laboratory notes he reported "slight dizziness, unrest, difficulty in concentration, visual disturbances, marked desire to laugh." At this point, his laboratory notes are discontinued. Later he describes what happened.

I asked my laboratory assistant to accompany me home as I believed that I should have a repetition of the disturbance of the previous Friday. While we were cycling home, however, it became clear that the symptoms were much stronger than the first time. I had great difficulty in speaking coherently, my field of vision swayed before me, and objects appeared distorted like images in curved mirrors. I had the impression of being unable to move from the spot, although my assistant told me afterwards that we had cycled at a good pace. . . . Once I was at home the physician was called.

---

[*]From Ayd FJ, Blackwell B: *Discoveries in Biological Psychiatry*. Philadelphia, PA, JB Lippincott, 1970, p. 91.

By the time the doctor arrived, the peak of the crisis had already passed. As far as I remember, the following were the most outstanding symptoms: vertigo; visual disturbances; the faces of those around me appeared as grotesque, colored masks; marked motoric unrest, alternating with paralysis; an intermittent heavy feeling in the head, limbs and the entire body, as if they were filled with lead; dry, constricted sensation in the throat; feeling of choking; clear recognition of my condition, in which state I sometimes observed, in the manner of an independent, neutral observer, that I shouted half insanely or babbled incoherent words. Occasionally I felt as if I were out of my body.

The doctor found a rather weak pulse but an otherwise normal circulation. . . . Six hours after ingestion of the [drug], my condition had already improved considerably. Only the visual disturbances were distorted, like the reflections in the surface of moving water. Moreover, all objects appeared in unpleasant, constantly changing colors, the predominant shades being sickly green and blue. When I closed my eyes, an unending series of colorful, very realistic and fantastic images surged in upon me. A remarkable feature was the manner in which all acoustic perceptions (e.g., the noise of a passing car) were transformed into optical effects, every sound evoking a corresponding colored hallucination constantly changing in shape and color like pictures in a kaleidoscope. At about 1 o'clock I fell asleep and awoke next morning feeling perfectly well.

Dr. Hofmann's Diagnosis: An "Extraordinary Disturbance" Caused by the Ingestion of a Hallucinogen

Discussion of "Dr. Hofmann"

The many symptoms, predominantly perceptual changes, are clearly related to the ingestion of a drug. In fact, the drug that Dr. Hofmann was working with was lysergic acid diethylamide, better known now as LSD. His description of his own reaction illustrates the characteristic features of Hallucinogen Intoxication (DSM-IV-TR, p. 253): illusions (e.g., faces appeared grotesque), depersonalization (e.g., "I felt as if I were out of my body"), hallucinations (e.g., "colored hallucination constantly changing in shape and color . . ."), and synesthesias (e.g., "acoustic perceptions . . . were transformed into optical effects"). He also describes another characteristic feature: all of the symptoms occur during a state of full wakefulness and alertness and with full recognition that the symptoms are the effect of the drug (e.g., "clear recognition of my condition, in which state I sometimes observed, in the manner of an independent, neutral observer").

The DSM-IV-TR criteria for Hallucinogen Intoxication also require certain physical symptoms, such as pupillary dilation, tachycardia, tremors, and incoordination. Although these are not reported by Dr. Hofmann, we can assume that some of them were present. Needless to say, the inability of Dr. Hofmann to continue working while experiencing the effect of the drug is evidence of maladaptive behavioral effects, also required to make the diagnosis.

HERVEY CLECKLEY (1905–1984)

In The Mask of Sanity,[*] *published in 1955, Cleckley attempted to clarify the confusing and paradoxical nature of Psychopathic Personality. According to him, people with this disorder are "outwardly intact, showing excellent peripheral function, but centrally deficient or disabled in such a way that abilities . . . cannot be utilized consistently for sane purposes or prevented from regularly working toward self-destructive and other seriously pathological results." The following case is adapted from his book.*

TOM

This young man, 21 years of age, does not look at all like a criminal type or a shifty delinquent. . . . Tom looks and is in robust physical health. His manner and appearance are pleasing. . . . There is nothing to suggest that he is putting on a bold front or trying to adopt any attitude or manner that will be misleading. Though he knows the examiner has evidence of

---

[*]From Cleckley H: *The Mask of Sanity*, 5th Edition. St. Louis, MO, CV Mosby, 1976, p. 64.

his almost incredible career, he gives such an impression that it seems for the moment likely he will be able to explain it all away.

This poised young man's immediate problem was serious, but not monumental. His family and legal authorities were in hope that if some [mental] disorder could be discovered in him, he might escape a jail sentence for stealing.

Evidence of his maladjustment became distinct in childhood. He appeared to be a reliable and manly fellow, but could never be counted upon to keep at any task or to give a straight account of any situation. He was frequently truant from school. . . . Though he was generously provided for, he stole some of his father's chickens from time to time, selling them at stores downtown. Pieces of table silver would be missed. These were sometimes recovered from those to whom he had sold them for a pittance or swapped them for odds and ends that seemed to hold no particular interest or value for him.

Often when truant from high school classes, Tom wandered more or less aimlessly, sometimes shooting at . . . chickens, setting fire to a rural privy on the outskirts of town, or perhaps loitering about a cigar store or a pool room, reading the comics, throwing rocks at squirrels in a park, perpetrating small thefts or swindles. He often charged things in stores to his father, stole cigarettes, candy, cigars, etc. . . . He lied so plausibly and with such equanimity, devised such ingenious alibis or simply denied all responsibility with such convincing appearances of candor that for many years his real career was poorly estimated. . . . Though he often fell in with groups or small gangs, he never for long identified himself with others in a common cause.

At 14 or 15, having learned to drive, Tom began to steal automobiles with some regularity. . . . After he had tried to sell a stolen car, his father consulted advisers and, on the theory that he might have some specific craving for automobiles, bought one for him as a therapeutic measure. On one occasion while out driving he deliberately parked his own car and, leaving it, stole an inferior model, which he left slightly damaged on the outskirts of a village some miles away. . . . Meanwhile, Tom continued to forge his father's name on small checks and steal change, pocketknives, textbooks, etc., at school. Occasionally, on the pretext of ownership he would sell a dog or a calf belonging to some member of the community.

Tom was sent to a federal institution in a distant state, where a well-organized program of rehabilitation and guidance was available. He soon impressed authorities at this place with his attitude and in the way he discussed his past mistakes and plans for a different future.

He found employment in a drydock at a nearby port and talked modestly, but convincingly, of the course he would now follow, expressing aims and plans few could greatly improve on. . . . His employers found him at first energetic, bright, and apparently enthusiastic about the work. Soon evidence of inexplicable irresponsibility emerged and accumulated. Sometimes he missed several days and brought simple, but convincing, excuses of illness. As the occasions multiplied, explanations so detailed and elaborate were made that it seemed only facts could have produced them. Later he sometimes left the job, stayed away for hours, and gave no account of his behavior except to say that he did not feel like working at the time.

Reliable information indicates that he has been arrested and imprisoned approximately 50 or 60 times. It is estimated that he would have been put in jails or police barracks for short or long periods of detention on approximately 150 other occasions if his family had not made good his small thefts, damages, etc., and paid fines for him.

Sometimes he was arrested for fomenting brawls in low resorts, provoking fights, or for such high-handed and disturbing behavior as to constitute public nuisance. Though not a very regular drinker or one who characteristically drank to sodden confusion or stupefaction, he exhibited unsociable and unprepossessing manners and conduct after taking even a few beers or highballs. In one juke-joint imbroglio, over the years, he is credited with having struck a fellow reveler on the head with a piece of iron.

Tom's mother had, over the years, suffered special anxiety and distress because of his unannounced absences. After kissing her goodbye, saying he was going downtown for a Coca-Cola or to a movie, he might not appear for several days or even for a couple of weeks! . . . This young man, has, apparently, never formed any substantial attachment to another person. Sexually he has been desultorily promiscuous under a wide variety of circumstances. A year or 2 earlier, he married a girl who had achieved considerable local recognition as a prostitute whose fee was moderate. He had previously shared her offerings during an evening (on a commercial basis) with friends or with brief acquaintances among whom he found himself. He soon left the bride and never showed signs of shame or chagrin about the character of the woman he had espoused or any responsibility toward her.

Cleckley's Diagnosis: Psychopathic Personality

Discussion of "Tom"

Tom illustrates all of the features required for a DSM-IV-TR diagnosis of Antisocial Personality Disorder (DSM-IV-TR, p. 706): current age over 18, evidence of Conduct Disorder before age 15 (truancy, stealing, lying, vandalism, delinquency, chronic violations of rules at home), and, since age 18, a pervasive pattern of irresponsible behavior and disregard for and violation of the rights of others (failure to sustain consistent work behavior, abandonment of his wife, stealing, lying, assaulting others) and lack of remorse.

One criticism of the DSM-III criteria for Antisocial Personality Disorder was that they put too much emphasis on overt antisocial acts that might result in legal difficulties and not enough on the psychological features of the disorder, such as absence of guilt feelings, loyalty to others, and empathy. Tom certainly demonstrates these psychological characteristics, which Cleckley believed were central to the concept of Psychopathic Personality.

These features were not included in the DSM-III, -III-R, and -IV and IV-TR criteria for Antisocial Personality Disorder for two reasons. First of all, they require more inferential judgments than do the largely behavioral symptoms listed in the criteria. Second, there is evidence that, for the most part, people who exhibit the behavioral disturbances required for the diagnosis of Antisocial Personality Disorder are, like Tom, undersocialized. Finally, in the DSM-IV field trial comparing alternative criteria sets, the more behavioral DSM-III-R criteria had as high correlations with external variables indicating validity (e.g., number of marriages and sexual partners, poor work history, number of arrests and convictions) as did criteria focusing on the characteristic psychological features of the disorder.

Index of Case Names

APPENDIX B

Cases by Special Interest

APPENDIX C

DSM-IV-TR Classification

NOS = Not Otherwise Specified.

An *x* appearing in a diagnostic code indicates that a specific code number is required.

An ellipsis (. . .) is used in the names of certain disorders to indicate that the name of a specific mental disorder or general medical condition should be inserted when recording the name (e.g., 293.0 Delirium Due to Hypothyroidism).

If criteria are currently met, one of the following severity specifiers may be noted after the diagnosis:

> Mild
> Moderate
> Severe

If criteria are no longer met, one of the following specifiers may be noted:

> In Partial Remission
> In Full Remission
> Prior History

Disorders Usually First Diagnosed in Infancy, Childhood, or Adolescence

MENTAL RETARDATION

Note: *These are coded on Axis II.*

317   Mild Mental Retardation
318.0   Moderate Mental Retardation
318.1   Severe Mental Retardation
318.2   Profound Mental Retardation
319   Mental Retardation, Severity Unspecified

LEARNING DISORDERS

315.00   Reading Disorder
315.1   Mathematics Disorder
315.2   Disorder of Written Expression
315.9   Learning Disorder NOS

MOTOR SKILLS DISORDER

315.4   Developmental Coordination Disorder

COMMUNICATION DISORDERS

315.31   Expressive Language Disorder
315.32   Mixed Receptive-Expressive Language Disorder
315.39   Phonological Disorder
307.0   Stuttering
307.9   Communication Disorder NOS

PERVASIVE DEVELOPMENTAL DISORDERS

299.00   Autistic Disorder
299.80   Rett's Disorder
299.10   Childhood Disintegrative Disorder
299.80   Asperger's Disorder
299.80   Pervasive Developmental Disorder NOS

ATTENTION-DEFICIT AND DISRUPTIVE BEHAVIOR DISORDERS

314.xx Attention-Deficit/Hyperactivity
Disorder
  .01 Combined Type
  .00 Predominantly Inattentive
      Type
  .01 Predominantly Hyperactive-
      Impulsive Type
314.9 Attention-Deficit/Hyperactivity
Disorder NOS
312.xx Conduct Disorder
  .81 Childhood-Onset Type
  .82 Adolescent-Onset Type
  .89 Unspecified Onset
313.81 Oppositional Defiant
Disorder
312.9 Disruptive Behavior
Disorder NOS

FEEDING AND EATING DISORDERS OF INFANCY OR EARLY CHILDHOOD

307.52 Pica
307.53 Rumination Disorder
307.59 Feeding Disorder of Infancy
or Early Childhood

TIC DISORDERS

307.23 Tourette's Disorder
307.22 Chronic Motor or Vocal Tic
Disorder
307.21 Transient Tic Disorder
Specify if: Single
Episode/Recurrent
307.20 Tic Disorder NOS

ELIMINATION DISORDERS

——.— Encopresis
787.6   With Constipation and
Overflow Incontinence
307.7   Without Constipation and
Overflow Incontinence

307.6 Enuresis (Not Due to a
General Medical Condition)
Specify type: Nocturnal Only/
Diurnal Only/Nocturnal and
Diurnal

OTHER DISORDERS OF INFANCY, CHILDHOOD, OR ADOLESCENCE

309.21 Separation Anxiety Disorder
Specify if: Early Onset
313.23 Selective Mutism
313.89 Reactive Attachment Disorder
of Infancy or Early Childhood
Specify type: Inhibited Type/
Disinhibited Type
307.3 Stereotypic Movement Disorder
Specify if: With Self-Injurious
Behavior
313.9 Disorder of Infancy, Childhood,
or Adolescence NOS

Delirium, Dementia, and Amnestic and Other Cognitive Disorders

DELIRIUM

293.0 Delirium Due to . . .
*[Indicate the General
Medical Condition]*
——.— Substance Intoxication
Delirium *(refer to
Substance-Related Disorders
for substance-specific codes)*
——.— Substance Withdrawal
Delirium *(refer to
Substance-Related Disorders
for substance-specific codes)*
——.— Delirium Due to Multiple
Etiologies *(code each of the
specific etiologies)*
780.09 Delirium NOS

DEMENTIA

294.xx Dementia of the Alzheimer's Type, With Early Onset *(also code 331.0 Alzheimer's disease on Axis III)*
.10   Without Behavioral Disturbance
.11   With Behavioral Disturbance

294.xx Dementia of the Alzheimer's Type, With Late Onset *(also code 331.0 Alzheimer's disease on Axis III)*
.10   Without Behavioral Disturbance
.11   With Behavioral Disturbance

290.xx Vascular Dementia
.40   Uncomplicated
.41   With Delirium
.42   With Delusions
.43   With Depressed Mood

   Specify if: With Behavioral Disturbance

Code presence or absence of a behavioral disturbance in the fifth digit for Dementia Due to a General Medical Condition:

   0 = Without Behavioral Disturbance
   1 = With Behavioral Disturbance

294.1x Dementia Due to HIV Disease *(also code 042 HIV on Axis III)*
294.1x Dementia Due to Head Trauma *(also code 854.00 head injury on Axis III)*
294.1x Dementia Due to Parkinson's Disease *(also code 332.0 Parkinson's disease on Axis III)*

294.1x Dementia Due to Huntington's Disease *(also code 333.4 Huntington's disease on Axis III)*
294.1x Dementia Due to Pick's Disease *(also code 331.1 Pick's disease on Axis III)*
294.1x Dementia Due to Creutzfeldt-Jakob Disease *(also code 046.1 Creutzfeldt-Jakob disease on Axis III)*
294.1x Dementia Due to . . . *[Indicate the General Medical Condition not listed above] (also code the general medical condition on Axis III)*
——.— Substance-Induced Persisting Dementia *(refer to Substance-Related Disorders for substance-specific codes)*
——.— Dementia Due to Multiple Etiologies *(code each of the specific etiologies)*
294.8 Dementia NOS

AMNESTIC DISORDERS

294.0 Amnestic Disorder Due to . . . *[Indicate the General Medical Condition]*
   Specify if: Transient/Chronic
——.— Substance-Induced Persisting Amnestic Disorder *(refer to Substance-Related Disorders for substance-specific codes)*
294.8 Amnestic Disorder NOS

OTHER COGNITIVE DISORDERS

294.9 Cognitive Disorder NOS

Mental Disorders Due to a General Medical Condition Not Elsewhere Classified

293.89 Catatonic Disorder Due to . . . *[Indicate the General Medical Condition]*

310.1 Personality Change Due to . . . *[Indicate the General Medical Condition]*
Specify type: Labile Type/Disinhibited Type/ Aggressive Type/Apathetic Type/ Paranoid Type/Other Type/ Combined Type/Unspecified Type

293.9 Mental Disorder NOS Due to . . . *[Indicate the General Medical Condition]*

Substance-Related Disorders

The following specifiers apply to Substance Dependence as noted:

[a]With Physiological Dependence/ Without Physiological Dependence
[b]Early Full Remission/Early Partial Remission/Sustained Full Remission/Sustained Partial Remission
[c]In a Controlled Environment
[d]On Agonist Therapy

The following specifiers apply to Substance-Induced Disorders as noted:

[I]With Onset During Intoxication/
[W]With Onset During Withdrawal

ALCOHOL-RELATED DISORDERS

Alcohol Use Disorders

303.90 Alcohol Dependence[a,b,c]
305.00 Alcohol Abuse

Alcohol-Induced Disorders

303.00 Alcohol Intoxication
291.81 Alcohol Withdrawal
Specify if: With Perceptual Disturbances
291.0 Alcohol Intoxication Delirium
291.0 Alcohol Withdrawal Delirium
291.2 Alcohol-Induced Persisting Dementia
291.1 Alcohol-Induced Persisting Amnestic Disorder
291.x Alcohol-Induced Psychotic Disorder
 .5 With Delusions[I,W]
 .3 With Hallucinations[I,W]
291.89 Alcohol-Induced Mood Disorder[I,W]
291.89 Alcohol-Induced Anxiety Disorder[I,W]
291.89 Alcohol-Induced Sexual Dysfunction[I]
291.89 Alcohol-Induced Sleep Disorder[I,W]

291.9 Alcohol-Related Disorder NOS

AMPHETAMINE (OR AMPHETAMINE-LIKE)– RELATED DISORDERS

Amphetamine Use Disorders

304.40 Amphetamine Dependence[a,b,c]
305.70 Amphetamine Abuse

Amphetamine-Induced Disorders

292.89 Amphetamine Intoxication
Specify if: With Perceptual Disturbances
292.0 Amphetamine Withdrawal
292.81 Amphetamine Intoxication Delirium

292.xx Amphetamine-Induced
      Psychotic Disorder
  .11   With Delusions[I]
  .12   With Hallucinations[I]
292.84 Amphetamine-Induced Mood
      Disorder[I,W]
292.89 Amphetamine-Induced Anxiety
      Disorder[I]
292.89 Amphetamine-Induced Sexual
      Dysfunction[I]
292.89 Amphetamine-Induced Sleep
      Disorder[I,W]

292.9 Amphetamine-Related Disorder
     NOS

CAFFEINE-RELATED DISORDERS

Caffeine-Induced Disorders

305.90 Caffeine Intoxication
292.89 Caffeine-Induced Anxiety
      Disorder[I]
292.89 Caffeine-Induced Sleep
      Disorder[I]
292.9 Caffeine-Related Disorder NOS

CANNABIS-RELATED DISORDERS

Cannabis Use Disorders
304.30 Cannabis Dependence[a,b,c]
305.20 Cannabis Abuse

Cannabis-Induced Disorders

292.89 Cannabis Intoxication
     Specify if: With Perceptual
     Disturbances
292.81 Cannabis Intoxication
      Delirium
292.xx Cannabis-Induced Psychotic
      Disorder
  .11   With Delusions[I]

  .12   With Hallucinations[I]
292.89 Cannabis-Induced Anxiety
      Disorder[I]

292.9 Cannabis-Related Disorder NOS

COCAINE-RELATED DISORDERS

Cocaine Use Disorders
304.20 Cocaine Dependence[a,b,c]
305.60 Cocaine Abuse

Cocaine-Induced Disorders

292.89 Cocaine Intoxication
     Specify if: With Perceptual
     Disturbances
292.0 Cocaine Withdrawal
292.81 Cocaine Intoxication Delirium
292.xx Cocaine-Induced Psychotic
      Disorder
  .11   With Delusions[I]
  .12   With Hallucinations[I]
292.84 Cocaine-Induced Mood
      Disorder[I,W]
292.89 Cocaine-Induced Anxiety
      Disorder[I,W]
292.89 Cocaine-Induced Sexual
      Dysfunction[I]
292.89 Cocaine-Induced Sleep
      Disorder[I,W]

292.9 Cocaine-Related Disorder
     NOS

HALLUCINOGEN-RELATED DISORDERS

Hallucinogen Use Disorders
304.50 Hallucinogen Dependence[b,c]
305.30 Hallucinogen Abuse

Hallucinogen-Induced Disorders

292.89 Hallucinogen Intoxication
292.89 Hallucinogen Persisting Perception Disorder (Flashbacks)
292.81 Hallucinogen Intoxication Delirium
292.xx Hallucinogen-Induced Psychotic Disorder
    .11 With Delusions[I]
    .12 With Hallucinations[I]
292.84 Hallucinogen-Induced Mood Disorder[I]
292.89 Hallucinogen-Induced Anxiety Disorder[I]

292.9 Hallucinogen-Related Disorder NOS

INHALANT-RELATED DISORDERS

Inhalant Use Disorders

304.60 Inhalant Dependence[b,c]
305.90 Inhalant Abuse

Inhalant-Induced Disorders

292.89 Inhalant Intoxication
292.81 Inhalant Intoxication Delirium
292.82 Inhalant-Induced Persisting Dementia
292.xx Inhalant-Induced Psychotic Disorder
    .11 With Delusions[I]
    .12 With Hallucinations[I]
292.84 Inhalant-Induced Mood Disorder[I]
292.89 Inhalant-Induced Anxiety Disorder[I]

292.9 Inhalant-Related Disorder NOS

NICOTINE-RELATED DISORDERS

Nicotine Use Disorder

305.1 Nicotine Dependence[a,b]

Nicotine-Induced Disorder

292.0 Nicotine Withdrawal

292.9 Nicotine-Related Disorder NOS

OPIOID-RELATED DISORDERS

Opioid Use Disorders

304.00 Opioid Dependence[a,b,c,d]
305.50 Opioid Abuse

Opioid-Induced Disorders

292.89 Opioid Intoxication
    Specify if: With Perceptual Disturbances
292.0 Opioid Withdrawal
292.81 Opioid Intoxication Delirium
292.xx Opioid-Induced Psychotic Disorder
    .11 With Delusions[I]
    .12 With Hallucinations[I]
292.84 Opioid-Induced Mood Disorder[I]
292.89 Opioid-Induced Sexual Dysfunction[I]
292.89 Opioid-Induced Sleep Disorder[I,W]

292.9 Opioid-Related Disorder NOS

PHENCYCLIDINE (OR PHENCYCLIDINE-LIKE)– RELATED DISORDERS

Phencyclidine Use Disorders

304.60 Phencyclidine Dependence[b,c]
305.90 Phencyclidine Abuse

Phencyclidine-Induced Disorders

292.89 Phencyclidine Intoxication
        Specify if: With Perceptual
        Disturbances
292.81 Phencyclidine Intoxication
        Delirium
292.xx Phencyclidine-Induced
        Psychotic Disorder
  .11   With Delusions[I]
  .12   With Hallucinations[I]
292.84 Phencyclidine-Induced Mood
        Disorder[I]
292.89 Phencyclidine-Induced Anxiety
        Disorder[I]
292.9   Phencyclidine-Related Disorder
        NOS

SEDATIVE-, HYPNOTIC-, OR ANXIOLYTIC-RELATED DISORDERS

Sedative, Hypnotic, or Anxiolytic Use Disorders

304.10 Sedative, Hypnotic, or
        Anxiolytic Dependence[a,b,c]
305.40 Sedative, Hypnotic, or
        Anxiolytic Abuse

Sedative-, Hypnotic-, or Anxiolytic-Induced Disorders

292.89 Sedative, Hypnotic, or
        Anxiolytic Intoxication
292.0   Sedative, Hypnotic, or
        Anxiolytic Withdrawal
        Specify if: With Perceptual
        Disturbances
292.81 Sedative, Hypnotic, or
        Anxiolytic Intoxication
        Delirium
292.81 Sedative, Hypnotic, or Anxio-
        lytic Withdrawal Delirium

292.82 Sedative-, Hypnotic-, or
        Anxiolytic-Induced Persisting
        Dementia
292.83 Sedative-, Hypnotic-, or
        Anxiolytic-Induced Persisting
        Amnestic Disorder
292.xx Sedative-, Hypnotic-, or
        Anxiolytic-Induced Psychotic
        Disorder
  .11   With Delusions[I,W]
  .12   With Hallucinations[I,W]
292.84 Sedative-, Hypnotic-, or
        Anxiolytic-Induced Mood
        Disorder[I,W]
292.89 Sedative-, Hypnotic-, or
        Anxiolytic-Induced Anxiety
        Disorder[W]
292.89 Sedative-, Hypnotic-, or
        Anxiolytic-Induced Sexual
        Dysfunction[I]
292.89 Sedative-, Hypnotic-, or
        Anxiolytic-Induced Sleep
        Disorder[I,W]

292.9   Sedative-, Hypnotic-, or
        Anxiolytic-Related
        Disorder NOS

POLYSUBSTANCE-RELATED DISORDER

304.80 Polysubstance
        Dependence[a,b,c,d]

OTHER (OR UNKNOWN) SUBSTANCE–RELATED DISORDERS

Other (or Unknown) Substance Use Disorders

304.90 Other (or Unknown)
        Substance Dependence[a,b,c,d]
305.90 Other (or Unknown)
        Substance Abuse

Other (or Unknown) Substance–Induced Disorders

292.89 Other (or Unknown)
 Substance Intoxication
 Specify if: With Perceptual
 Disturbances

292.0 Other (or Unknown) Substance
 Withdrawal
 Specify if: With Perceptual
 Disturbances

292.81 Other (or Unknown)
 Substance–Induced Delirium

292.82 Other (or Unknown)
 Substance–Induced Persisting
 Dementia

292.83 Other (or Unknown)
 Substance–Induced Persisting
 Amnestic Disorder

292.xx Other (or Unknown)
 Substance–Induced Psychotic
 Disorder
 .11 With Delusions[I,W]
 .12 With Hallucinations[I,W]

292.84 Other (or Unknown)
 Substance–Induced Mood
 Disorder[I,W]

292.89 Other (or Unknown)
 Substance–Induced Anxiety
 Disorder[I,W]

292.89 Other (or Unknown)
 Substance–Induced Sexual
 Dysfunction[I]

292.89 Other (or Unknown) Substance–
 Induced Sleep Disorder[I,W]

292.9 Other (or Unknown) Substance–
 Related Disorder NOS

Schizophrenia and Other Psychotic Disorders

295.xx Schizophrenia

The following Classification of Longitudinal Course applies to all subtypes of Schizophrenia:

Episodic With Interepisode Residual
 Symptoms (*specify if:* With
 Prominent Negative
 Symptoms)/Episodic With No
 Interepisode Residual Symptoms
Continuous (*specify if:* With Prominent
 Negative Symptoms)
Single Episode In Partial Remission
 (*specify if:* With Prominent
 Negative Symptoms)/Single
 Episode In Full Remission
Other or Unspecified Pattern
 .30 Paranoid Type
 .10 Disorganized Type
 .20 Catatonic Type
 .90 Undifferentiated Type
 .60 Residual Type

295.40 Schizophreniform Disorder
 Specify if: Without Good
 Prognostic Features/With Good
 Prognostic Features

295.70 Schizoaffective Disorder
 Specify type: Bipolar Type/
 Depressive Type

297.1 Delusional Disorder
 Specify type: Erotomanic Type/
 Grandiose Type/Jealous Type/
 Persecutory Type/Somatic Type/
 Mixed Type/Unspecified Type

298.8 Brief Psychotic Disorder
 Specify if: With Marked
 Stressor(s)/Without Marked
 Stressor(s)/With Postpartum
 Onset

297.3 Shared Psychotic Disorder

293.xx Psychotic Disorder Due to . . .
 *[Indicate the General Medical
 Condition]*
 .81 With Delusions
 .82 With Hallucinations

—.— Substance-Induced Psychotic Disorder *(refer to Substance-Related Disorders for substance-specific codes)*
Specify if: With Onset During Intoxication/With Onset During Withdrawal

298.9 Psychotic Disorder NOS

Mood Disorders

Code current state of Major Depressive Disorder or Bipolar I Disorder in fifth digit:

1 = Mild
2 = Moderate
3 = Severe Without Psychotic Features
4 = Severe With Psychotic Features
　　Specify: Mood-Congruent Psychotic Features/Mood-Incongruent Psychotic Features
5 = In Partial Remission
6 = In Full Remission
0 = Unspecified

The following specifiers apply (for current or most recent episode) to Mood Disorders as noted:

[a]Severity/Psychotic/Remission Specifiers/[b]Chronic/[c]With Catatonic Features/[d]With Melancholic Features/[e]With Atypical Features/[f]With Postpartum Onset

The following specifiers apply to Mood Disorders as noted:

[g]With or Without Full Interepisode Recovery/ [h]With Seasonal Pattern/[i]With Rapid Cycling

DEPRESSIVE DISORDERS

296.xx Major Depressive Disorder
　.2x Single Episode[a,b,c,d,e,f]
　.3x Recurrent[a,b,c,d,e,f,g,h]

300.4 Dysthymic Disorder
Specify if: Early Onset/Late Onset
Specify: With Atypical Features
311 Depressive Disorder NOS

BIPOLAR DISORDERS

296.xx Bipolar I Disorder,
　.0x Single Manic Episode[a,c,f]
Specify if: Mixed
　.40 Most Recent Episode Hypomanic[g,h,i]
　.4x Most Recent Episode Manic[a,c,f,g,h,i]
　.6x Most Recent Episode Mixed[a,c,f,g,h,i]
　.5x Most Recent Episode Depressed[a,b,c,d,e,f,g,h,i]
　.7 Most Recent Episode Unspecified[g,h,i]
296.89 Bipolar II Disorder[a,b,c,d,e,f,g,h,i]
Specify (current or most recent episode): Hypomanic/Depressed
301.13 Cyclothymic Disorder
296.80 Bipolar Disorder NOS

293.83 Mood Disorder Due to . . . *[Indicate the General Medical Condition]*
Specify type: With Depressive Features/With Major Depressive–Like Episode/With Manic Features/ With Mixed Features
—.— Substance-Induced Mood Disorder *(refer to Substance-Related Disorders for substance-specific codes)*
Specify type: With Depressive Features/With Manic Features/ With Mixed Features
Specify if: With Onset During Intoxication/With Onset During Withdrawal

296.90 Mood Disorder NOS

Anxiety Disorders

300.01 Panic Disorder Without
        Agoraphobia
300.21 Panic Disorder With
        Agoraphobia
300.22 Agoraphobia Without History
        of Panic Disorder
300.29 Specific Phobia
        Specify type: Animal Type/
        Natural Environment Type/
        Blood-Injection-Injury Type/
        Situational Type/Other Type
300.23 Social Phobia
        Specify if: Generalized
300.3   Obsessive-Compulsive Disorder
        Specify if: With Poor Insight
309.81 Posttraumatic Stress Disorder
        Specify if: Acute/Chronic
        Specify if: With Delayed Onset
308.3   Acute Stress Disorder
300.02 Generalized Anxiety Disorder
293.84 Anxiety Disorder Due to . . .
        *[Indicate the General Medical
        Condition]*
        Specify if: With Generalized
        Anxiety/With Panic Attacks/With
        Obsessive-Compulsive Symptoms
——.—   Substance-Induced Anxiety
        Disorder *(refer to Substance-
        Related Disorders for substance-
        specific codes)*
        Specify if: With Generalized
        Anxiety/With Panic Attacks/With
        Obsessive-Compulsive Symptoms/
        With Phobic Symptoms
        Specify if: With Onset During
        Intoxication/With Onset During
        Withdrawal
300.00 Anxiety Disorder NOS

Somatoform Disorders

300.81 Somatization Disorder
300.82 Undifferentiated Somatoform
        Disorder

300.11 Conversion Disorder
        Specify type: With Motor
        Symptom or Deficit/With Sensory
        Symptom or Deficit/With Seizures
        or Convulsions/With Mixed
        Presentation
307.xx Pain Disorder
   .80   Associated With
           Psychological Factors
   .89   Associated With Both
           Psychological Factors and a
           General Medical Condition
        Specify if: Acute/Chronic
300.7   Hypochondriasis
        Specify if: With Poor Insight
300.7   Body Dysmorphic Disorder
300.82 Somatoform Disorder NOS

Factitious Disorders

300.xx Factitious Disorder
   .16   With Predominantly
           Psychological Signs and
           Symptoms
   .19   With Predominantly Physical
           Signs and Symptoms
   .19   With Combined Psychological
           and Physical Signs and
           Symptoms
300.19 Factitious Disorder NOS

Dissociative Disorders

300.12 Dissociative Amnesia
300.13 Dissociative Fugue
300.14 Dissociative Identity Disorder
300.6   Depersonalization Disorder
300.15 Dissociative Disorder NOS

Sexual and Gender Identity Disorders

SEXUAL DYSFUNCTIONS

The following specifiers apply to all primary Sexual Dysfunctions:

Lifelong Type/Acquired Type
Generalized Type/Situational Type
Due to Psychological Factors/Due to
Combined Factors

Sexual Desire Disorders

302.71 Hypoactive Sexual Desire
Disorder
302.79 Sexual Aversion Disorder

Sexual Arousal Disorders

302.72 Female Sexual Arousal
Disorder
302.72 Male Erectile Disorder

Orgasmic Disorders

302.73 Female Orgasmic Disorder
302.74 Male Orgasmic Disorder
302.75 Premature Ejaculation

Sexual Pain Disorders

302.76 Dyspareunia (Not Due to a
General Medical Condition)
306.51 Vaginismus (Not Due to a
General Medical Condition)

Sexual Dysfunction Due to a General Medical Condition

625.8 Female Hypoactive Sexual
Desire Disorder Due to . . .
*[Indicate the General Medical
Condition]*

608.89 Male Hypoactive Sexual
Desire Disorder Due to . . .
*[Indicate the General Medical
Condition]*
607.84 Male Erectile Disorder Due
to . . . *[Indicate the General
Medical Condition]*
625.0 Female Dyspareunia Due to . . .
*[Indicate the General Medical
Condition]*
608.89 Male Dyspareunia Due to . . .
*[Indicate the General Medical
Condition]*
625.8 Other Female Sexual
Dysfunction Due to . . . *[Indicate
the General Medical Condition]*
608.89 Other Male Sexual Dysfunction
Due to . . . *[Indicate the
General Medical Condition]*
——.— Substance-Induced Sexual
Dysfunction *(refer to
Substance-Related Disorders
for substance-specific codes)*
Specify if: With Impaired Desire/
With Impaired Arousal/
With Impaired Orgasm/
With Sexual Pain
Specify if: With Onset During
Intoxication

302.70 Sexual Dysfunction NOS

PARAPHILIAS

302.4 Exhibitionism
302.81 Fetishism
302.89 Frotteurism
302.2 Pedophilia
Specify if: Sexually Attracted to
Males/Sexually Attracted to Females/
Sexually Attracted to Both
Specify if: Limited to Incest
Specify type: Exclusive Type/
Nonexclusive Type
302.83 Sexual Masochism
302.84 Sexual Sadism

302.3   Transvestic Fetishism
        Specify if: With Gender Dysphoria
302.82 Voyeurism
302.9   Paraphilia NOS

GENDER IDENTITY DISORDERS

302.xx Gender Identity Disorder ·
  .6   in Children
  .85   in Adolescents or Adults
          Specify if: Sexually Attracted to
          Males/Sexually Attracted to Females/
          Sexually Attracted to Both/
          Sexually Attracted to Neither
302.6   Gender Identity Disorder NOS

302.9   Sexual Disorder NOS

Eating Disorders

307.1   Anorexia Nervosa
        Specify type: Restricting Type;
        Binge-Eating/Purging Type
307.51 Bulimia Nervosa
        Specify type: Purging Type/
        Nonpurging Type
307.50 Eating Disorder NOS

Sleep Disorders

PRIMARY SLEEP DISORDERS

Dyssomnias

307.42 Primary Insomnia
307.44 Primary Hypersomnia
        Specify if: Recurrent
347   Narcolepsy
780.59 Breathing-Related Sleep
        Disorder
307.45 Circadian Rhythm Sleep
        Disorder
        Specify type: Delayed Sleep
        Phase Type/Jet Lag Type/Shift
        Work Type/Unspecified Type
307.47 Dyssomnia NOS

Parasomnias

307.47 Nightmare Disorder
307.46 Sleep Terror Disorder
307.46 Sleepwalking Disorder
307.47 Parasomnia NOS

SLEEP DISORDERS RELATED TO ANOTHER MENTAL DISORDER

307.42 Insomnia Related to . . .
        *[Indicate the Axis I or Axis II
        Disorder]*
307.44 Hypersomnia Related to . . .
        *[Indicate the Axis I or Axis II
        Disorder]*

OTHER SLEEP DISORDERS

780.xx Sleep Disorder Due to . . .
        *[Indicate the General Medical
        Condition]*
  .52   Insomnia Type
  .54   Hypersomnia Type
  .59   Parasomnia Type
  .59   Mixed Type
——.—   Substance-Induced Sleep
        Disorder *(refer to Substance-
        Related Disorders for substance-
        specific codes)*
        Specify type: Insomnia Type/
        Hypersomnia Type/Parasomnia
        Type/Mixed Type
        Specify if: With Onset During
        Intoxication/With Onset During
        Withdrawal

Impulse-Control Disorders Not Elsewhere Classified

312.34 Intermittent Explosive Disorder
312.32 Kleptomania
312.33 Pyromania
312.31 Pathological Gambling
312.39 Trichotillomania
312.30 Impulse-Control Disorder NOS

Adjustment Disorders

309.xx Adjustment Disorder
  .0   With Depressed Mood
  .24   With Anxiety
  .28   With Mixed Anxiety and
        Depressed Mood
  .3   With Disturbance of Conduct
  .4   With Mixed Disturbance of
        Emotions and Conduct
  .9   Unspecified
      Specify if: Acute/Chronic

Personality Disorders

Note: *These are coded on Axis II.*
301.0   Paranoid Personality Disorder
301.20 Schizoid Personality Disorder
301.22 Schizotypal Personality Disorder
301.7   Antisocial Personality Disorder
301.83 Borderline Personality Disorder
301.50 Histrionic Personality Disorder
301.81 Narcissistic Personality Disorder
301.82 Avoidant Personality Disorder
301.6   Dependent Personality Disorder
301.4   Obsessive-Compulsive Personality Disorder
301.9   Personality Disorder NOS

Other Conditions That May Be a Focus of Clinical Attention

PSYCHOLOGICAL FACTORS AFFECTING MEDICAL CONDITION

316   *. . . [Specified Psychological Factor] Affecting . . . [Indicate the General Medical Condition]*

Choose name based on nature of factors:
Mental Disorder Affecting Medical Condition
Psychological Symptoms Affecting Medical Condition
Personality Traits or Coping Style Affecting Medical Condition
Maladaptive Health Behaviors Affecting Medical Condition
Stress-Related Physiological Response Affecting Medical Condition
Other or Unspecified Psychological Factors Affecting Medical Condition

MEDICATION-INDUCED MOVEMENT DISORDERS

332.1 Neuroleptic-Induced Parkinsonism
333.92 Neuroleptic Malignant Syndrome
333.7 Neuroleptic-Induced Acute Dystonia
333.99 Neuroleptic-Induced Acute Akathisia
333.82 Neuroleptic-Induced Tardive Dyskinesia
333.1 Medication-Induced Postural Tremor
333.90 Medication-Induced Movement Disorder NOS

OTHER MEDICATION-INDUCED DISORDER

995.2 Adverse Effects of Medication NOS

RELATIONAL PROBLEMS

V61.9   Relational Problem Related to
         a Mental Disorder or General
         Medical Condition
V61.20   Parent-Child Relational
         Problem
V61.10   Partner Relational Problem
V61.8   Sibling Relational Problem
V62.81   Relational Problem NOS

PROBLEMS RELATED TO ABUSE OR NEGLECT

V61.21   Physical Abuse of Child
         (code 995.54 if focus of
         attention is on victim)
V61.21   Sexual Abuse of Child
         (code 995.53 if focus of
         attention is on victim)
V61.21   Neglect of Child
         (code 995.52 if focus of
         attention is on victim)
——.—   Physical Abuse of Adult
V61.12   (if by partner)
V62.83   (if by person other than
         partner)
         (code 995.81 if focus of
         attention is on victim)
——.—   Sexual Abuse of Adult
V61.12   (if by partner)
V62.83   (if by person other than
         partner)
         (code 995.83 if focus of
         attention is on victim)

ADDITIONAL CONDITIONS THAT MAY BE A FOCUS OF CLINICAL ATTENTION

V15.81   Noncompliance With
         Treatment
V65.2   Malingering
V71.01   Adult Antisocial Behavior

V71.02   Child or Adolescent Antisocial
         Behavior
V62.89   Borderline Intellectual
         Functioning
         Note: This is coded on Axis II.
780.9   Age-Related Cognitive Decline
V62.82   Bereavement
V62.3   Academic Problem
V62.2   Occupational Problem
313.82   Identity Problem
V62.89   Religious or Spiritual Problem
V62.4   Acculturation Problem
V62.89   Phase of Life Problem

Additional Codes

300.9   Unspecified Mental Disorder
         (nonpsychotic)
V71.09   No Diagnosis or Condition on
         Axis I
799.9   Diagnosis or Condition
         Deferred on Axis I
V71.09   No Diagnosis on Axis II
799.9   Diagnosis Deferred on Axis II

Multiaxial System

Axis I   Clinical Disorders
          Other Conditions That May Be
          a Focus of Clinical Attention

Axis II   Personality Disorders
          Mental Retardation

Axis III General Medical Conditions

Axis IV   Psychosocial and
          Environmental Problems

Axis V   Global Assessment of
          Functioning

Index of Cases by DSM-IV-TR Diagnosis

Case history titles appear in *italic* type.